Comparative Effectiveness Review
Number 133

Transitional Care Interventions To Prevent Readmissions for People With Heart Failure

Prepared for:
Agency for Healthcare Research and Quality
U.S. Department of Health and Human Services
540 Gaither Road
Rockville, MD 20850
www.ahrq.gov

Contract No. 290-2012-00008-I

Prepared by:
Research Triangle Institute–University of North Carolina Evidence-based Practice Center
Research Triangle Park, NC

Investigators:
Cynthia Feltner, M.D., M.P.H.
Christine D. Jones, M.D., M.S.
Crystal W. Cené, M.D., M.P.H.
Zhi-Jie Zheng, M.D., M.P.H., Ph.D.
Carla A. Sueta, M.D., Ph.D.
Emmanuel J.L. Coker-Schwimmer, M.P.H.
Marina Arvanitis, M.D.
Kathleen N. Lohr, Ph.D., M.Phil., M.A.
Jennifer Cook Middleton, Ph.D.
Daniel E. Jonas, M.D., M.P.H.

AHRQ Publication No. 14-EHC021-EF
May 2014

This report is based on research conducted by the Research Triangle Institute–University of North Carolina Evidence-based Practice Center (EPC) under contract to the Agency for Healthcare Research and Quality (AHRQ), Rockville, MD (Contract No. 290-2012-00008-I). The findings and conclusions in this document are those of the authors, who are responsible for its contents; the findings and conclusions do not necessarily represent the views of AHRQ. Therefore, no statement in this report should be construed as an official position of AHRQ or of the U.S. Department of Health and Human Services.

The information in this report is intended to help health care decisionmakers—patients and clinicians, health system leaders, and policymakers, among others—make well informed decisions and thereby improve the quality of health care services. This report is not intended to be a substitute for the application of clinical judgment. Anyone who makes decisions concerning the provision of clinical care should consider this report in the same way as any medical reference and in conjunction with all other pertinent information, i.e., in the context of available resources and circumstances presented by individual patients.

This report may be used, in whole or in part, as the basis for development of clinical practice guidelines and other quality enhancement tools, or as a basis for reimbursement and coverage policies. AHRQ or U.S. Department of Health and Human Services endorsement of such derivative products may not be stated or implied.

This report may periodically be assessed for the urgency to update. If an assessment is done, the resulting surveillance report describing the methodology and findings will be found on the Effective Health Care Program Web site at www.effectivehealthcare.ahrq.gov. Search on the title of the report.

This document is in the public domain and may be used and reprinted without permission. Citation of the source is appreciated.

Persons using assistive technology may not be able to fully access information in this report. For assistance contact EffectiveHealthCare@ahrq.hhs.gov.

Suggested citation: Feltner C, Jones CD, Cené CW, Zheng Z-J, Sueta CA, Coker-Schwimmer EJL, Arvanitis M, Lohr KN, Middleton JC, Jonas DE. Transitional Care Interventions To Prevent Readmissions for People With Heart Failure. Comparative Effectiveness Review No. 133. (Prepared by the Research Triangle Institute–University of North Carolina Evidence-based Practice Center under Contract No. 290-2012-00008-I). AHRQ Publication No. 14-EHC021-EF. Rockville, MD: Agency for Healthcare Research and Quality; May 2014. www.effectivehealthcare.ahrq.gov/reports/final.cfm.

Preface

The Agency for Healthcare Research and Quality (AHRQ), through its Evidence-based Practice Centers (EPCs), sponsors the development of systematic reviews to assist public- and private-sector organizations in their efforts to improve the quality of health care in the United States. These reviews provide comprehensive, science-based information on common, costly medical conditions, and new health care technologies and strategies.

Systematic reviews are the building blocks underlying evidence-based practice; they focus attention on the strength and limits of evidence from research studies about the effectiveness and safety of a clinical intervention. In the context of developing recommendations for practice, systematic reviews can help clarify whether assertions about the value of the intervention are based on strong evidence from clinical studies. For more information about AHRQ EPC systematic reviews, see www.effectivehealthcare.ahrq.gov/reference/purpose.cfm.

AHRQ expects that these systematic reviews will be helpful to health plans, providers, purchasers, government programs, and the health care system as a whole. Transparency and stakeholder input are essential to the Effective Health Care Program. Please visit the Web site (www.effectivehealthcare.ahrq.gov) to see draft research questions and reports or to join an email list to learn about new program products and opportunities for input.

We welcome comments on this systematic review. They may be sent by mail to the Task Order Officer named below at: Agency for Healthcare Research and Quality, 540 Gaither Road, Rockville, MD 20850, or by email to epc@ahrq.hhs.gov.

Richard G. Kronick, Ph.D.
Director
Agency for Healthcare Research and Policy

Yen-pin Chiang, Ph.D.
Acting Director
Center for Outcomes and Evidence
Agency for Healthcare Research and Quality

Stephanie Chang, M.D., M.P.H.
Director, EPC Program
Center for Outcomes and Evidence
Agency for Healthcare Research and Quality

Christine Chang, M.D., M.P.H.
Task Order Officer
Center for Outcomes and Evidence
Agency for Healthcare Research and Quality

Acknowledgments

The authors gratefully acknowledge the continuing support of our AHRQ Task Order Officer, Christine Chang, M.D., M.P.H., and our Associate Editor, Donna Dryden, Ph.D. We extend our appreciation to our Key Informants and members of our Technical Expert Panel (listed below), all of whom provided thoughtful advice and input during our research process. The investigators deeply appreciate the considerable support, commitment, and contributions of the EPC team staff at RTI International and the University of North Carolina at Chapel Hill. We express our gratitude to the following individuals for their contributions to this project: Carol Woodell, B.S.P.H., our Project Manager; Meera Viswanathan, Ph.D., Director of the RTI-UNC EPC; Timothy S. Carey, M.D., M.P.H., Director of the Cecil G. Sheps Center for Health Services Research at UNC; Rachael Posey, M.S.L.S., our EPC Librarian; Ellen Shanahan, M.A., our research associate; Claire Baker and Cassandra Rowe, B.A., our Research Assistants; Laura Small, editor; and Loraine Monroe, our EPC Publications Specialist.

Key Informants

In designing the study questions, the EPC consulted several Key Informants who represent the end-users of research. The EPC sought the Key Informant input on the priority areas for research and synthesis. Key Informants are not involved in the analysis of the evidence or the writing of the report. Therefore, in the end, study questions, design, methodological approaches, and/or conclusions do not necessarily represent the views of individual Key Informants.

Key Informants must disclose any financial conflicts of interest greater than $10,000 and any other relevant business or professional conflicts of interest. Because of their role as end-users, individuals with potential conflicts may be retained. The TOO and the EPC work to balance, manage, or mitigate any conflicts of interest.

The list of Key Informants who participated in developing this report follows:

Kenneth S. Fink, M.D., M.G.A., M.P.H.
Med-Quest Division, Hawaii State
Medicaid
Kapolei, HI

Jalal Ghali, M.D.
Division of Cardiology
Mercer University School of Medicine
Macon, GA

Mariell Jessup, M.D.
Professor of Medicine, University of
Pennsylvania School of Medicine
Medical Director,
Penn Heart and Vascular Center
Philadelphia, PA

Carol Levine, M.A.
Families and Health Care Project
United Hospital Fund
New York, NY

JoAnn Lindenfeld, M.D.
Cardiac Transplant Program
University of Colorado
Aurora, CO

Timothy J. Wilt, M.D., M.P.H.
Minneapolis VA Center for Chronic
Disease Outcomes Research
University of Minnesota School of
Medicine
Minneapolis, MN

Clyde W. Yancy, M.D., M.Sc., FACC,
FAHA, M.A.C.P.
Division of Cardiology
Northwestern University
Chicago, IL

Judy Zerzan, M.D., M.P.H.
Colorado Department of Health
Care Policy and Financing
Denver, CO

Technical Expert Panel

In designing the study questions and methodology at the outset of this report, the EPC consulted several technical and content experts. Broad expertise and perspectives were sought. Divergent and conflicted opinions are common and perceived as healthy scientific discourse that results in a thoughtful, relevant systematic review. Therefore, in the end, study questions, design, methodologic approaches, and/or conclusions do not necessarily represent the views of individual technical and content experts.

Technical Experts must disclose any financial conflicts of interest greater than $10,000 and any other relevant business or professional conflicts of interest. Because of their unique clinical or content expertise, individuals with potential conflicts may be retained. The TOO and the EPC work to balance, manage, or mitigate any potential conflicts of interest identified.

The list of Technical Experts who participated in developing this report follows:

Darren A. DeWalt, M.D., M.P.H.[a]
University of North Carolina at
Chapel Hill School of Medicine
Chapel Hill, NC

Paul A. Heidenreich, M.D., M.S.,
FACC[a]
Cardiovascular Research Institute
Stanford University School of Medicine
Palo Alto, CA

Mariell Jessup, M.D.[a]
Professor of Medicine,
University of Pennsylvania
School of Medicine
Medical Director,
Penn Heart and Vascular Center
Philadelphia, PA

Devan Kansagara, M.D., M.C.R.,
FACP[a]
Portland VA Evidence-based Synthesis
Program
Oregon Health and Science University
Portland, OR

Gowri Raman, M.D., M.S.[a]
Assistant Professor of Medicine,
Tufts University School of Medicine
Scientific Staff, Center for Clinical
Evidence Synthesis
Tufts Medical Center
Boston, MA

Juliana Tiongson, M.P.H.
Center for Medicare &
Medicaid Innovation
Baltimore, MD

Timothy J. Wilt, M.D., M.P.H.[a]
Minneapolis VA Center for Chronic
Disease Outcomes Research
University of Minnesota School of
Medicine
Minneapolis, MN

Clyde W. Yancy, M.D., M.Sc.,
FACC, FAHA, M.A.C.P.
Division of Cardiology
Northwestern University
Chicago, IL

[a]Indicates Technical Expert Panel member also provided Peer Review commentary and feedback.

Peer Reviewers

Before publication of the final evidence report, EPCs sought input from independent Peer Reviewers without financial conflicts of interest. However, the conclusions and synthesis of the scientific literature presented in this report do not necessarily represent the views of individual reviewers.

Peer Reviewers must disclose any financial conflicts of interest greater than $10,000 and any other relevant business or professional conflicts of interest. Because of their unique clinical or content expertise, individuals with potential nonfinancial conflicts may be retained. The TOO and the EPC work to balance, manage, or mitigate any potential nonfinancial conflicts of interest identified.

The list of Peer Reviewers follows:

Jalal Ghali, M.D.
Division of Cardiology
Mercer University School of Medicine
Macon, GA

Joseph Lau, M.D.
Brown University Center for Evidence-based Medicine
Providence, RI

Christopher O. Phillips, M.D., M.P.H., FACP
Director, Clinical Outcomes Research and Evaluation
Associate Professor of Medicine and Epidemiology
Department of General Internal Medicine
Morehouse School of Medicine
Atlanta, GA

Ileana Piña, M.D., M.P.H.
Albert Einstein College of Medicine of Yeshiva University
Montefiore Medical Center
Bronx, NY

Michael W. Rich, M.D.
Washington University in St. Louis School of Medicine
St. Louis, MO

Barbara Riegel, D.N.Sc., R.N., FAAN, FAHA
University of Pennsylvania School of Nursing
Philadelphia, PA

Transitional Care Interventions To Prevent Readmissions for People With Heart Failure

Structured Abstract

Objectives. To conduct a systematic review and meta-analysis of the efficacy, comparative effectiveness, and harms of transitional care interventions that aim to reduce readmissions and mortality for adults hospitalized with heart failure (HF). We also sought to describe the components of interventions that showed efficacy.

Data sources. MEDLINE®, Cochrane Library, CINAHL®, ClinicalTrials.gov, and World Health Organization International Clinical Trials Registry Platform (January 1, 1990, to early May 2013).

Review methods. Two investigators independently selected, extracted data from, and rated risk of bias of relevant randomized controlled trials. We conducted meta-analyses using random-effects models to estimate pooled effects. We graded strength of evidence (SOE) based on established guidance.

Results. We included 47 trials. Most included patients with moderate to severe HF; mean ages of patients were in the 70s. Few trials reported 30-day readmission rates. A high-intensity home-visiting program reduced all-cause readmission and the composite endpoint (all-cause readmission or death) at 30 days (low SOE). Over 3 to 6 months, home-visiting programs reduced all-cause readmission (high SOE), HF-specific readmission (moderate SOE), and the composite endpoint (moderate SOE). Multidisciplinary (MDS)-HF clinic interventions reduced all-cause readmission (high SOE). Structured telephone support (STS) interventions reduced HF-specific readmission (high SOE) but not all-cause readmissions (moderate SOE). Home-visiting programs, MDS-HF clinics, and STS interventions produced a mortality benefit (moderate SOE). Neither telemonitoring nor nurse-led clinic interventions reduced readmissions or mortality.

Components of interventions showing efficacy for reducing all-cause readmissions or mortality include: HF education, emphasizing self-care; HF pharmacotherapy, emphasizing promotion of adherence and evidence-based HF pharmacotherapy; and a streamlined mechanism to contact care delivery personnel (e.g., patient hotline). In general, categories of interventions that reduced all-cause readmissions or mortality were more likely to be of higher intensity, to be delivered face to face, and to be provided by MDS teams.

Conclusions. Home-visiting programs and MDS-HF clinic interventions reduced all-cause readmission and mortality; STS reduced HF-specific readmission and mortality but not all-cause readmission. These interventions should receive the greatest consideration by systems or providers seeking to implement transitional care interventions for people with HF. We found no evidence assessing harms of transitional care interventions, such as increased caregiver burden.

Contents

Executive Summary ES-1

Introduction 1
  Background 1
    Epidemiology of Heart Failure in the United States.. 1
    Heart Failure and Preventable Readmissions.. 1
    Transitional Care for People With Heart Failure 2
  Existing Guidelines and Current Practice 3
    Existing Guidelines.. 3
    Current Practice 3
  Rationale for Evidence Review... 3
  Scope and Key Questions 4
  Analytic Framework 5

Organization of This Report 6

Methods..7
  Topic Refinement and Review Protocol 7
  Literature Search Strategy... 7
    Search Strategy 7
    Inclusion and Exclusion Criteria 8
    Study Selection 8
    Data Extraction 10
  Risk-of-Bias Assessment of Individual Studies... 10
  Categorization of Interventions.. 11
  Data Synthesis... 12
  Strength of the Body of Evidence 14
  Applicability 15
  Peer Review and Public Commentary 15

Results 16
  Literature Search and Screening 16
  Characteristics of Included Studies... 17
    Home-Visiting Programs 17
    Structured Telephone Support 21
    Telemonitoring.. 23
    Clinic-Based Interventions... 26
    Primarily Educational Interventions 28
    Other Interventions 30
  KQ 1. Transitional Care Interventions and Health Care Utilization Outcomes 31
    Key Points: All-Cause Readmissions 31
    Key Points: Heart Failure-Specific Readmissions... 32
    Key Points: Composite All-Cause Readmission or Death...................................... 32
    Key Points: Emergency Room Visits, Acute Care Visits, Hospital Days 32
    Key Points: Comparative Effectiveness... 32
    Detailed Synthesis: Transitional Care Interventions Compared With Usual Care ... 33
    Detailed Synthesis: Comparative Effectiveness of Transitional Care Interventions ... 42
  KQ 2: Transitional Care Interventions and Health and Social Outcomes 42
    Key Points: Mortality.. 42

Key Points: Quality of Life and Function 43
Key Points: Caregiver and Self-Care Burden 43
Key Points: Comparative Effectiveness.. 43
Detailed Synthesis: Transitional Care Interventions Compared With Usual Care 43
Detailed Synthesis: Comparative Effectiveness of Transitional Care Interventions 49
KQ 3. Components of Effective Interventions 49
KQ 3a. Intervention Components 50
KQ 3b. Necessity of Particular Components in Effective Interventions 58
KQ 3c. Benefits of Particular Components in Multicomponent Interventions..................... 58
KQ 4. Intensity, Delivery Personnel, Method of Communication 58
Key Points: Intensity... 59
Key Points: Delivery Personnel 59
Key Points: Method of Communication 59
Detailed Synthesis.. 59
KQ 5. Subgroups.. 65
Key Points 65
Detailed Synthesis.. 65
Discussion..67
Key Findings and Strength of Evidence 67
Reducing Readmissions and Mortality 67
Utilization Outcomes 71
Quality of Life... 71
Components of Effective Interventions 71
Intensity, Delivery Personnel, and Mode of Delivery 72
Findings in Relation to What Is Already Known 73
Applicability... 74
Implications for Clinical and Policy Decisionmaking... 75
Limitations of the Comparative Effectiveness Review Process 76
Limitations of the Evidence Base 77
Research Gaps... 78
Conclusions... 79
References 81
Abbreviations and Acronyms 88
Glossary of Terms.. 91

Tables
Table A. Categories and definitions of transitional care interventions.................................... ES-7
Table B. Summary of key findings and strength of evidence, by outcome and intervention
category ES-11
Table C. Summary of key findings and strength of evidence for transitional care
interventions: readmission rates and mortality ES-12
Table D. Evidence gaps for future research, by Key Question... ES-19
Table 1. Inclusion/exclusion criteria for studies of transitional care interventions for patients
hospitalized for heart failure 9
Table 2. Categories and definitions of transitional care interventions..................................... 12
Table 3. Definitions of the grades of overall strength of evidence 14

Table 4. Characteristics of trials assessing home-visiting programs 17
Table 5. Characteristics of trials assessing structured telephone support 21
Table 6. Characteristics of trials assessing telemonitoring 24
Table 7. Characteristics of trials assessing outpatient clinic-based interventions 27
Table 8. Characteristics of trials assessing primarily educational interventions 29
Table 9. Characteristics of trials assessing other interventions 30
Table 10. Hospital days accumulated over 6 months: Home visiting versus usual care 41
Table 11. Quality of life or function measures used in the included trials 46
Table 12. Results of quality of life and function: Home visiting versus usual care 46
Table 13. Results of quality of life and function: Structured telephone care versus usual care ... 48
Table 14. KQ 3—Components of effective interventions: All-cause readmissions or composite
(all-cause readmission or death) outcome 51
Table 15. KQ 3—Components of effective interventions: Mortality 55
Table 16. Intensity, delivery personnel, and method of communication in trials assessing home-
visiting programs compared with usual care 60
Table 17. Intensity, delivery personnel, and method of communication in trials assessing
structured telephone support compared with usual care 61
Table 18. Intensity, delivery personnel, and method of communication in trials assessing
telemonitoring compared with usual care 62
Table 19. Intensity, delivery personnel, and method of communication in trials assessing
primarily educational interventions compared with usual care 63
Table 20. Summary of key findings and strength of evidence, by intervention category and
outcome 68
Table 21. Summary of key findings and strength of evidence for transitional care interventions:
Readmission, composite endpoint, and mortality 68
Table 22. Evidence gaps for future research, by Key Question 78

Figures

Figure A. Analytic framework for transitional care interventions to prevent readmissions in
people with heart failure ES-4
Figure B. Disposition of articles about transitional care interventions for patients hospitalized
for heart failure ES-10
Figure 1. Analytic framework for transitional care interventions to prevent readmissions in
people with heart failure 6
Figure 2. Disposition of articles about transitional care interventions for patients hospitalized
for heart failure 17
Figure 3. All-cause readmission for transitional care interventions compared with usual care, by
intervention category and outcome timing: Meta-analysis and forest plot of individual trials 33
Figure 4. HF-specific readmission for transitional care interventions compared with usual care,
by intervention category and outcome timing: Meta-analysis and forest plot of individual
trials 36
Figure 5. Composite all-cause readmission or death for transitional care interventions compared
with usual care, by intervention category and outcome timing: Meta-analysis and forest plot of
individual trials 38
Figure 6. Mortality among patients receiving transitional care interventions compared with usual
care, by intervention category and outcome timing: Meta-analysis and forest plot of individual
trials 44

Appendixes

Appendix A. Literature Search Strategies

Appendix B. Studies Excluded After Full-Text Level Review

Appendix C. Characteristics of Interventions

Appendix D. Risk of Bias Assessments for Included Studies

Appendix E. Meta-Analysis and Forest Plots of Individual Trials

Appendix F. Meta-Analysis and Forest Plots of Individual Trials: Sensitivity Analyses

Appendix G. Strength of Evidence Tables

Executive Summary

Background

Heart failure (HF) is a major public health problem and a leading cause of hospitalization and health care costs in the United States. It is the most common principal discharge diagnosis among Medicare beneficiaries and the third highest for hospital reimbursements, according to 2005 data from the Centers for Medicare & Medicaid Services (CMS).[1] Up to 25 percent of patients hospitalized with HF are readmitted within 30 days.[2-5]

In an effort to reduce the frequency of rehospitalization of Medicare patients, in October 2012 CMS began lowering reimbursements to hospitals with excessive risk-standardized readmission rates as part of the Hospital Readmissions Reduction Program authorized by the Affordable Care Act.[6] This policy provides incentives for hospitals to develop effective transition programs to reduce readmission rates for people with HF.

In 2010, nearly 7 million Americans 18 years of age and older had an HF diagnosis; by 2030, an additional 3 million Americans will have the condition.[7,8] The incidence of HF increases with age; it affects 1 of every 100 people 65 years of age and older.[9] Coronary disease and uncontrolled hypertension are the two highest population-attributable risks for HF.[10] Survival after HF diagnosis has improved over time, as shown by data from the Framingham Heart Study.[11,12] However, the death rate remains high: 50 percent of people diagnosed with HF die within 5 years after diagnosis.[11,12] Among Medicare beneficiaries, more than 30 percent of patients with HF die within 1 year after hospitalization.[13] National data show no evidence that readmission rates for HF patients have fallen during the past two decades, despite the observation that HF hospitalizations in the United States have declined by almost 30 percent during the past decade. Readmission rates vary by both geographic location and insurance coverage.[14,15]

In 2007, the Medicare Payment Advisory Commission called for hospital-specific public reporting of readmission rates, identifying HF as a priority condition. The Commission stated that readmissions for HF were common, costly, and often preventable.[16] An estimated 12.5 percent of readmissions for HF were potentially preventable.[17]

Readmissions following an index hospitalization for HF are related to various conditions. An analysis of Medicare claims data for 2007–09 reported that 35.2 percent of readmissions within 30 days were for HF; the remainder of readmissions were for diverse indications (e.g., renal disorders, pneumonia, arrhythmias, and septicemia or shock).[5]

The relationship between readmission rates and other important outcomes (e.g., mortality, emergency room [ER] visits) is unclear. Some data suggest that hospitals with the lowest mortality rates among patients with HF tend to have higher readmission rates.[18] Some predict that interventions aimed at reducing readmissions may increase use of other health care services, such as ER observational visits.[19]

Transitional Care Interventions for People With Heart Failure

Interventions designed to prevent readmission among patients with HF are often referred to as "transitional care interventions."[20,21] Naylor and colleagues defined transitional care as "a broad range of time-limited services designed to ensure health care continuity, avoid preventable poor outcomes among at-risk populations, and promote the safe and timely transfer of patients from one level of care to another or from one type of setting to another" (p. 747).[20] Transitional care interventions overlap other forms of care (primary care, care coordination, discharge planning, disease management, and case management); however, they aim specifically to avoid poor clinical outcomes arising from uncoordinated care.[22]

No clear set of intervention components defines transitional care interventions. They tend to focus on the following: patient or caregiver education (including education on self-care—e.g., self-titrating diuretics), medication reconciliation, coordination with outpatient providers, arrangements for future care (e.g., home health, outpatient followup), and symptom monitoring or reinforcement of education during the transition (e.g., home visits, telephone support, or additional outpatient visits).

No clear consensus exists about when the transition period ends. Although evaluating 30-day readmissions is important for certain stakeholders (hospitals, payers, quality improvement organizations, health care providers), outcomes beyond this period are clinically important and may benefit from overall improvements in care. Outcomes far away from the index hospitalization probably reflect the natural history of HF or an unrelated illness, whereas a higher proportion of earlier readmissions are thought to be preventable.

Existing Guidance

The 2013 American Heart Association/American College of Cardiology (AHA/ACC) Heart Failure guidelines addressed postdischarge HF interventions.[23] These guidelines focus on the importance of optimizing HF pharmacotherapy before discharge, providing HF education before discharge (including education on self-care), and addressing barriers to care. Specifically, the following components were noted as reasonable postdischarge care options: a followup visit within 7 to 14 days of discharge, a telephone followup within 3 days of discharge, or both.[24] The AHA/ACC guidelines also recommend initiating multidisciplinary (MDS)-HF disease management programs for patients at high risk for readmission. The 2010 Heart Failure Society of America guidelines are similar; their guidance emphasizes particular components of discharge planning.[25,26] No specific guidance is given on the optimal components of transitional care interventions aimed at preventing readmissions for patients with HF.

Several national performance measures pertain to the standard of care for hospital discharge of HF patients. The Joint Commission performance measures mandate that all patients with HF receive comprehensive written discharge instructions or other educational materials that address activity level, diet, discharge medications, followup appointment, weight monitoring, and planned actions to take should symptoms worsen.[27] These measures are publicly reported by hospitals. In 2011, the ACC/AHA/AMA (American Medical Association) Performance Consortium added a documented postdischarge appointment to the list of recommended HF performance measures.[28] Required documentation includes location, date, and time for a followup office visit or home health care visit.

Scope and Key Questions

An assessment of the efficacy, comparative effectiveness, and harms of transitional care interventions is needed to support evidence-based policy and clinical decisionmaking. Despite advances in the quality of acute and chronic HF disease management, gaps remain in knowledge about effective interventions to support the transition of care for patients with HF. To address these issues, we conducted a systematic review and meta-analysis of investigations of transitional care interventions for adults with HF.

Our report focuses mainly on transitional care interventions that aim to reduce 30-day readmission and mortality rates for patients hospitalized with HF. We also include readmissions measured over 3 to 6 months because these are common, costly, and potentially preventable. We examine several related issues, including other health care use (e.g., ER visits), quality of life, and potential harms such as increased caregiver burden. We include these outcomes because they may provide information on the unintended consequences of interventions aimed at preventing readmissions. Specifically, we address the following five Key Questions (KQs):

KQ 1: Among adults who have been admitted for heart failure, do transitional care interventions increase or decrease the following health care utilization rates?

    a. Readmission rates
    b. Emergency room visits
    c. Acute care visits
    d. Hospital days (of subsequent readmissions)

KQ 2: Among adults who have been admitted for heart failure, do transitional care interventions increase or decrease the following health and social outcomes?
    a. Mortality rate
    b. Functional status
    c. Quality of life
    d. Caregiver burden
    e. Self-care burden

KQ 3: This question has three parts:
    a. What are the components of effective interventions?
    b. Among effective interventions, are particular components necessary?
    c. Among multicomponent interventions, do particular components add benefit?

KQ 4: This question has three parts:
    a. Does the effectiveness of interventions differ based on intensity (e.g., duration, frequency, or periodicity) of the interventions?
    b. Does the effectiveness of interventions differ based on delivery personnel (e.g., nurse, pharmacist)?
    c. Does the effectiveness of interventions differ based on method of communication (e.g., face-to-face, telephone, Internet)?

KQ 5: Do transitional care interventions differ in effectiveness or harms for subgroups of patients based on age, sex, race, ethnicity, disease severity (left ventricular ejection fraction or New York Heart Association classification), coexisting conditions, or socioeconomic status?

Analytic Framework

We developed an analytic framework to guide the systematic review process (Figure A).

Figure A. Analytic framework for transitional care interventions to prevent readmissions in people with heart failure

KQ = Key Question.

Methods

Literature Search Strategy

We searched MEDLINE®, the Cochrane Library, and the Cumulative Index to Nursing and Allied Health Literature (CINAHL)® for English-language and human-only studies published from July 1, 2007, to May 9, 2013, and used a previous Agency for Healthcare Research and Quality (AHRQ) Technology Assessment on a similar topic to identify randomized controlled trials (RCTs) published before July 1, 2007.[29] We also searched the same electronic databases for relevant nonrandomized trials or prospective cohort studies from 1990 to May 5, 2013, that measured caregiver or self-care burden. We updated the database searches through October 29, 2013, while the report was undergoing peer review. An experienced Evidence-based Practice Center (EPC) librarian conducted the searches and another EPC librarian peer-reviewed them.

We also manually searched reference lists of pertinent reviews, included trials, and background articles on this topic to look for any relevant citations that our searches might have missed. We searched for unpublished studies relevant to this review using ClinicalTrials.gov and the World Health Organization's International Clinical Trials Registry Platform. We updated these searches through February 5, 2014.

Eligibility Criteria

We developed inclusion and exclusion criteria with respect to populations, interventions, comparators, outcomes, timing, and setting (PICOTS) and study designs. Briefly, we included studies of adults with HF requiring inpatient admission that recruited subjects during or immediately following (i.e., within 1 week) the index hospitalization. We ultimately included one trial (after verification with trial investigators) that enrolled most participants during an inpatient admission but allowed enrollment up to 2 weeks following an inpatient admission.[30]

We required studies to compare a transitional care intervention aimed at reducing readmissions with another transitional care intervention or with usual care (i.e., routine care or standard care, as defined by the primary studies). We required that transitional care interventions include one or more of the following components: education to patient, caregiver, or both delivered predischarge, postdischarge, or both; discharge planning; appointment scheduling before discharge; increased planned or scheduled outpatient clinic visits (primary care, MDS-HF); home visits; telemonitoring (including remote clinical visits); telephone support; transition coach or case management; or interventions to increase provider continuity.

This review focuses on the primary outcomes of readmission rates and mortality. Specifically, we included the following primary outcomes: all-cause readmission, HF-specific readmission, composite all-cause readmission or death, and all-cause mortality. We also evaluated the following outcomes when studies assessing readmission rates or mortality reported them: ER visits, acute care visits, hospital days (of subsequent readmissions), quality of life, functional status, and caregiver or self-care burden. We required a length of followup of at least 30 days, and we included outcomes occurring no more than 6 months from the index hospitalization. We included only studies that assessed interventions applicable to patients who were discharged to home (and not another health care facility).

RCTs were eligible for all KQs. For caregiver burden and self-care burden outcomes, nonrandomized controlled trials or prospective cohort studies with an eligible comparison group were also eligible.

Study Selection

Two members of the research team independently reviewed each title and abstract (identified through searches) to determine eligibility. Studies marked for possible inclusion by either reviewer and those that lacked adequate information to determine eligibility underwent a full-text review. Two members of the team independently reviewed each full-text article to determine eligibility. If the reviewers disagreed, they resolved conflicts by discussion and consensus or by consulting a senior member of the team.

Data Extraction

We designed and used structured data extraction forms to gather pertinent information from each article, including characteristics of study populations, settings, interventions, comparators, study designs, methods, and results. One investigator extracted the relevant data from each included article; a second member of the team reviewed all data abstractions for completeness and accuracy.

Risk-of-Bias Assessment of Individual Studies

To assess the risk of bias (internal validity) of studies, we used predefined criteria based on the AHRQ "Methods Guide for Effectiveness and Comparative Effectiveness Reviews" (Methods Guide).[31] We assessed selection bias, confounding, performance bias, detection bias, and attrition bias. We included questions about adequacy of randomization, allocation concealment, similarity of groups at baseline, masking, attrition, use of intention-to-treat (ITT) analysis, methods of handling missing data, reliability and validity of outcome measures, and treatment fidelity. When assessing measurement bias related to readmission ascertainment, we considered whether studies had access to all potential readmission data as opposed to readmissions collected only from a single institution's database. We rated the studies as low, medium, high, or unclear risk of bias.[31] Two independent reviewers assessed the risk of bias for each study. Disagreements between the two reviewers were resolved by discussion and consensus or by consulting a third member of the team.

Categorization of Interventions

We grouped studies of similar interventions for our evidence synthesis. We categorized intervention types based primarily on the mode and environment of delivery (Table A). We believed that this method of categorization would best address the needs of multiple stakeholders who may be interested in interventions that could be implemented in specific health care settings. One investigator categorized the intervention, and a second team member reviewed the categorization. Disagreements were resolved by consensus. Most of the studies included components delivered both during hospitalization and after discharge.

Table A. Categories and definitions of transitional care interventions

Category	Definition
Home-visiting programs	Home visits by clinicians, such as nurses or pharmacists, who deliver education, reinforce self-care instructions, perform physical examinations, or provide other care (e.g., physical therapy, medication reconciliation). These interventions are often referred to as nurse case-management interventions, but they also can include home visits by a pharmacist or multidisciplinary team.
Structured telephone support	Monitoring, education, and/or self-care management (or various combinations) using simple telephone technology after discharge in a structured format (e.g., series of scheduled calls with a specific goal, structured questioning, or use of decision support software).
Telemonitoring	Remote monitoring of physiological data (e.g., electrocardiogram, blood pressure, weight, pulse oximetry, respiratory rate) with digital, broadband, satellite, wireless, or Bluetooth transmission to a monitoring center, with or without remote clinical visits (e.g., video monitoring).
Outpatient clinic-based interventions	Services provided in one of several different types of outpatient clinics—multidisciplinary-HF, nurse-led HF, or primary care clinic. The clinic-based intervention can be managed by a nurse or other provider and may also offer unstructured telephone support (e.g., patient hotline) outside clinic hours.
Primarily educational interventions	Patient education (and self-care training) delivered before discharge or upon discharge by various delivery personnel or modes of delivery: in person, interactive CD-ROM, video education. Interventions in this category do not feature telemonitoring, home visiting, or structured telephone support. They are not delivered primarily through a clinic-based intervention (described above). Followup telephone calls may occur to ascertain outcomes (e.g., readmission rates) but not to monitor patients' physiological data.
Other	Unique interventions or interventions that did not fit into any of the other categories (e.g., individual peer support for HF patients).

CD-ROM = compact disc read-only memory; HF = heart failure.

Data Synthesis

We conducted meta-analyses using random-effects models to estimate pooled effects. For binary outcomes, we calculated relative risks (RRs) and 95% confidence intervals (CIs). For continuous outcomes (e.g., scales of quality of life or functional status) measured with the same scale, we report the weighted mean difference between intervention and control subjects. When we combined multiple scales in one meta-analysis, we used the standardized mean difference, Cohen's d. A Cohen's d of zero means that the intervention and control groups have equivalent effects; a small effect size is 0.20, medium effect size is 0.50, and large effect size is 0.80.[32] For readmission rates, we conducted meta-analyses of studies that reported the number of people readmitted in each group (and not the total number of readmissions per group). We stratified analyses for each intervention category by timing; specifically, we separated rates reported at 30 days from those beyond 30 days, including combining rates reported over 3 to 6 months. We did not include studies rated as high or unclear risk of bias in our main analyses, but we included them in sensitivity analyses for KQ 1 and KQ 2. We calculated the chi-squared statistic and the I^2 statistic (the proportion of variation in study estimates attributable to heterogeneity) to assess statistical heterogeneity in effects between studies.[33,34] When quantitative synthesis was not appropriate (e.g., because of clinical heterogeneity, insufficient numbers of similar studies, or insufficiency or variation in outcome reporting), we synthesized the data qualitatively.

In addition, we calculated the number needed to treat (NNT) for readmission and mortality outcomes. We derived the NNTs from the RRs and the median usual care event rates reported in included trials, using the methods described in the Cochrane Handbook.[35]

The aim of KQ 3 was to describe the components of effective interventions; KQ 3 is intended as a descriptive question to provide information about the interventions that work to providers, health systems, and others who may want to implement transitional care interventions. For KQ 3, we synthesized the evidence qualitatively by first extracting detailed information on intervention components, content, and processes and then describing common components and combinations of components that were effective in reducing all-cause readmissions or mortality. KQ 3 asks primarily: "What are the components of effective interventions?" and "Are particular components necessary?" We considered "necessary" to mean that a particular component (e.g., inpatient education) was included in every effective intervention but was not necessarily sufficient (i.e., the component could be included in some interventions that were not efficacious). We defined effective interventions as: (1) intervention categories (defined in Table A, above) that reduced all-cause readmissions (from our meta-analyses for KQ 1) or the composite endpoint; (2) intervention categories that reduced mortality in our meta-analyses; (3) individual trials in other categories that were efficacious for reducing all-cause readmissions, mortality, or the composite endpoint.

For KQ 4, we assessed whether the efficacy of interventions differed based on intensity, delivery personnel, and method of communication both across intervention categories and within categories of interventions. We conducted meta-analyses stratified by intensity, delivery personnel, and method of communication within each intervention category when appropriate (e.g., when these factors varied).

Given the heterogeneity of included interventions, we were unable to develop a single measure of intensity to apply to all interventions. We categorized the intensity of each intervention as low, medium, or high using the duration, frequency, and periodicity of patient contact. We also considered resource use as a dimension of intensity, such as the total number of intervention components. We reserved the low-intensity category for interventions that included one episode of patient contact or that required few resources (e.g., no additional components, such as time spent coordinating care).

We considered the majority of interventions to be medium or high intensity; most were multicomponent and included repeated patient contacts. For KQ 4, we included only studies rated as low or medium risk of bias.

Strength of the Body of Evidence

We graded the strength of evidence (SOE) to answer KQs using the guidance established for the EPC program.[36] We graded the SOE for the following outcomes: all-cause readmissions, HF-specific readmissions, a composite endpoint (all-cause readmission or mortality), mortality, ER visits, length of hospital stay (for all-cause readmissions), quality of life, and functional status.

Developed to grade the overall strength of a body of evidence, the approach incorporates four key domains: risk of bias (including study design and aggregate quality), consistency, directness, and precision of the evidence.[36] It also considers optional domains. Two reviewers assessed each domain for each key outcome and determined an overall SOE grade based on domain ratings. In the event of disagreements on the domain rating or overall grade, we resolved differences by discussion or by consulting a third investigator.

SOE grades are specified as high, moderate, low, or insufficient to convey the confidence we have that the effect estimates reported lie close to the true effect of an intervention. "Insufficient" indicates that evidence is unavailable, does not permit estimation of an effect, or does not permit us to draw a conclusion with at least a low level of confidence.

Applicability

We assessed applicability of the evidence following guidance from the Methods Guide.[37] We used the PICOTS framework to explore factors that affect applicability.

Results

We included 53 published articles reporting on 47 studies; all were RCTs (Figure B).

We grouped trials of similar interventions based primarily on the mode and environment of delivery (Table A): home-visiting programs (15 RCTs), structured telephone support (STS) (13 trials), telemonitoring (8 trials), outpatient clinic-based interventions (7 trials), and primarily educational interventions (4 trials). We also included two unique interventions in an "other" category; one featured "individual peer support" and one emphasized cognitive training for patients with coexisting mild cognitive impairment.

Most trials compared a transitional care intervention with usual care; only two trials (both rated high risk of bias) directly compared more than one transitional care intervention. Usual care was somewhat heterogeneous across trials and often not well described.

In general, trials included adults with moderate to severe HF. The mean age of subjects was generally in the 70s; very few trials enrolled patients who were, on average, younger or older. Across most included trials, the majority of patients were prescribed an angiotensin-converting enzyme inhibitor (ACEI) or angiotensin receptor blocker (ARB) (when information was reported). However, the percentages of patients across trials who were prescribed beta-blockers at discharge varied widely. Included trials were conducted in a mix of settings, including academic medical centers, Department of Veterans Affairs (VA) hospital settings, and community hospitals.

Figure B. Disposition of articles about transitional care interventions for patients hospitalized for heart failure

Number of records found through database searching after duplicates removed 2,280 MEDLINE: 1,670 CINAHL: 135 Cochrane Library: 475	Number of additional records identified through other sources 139 Hand searches of references: 139 Gray literature: 0

Total number of records after duplicates removed
2,419

Number of records screened
2,419 → Number of records excluded
2,017

Number of full-text articles assessed for eligibility
402 → Number of full-text articles excluded, with reasons
349

Ineligible publication type: 41
Ineligible design: 62
Ineligible population: 145
Ineligible or no intervention: 30
Ineligible comparator: 4
Ineligible outcomes: 33
Ineligible timing: 34

Number of studies (articles) included in qualitative synthesis of systematic review
47 (53)

Number of studies included in quantitative synthesis of systematic review
45

Efficacy for Reducing Readmissions and Mortality

Table B summarizes our key findings by intervention category, main outcomes (readmission rates, mortality rate, or the composite of all-cause readmissions or death), and timing of measurement of outcomes (30 days, 3–6 months). It documents our results when data met the following three criteria: (1) sufficient evidence to grade the SOE and to draw a conclusion that evidence either supports benefit (+) or does not (-); (2) insufficient (I) evidence to make a determination (e.g., only one trial reporting an outcome of interest); or (3) no included trials that reported an outcome (NR).

Table C presents more detailed results, including RRs and 95% CIs as well as NNTs (when applicable) for comparisons that included at least one trial reporting an outcome of interest.

Table B. Summary of key findings and strength of evidence, by outcome and intervention category

Intervention Category	All-Cause Readmissions		HF Readmissions		Composite Endpoint		Mortality	
	30 Days	3 to 6 Months	30 Days	3 to 6 Months	30 Days	3 to 6 Months	30 Days	3 to 6 Months
Home-visiting programs	+ low[a]	+ high	NR	+ mod	+ low	+ mod	I	+ Mod
Structured telephone support	I	- mod	I	+ high	NR	- low	NR	+ Mod
Telemonitoring	I	- mod	NR	- mod	NR	NR	NR	- Low
MDS-HF clinic interventions	NR	+ high	NR	I	NR	- mod	NR	+ Mod
Nurse-led clinic interventions	NR	- low	NR	I	NR	I	NR	- Low
Primary care clinic interventions	NR	I	NR	NR	NR	NR	NR	I
Primarily educational interventions	NR	I	NR	I	NR	- low	NR	- Low
Other interventions	I	NR	NR	NR	NR	NR	I	NR

[a]Two home-visiting programs reported all-cause readmission at 30 days. The intervention studied by Naylor and colleagues[38] was of higher intensity and showed efficacy. The lower intensity intervention studied by Jaarsma and colleagues[39] did not show efficacy at 30 days (low SOE). The "+" here refers to high intensity home-visiting programs.

Note: Low, mod, high, and I represent our strength-of-evidence grades: mod = moderate, I = insufficient; + indicates that we found benefit (i.e., statistically significant reduction in readmission rate or mortality compared with usual care), - indicates that we found no benefit (i.e., no statistically significant reduction in the outcome). HF = heart failure; MDS = multidisciplinary; NR = not reported (no trials in this category reported an eligible outcome at this timepoint).

Table C. Summary of key findings and strength of evidence for transitional care interventions: readmission rates and mortality

Intervention Category	Outcome	Outcome Timing	N Trials; N Subjects	Relative Risk (95% CI)[a]	Numbers Needed To Treat	Strength of Evidence
Home-visiting programs	All-cause readmission	30 days	2; 418	High intensity (1 study): 0.34 (0.19 to 0.62) Lower intensity (1 study): 0.89 (0.43 to 1.85)	6 for high intensity NA[b] for lower intensity programs	Low[c] for benefit
	All-cause readmission	3 to 6 months	9; 1,563	0.75 (0.68 to 0.86)	9	High for benefit
	HF-specific readmission	3 to 6 months	1; 282	0.51 (0.31 to 0.82)	7	Moderate[d] for benefit
	Composite endpoint[e]	30 days	1; 239	Hazard ratio (SE): 0.869 (0.033) vs. 0.737 (0.041)	NA	Low[f] for benefit
	Composite endpoint	3 to 6 months	4; 824	Hazard ratio (SE): 0.071 (0.045) vs. 0.558 (0.047) 0.78 (0.65 to 0.94)	10	Moderate[g] for benefit
	Mortality	30 days	1; 239	1.03 (0.15 to 7.16)	NA	Insufficient
	Mortality	3 to 6 months	8; 1,693	0.77 (0.60 to 0.997)	33	Moderate for benefit
Structured telephone support	All-cause readmission	30 days	1; 134	0.80 (0.38 to 1.65)	NA	Insufficient
	All-cause readmission	3 to 6 months	8; 2,166	0.92 (0.77 to 1.10)	NA	Moderate for no benefit
	HF-specific readmission	30 days	1; 134	0.63 (0.24 to 1.87)	NA	Insufficient
	HF-specific readmission	3 to 6 months	7; 1,790	0.74 (0.61 to 0.90)	14	High for benefit
	Composite endpoint	3 to 6 months	3; 977	0.81 (0.58 to 1.12)	NA	Low for no benefit
	Mortality	3 to 6 months	7; 2,011	0.74 (0.56 to 0.97)	27	Moderate for benefit
Telemonitoring	All-cause readmission	30 days	1; 168	1.02 (0.64 to 1.63)	NA	Insufficient
	All-cause readmission	3 to 6 months	3; 434	1.11 (0.87 to 1.42)	NA	Moderate[h] for no benefit
	HF-specific readmission	3 to 6 months	1; 182	1.70 (0.82 to 3.51)	NA	Moderate[h] for no benefit
	Mortality	3 to 6 months	3; 564	0.93 (0.25 to 3.48)	NA	Low for no benefit
MDS-HF clinic	All-cause readmission	3 to 6 months	2; 336	0.70 (0.55 to 0.89)	8	High for benefit
	HF-specific readmission	3 to 6 months	1; 106	0.70 (0.29 to 1.70)	NA	Insufficient
	Composite endpoint	3 to 6 months	2; 306	0.80 (0.43 to 1.01)	NA	Moderate for no benefit
	Mortality	3 to 6 months	3; 536	0.56 (0.34 to 0.92)	18	Moderate for benefit

Table C. Summary of key findings and strength of evidence for transitional care interventions: Readmission rates and mortality (continued)

Intervention Category	Outcome	Outcome timing	N Trials; N Subjects	Relative Risk (95% CI)[a]	Numbers Needed to Treat	Strength of Evidence
Nurse-led clinic	All-cause readmission	3 to 6 months	2; 264	0.88 (0.57 to 1.37)	NA	Low for no benefit
	HF-specific readmission	3 to 6 months	1; 158	0.95 (0.68 to 1.32)	NA	Insufficient
	Composite endpoint	3 to 6 months	1; 106	0.66 (0.43 to 1.01)	NA	Insufficient
	Mortality	3 to 6 months	2; 264	0.59 (0.12 to 3.03)	NA	Low for no benefit
Primary care clinic intervention	All-cause readmission	3 to 6 months	1; 443	1.27 (1.05 to 1.54)	NA	Insufficient
	Mortality	3 to 6 months	1; 443	1.52 (0.88 to 2.63)	NA	Insufficient
Primarily educational interventions	All-cause readmission	3 to 6 months	1; 200	1.14 (0.84 to 1.54)	NA	Insufficient
	HF-specific readmission	3 to 6 months	1; 223	0.53 (0.31 to 0.90)	NA	Insufficient
	Composite endpoint	3 to 6 months	2; 423	0.92 (0.58 to 1.47)	NA	Low
	Mortality	3 to 6 months	2; 423	1.20 (0.52 to 2.76)	NA	Low
Other (cognitive training)	All-cause readmission	30 days	1; 125	1.15 (0.71 to 2.28)	NA	Insufficient
	Mortality	30 days	1; 125	0.07 (0.00 to 1.12)	NA	Insufficient

[a]Entries in this column are RRs from our meta-analyses or RR calculations unless otherwise specified. RRs less than 1 favor interventions over controls.

[b]NA entry for NNT indicates that the relative risk (95% CI) was not statistically significant, so we did not calculate an NNT. NA for hazard ratios indicates that we could not calculate an NNT with the data provided by the investigators

[c]Two home-visiting programs reported all-cause readmission at 30 days; the higher intensity intervention showed efficacy but the lower intensity intervention did not. .

[d]Although only 1 trial reported total number of people readmitted per group, we considered the findings consistent because 1 other trial reported on the number of readmissions per group and found a similar effect.

[e]The composite endpoint comprises all-cause readmission or death.

[f] Although only a single trial reported the number of people alive and not readmitted at 30 days and 3 months, we considered the consistency of similar programs reducing 3-month readmission rates when grading the SOE for this intervention at 30 days.

[g] Although evidence was limited to 1 trial, consistency for the 30-day outcome was unknown, and evidence was imprecise, we upgraded the SOE because this intervention category demonstrated no effect on mortality at 3 or 6 months, thus increasing our confidence in the results of this single trial.

[h] Although only a single trial reported on the number of people readmitted, we considered this finding consistent given that 4 other telemonitoring trials reported the total number of readmissions per group (rather than the number of people readmitted); all-cause readmissions did not differ between people receiving telemonitoring and those receiving usual care at 30 days, 3 months, or 6 months.

CI = confidence level; MDS-HF = multidisciplinary heart failure; N = number; NA = not applicable; NNT = number needed to treat; RR = relative risk; SE = standard error; SOE = strength of evidence.

We found very little evidence on whether interventions reduce 30-day readmissions. Most trials reported rates over 3 to 6 months. A high-intensity home-visiting program reduced all-cause readmission and the composite endpoint (all-cause readmission or death) at 30 days (low SOE).[38] Despite having only a single trial of home visiting that reported rates at 30 days, we took into consideration, when grading the SOE, that similar interventions in this category consistently reduced readmission rates over 3 to 6 months. Evidence was insufficient to determine whether the following intervention types reduced 30-day all-cause readmissions (1 trial each, unknown consistency; none showed efficacy): STS, telemonitoring, and cognitive training. We found no eligible trials of other types of interventions that reported 30-day all-cause readmission rates.

For outcomes measured over 3 to 6 months, we found strong evidence of efficacy for improving at least one of our primary outcomes for home-visiting programs, STS, and MDS-HF clinic interventions. Specifically, we found that home-visiting programs and MDS-HF clinic interventions reduced all-cause readmission rates (high SOE for both). Home-visiting programs also reduced HF-specific readmission rates and the composite endpoint (moderate SOE for both outcomes). STS reduced HF-specific readmission rates (high SOE) but not all-cause readmission (moderate SOE). Three interventions produced a mortality benefit (all moderate SOE): home-visiting programs, MDS-HF clinic interventions, and STS.

For all-cause readmission over 3 to 6 months, NNTs were 9 for home-visiting programs and 8 for MDS-HF clinic interventions (Table C). For example, an NNT of 9 signifies that nine people with HF would need to receive a home-visiting program following discharge (rather than usual care) to prevent one additional person from being readmitted over 3 to 6 months. For mortality, NNTs were 33, 27, and 18, respectively, for home-visiting programs, STS, and MDS-HF clinic interventions.

Our meta-analyses found that telemonitoring and primarily educational interventions were not efficacious for any primary outcomes. In addition, home-visiting programs were not efficacious for reducing mortality at 30 days (low SOE). STS interventions were not efficacious for reducing all-cause readmissions (low SOE). Evidence was insufficient to determine the efficacy of the following interventions in reducing readmission rates: most primarily educational interventions, nurse-led HF clinic interventions, primary care clinic interventions, peer support interventions, and cognitive training interventions (for people with HF and coexisting mild cognitive impairment).

Some experts have cautioned that inappropriate focus on reduction of readmission rates could negatively affect patient care and perhaps increase mortality. We found no evidence of such an effect—i.e., no interventions that reduced readmission rates but increased mortality.

Other Utilization Outcomes

Few trials reported on ER visits or hospital days of subsequent readmissions; when these were reported, few trials reported measures in the same manner or at similar timepoints. No trial reported the number of acute outpatient (non-ER) visits.

We generally found insufficient evidence to determine whether transitional care interventions increased or decreased ER visits. The one exception was that STS interventions had no effect on the rate of ER visits over 3 to 6 months (low SOE).

Two intervention types significantly reduced the total number of all-cause hospital days (of subsequent readmissions) over 3 to 6 months: STS (moderate SOE) and home-visiting programs (low SOE). Evidence was generally insufficient to determine whether other transitional care interventions increased or decreased hospital days of subsequent readmissions.

Quality of Life

Few trials measured quality of life or function using the same measures at similar timepoints. We found that improvement in HF-specific quality of life (as measured by the Minnesota Living With Heart Failure questionnaire) was greater for home-visiting programs than usual care over 3 months (low SOE) but not at 6 months (low SOE). STS interventions did not improve HF-specific quality of life at 3 or 6 months. Evidence was insufficient to determine whether other intervention categories improved quality of life.

Components of Effective Interventions

The two categories of interventions that reduced all-cause readmissions and the composite outcome—namely, home-visiting programs and MDS-HF clinic interventions—are multicomponent complex interventions. We found no single-component intervention that reduced all-cause readmissions. As a whole, these two categories of interventions shared the following components:

- HF education emphasizing self-care, recognition of symptoms, and weight monitoring.
- HF pharmacotherapy emphasizing patient education about medications, promotion of adherence to medication regimens, and promotion of evidence-based HF pharmacotherapy before discharge, during followup, or both.
- Face-to-face contact following discharge via home-visiting personnel, MDS-HF clinic personnel, or both. In most cases, this contact occurred within 7 days of discharge.
- Streamlined mechanisms to contact care delivery personnel (clinic personnel or visiting nurses or pharmacists) outside of scheduled visits (e.g., patient hotline).
- Mechanisms for postdischarge medication adjustment. In most cases, home-visiting personnel either directly recommended medication adjustment or assisted with coordination of care (e.g., with primary care provider or cardiologist) to facilitate timely medication adjustment based on a patient's needs (rather than advising patients to call for help themselves).

Three categories of interventions reduced mortality rates over 3 to 6 months: home-visiting programs, STS, and MDS-HF clinic interventions. All are multicomponent complex interventions. As a whole, these three categories of interventions shared the following components:

- HF education emphasizing self-care, recognition of symptoms, and weight monitoring.
- A series of scheduled structured visits (via telephone or clinic followup) that focused on reinforcing education and monitoring for HF symptoms.
- A mechanism to contact providers easily outside of scheduled visits (e.g., patient hotline).

Separating out individual components from the overall categories (or "bundles") of interventions that showed efficacy was not possible.

Intensity, Delivery Personnel, and Mode of Delivery

In general, intervention categories that included higher intensity interventions (i.e., home-visiting programs, STS, MDS-HF clinic interventions) reduced all-cause readmissions or mortality, whereas categories with lower intensity interventions (i.e., primarily educational interventions, nurse-led HF clinic interventions) did not. Within most categories, evidence was insufficient to draw definitive conclusions about whether higher or lower intensity interventions were more or less efficacious in reducing all-cause readmissions or mortality. The one exception was home-visiting programs: a high-intensity program was efficacious in reducing all-cause readmission at 30 days, whereas a low-intensity program was not. Subgroup analyses found no significant difference in efficacy based on intensity for home-visiting programs or STS over 3 to 6 months. Subgroup analyses were not possible for other categories of interventions because of either lack of variation or too few trials reporting outcomes at similar timepoints.

The two categories of interventions that reduced all-cause readmissions and mortality (home-visiting programs and MDS-HF clinic interventions) were more likely to include teams of providers delivering the intervention (e.g., home visits that a nurse and pharmacist conducted together) than interventions that did not show efficacy (e.g., telemonitoring, primarily educational interventions). STS interventions (delivered primarily by nurses and pharmacists) were efficacious in reducing mortality but did not reduce all-cause readmissions. Within categories, evidence was insufficient to draw definitive conclusions about whether specific delivery personnel were more or less efficacious for reducing all-cause readmissions or mortality.

Across intervention categories, interventions were primarily delivered face to face or via technology (telephone, telemonitoring, video visits). The two categories of interventions delivered primarily face to face (i.e., home-visiting programs and MDS-HF clinic interventions) reduced all-cause readmission. For these two categories, method of delivery did not vary within each category. STS reduced mortality; some of these interventions included a face-to-face component (e.g., predischarge educational intervention). In general, interventions primarily delivered remotely (i.e., telemonitoring, STS) did not reduce all-cause readmissions. Only STS interventions varied in the method of communication; our subgroup analyses for reduction in all-cause readmissions and mortality found no statistically significant difference by method of communication at any outcome timepoint.

Discussion

We found very little evidence on whether interventions reduced 30-day readmissions; most trials reported rates over 3 to 6 months. One home-visiting trial showed efficacy in reducing both 30-day all-cause readmission and the 30-day composite outcome.[38] For improving all-cause readmission rates over 3 to 6 months, we found strong evidence of efficacy for home-visiting programs and MDS-HF clinic interventions. Three categories of interventions were efficacious in reducing mortality rates over 3 to 6 months (moderate SOE for each category): home-visiting programs, STS interventions, and MDS-HF clinic interventions.

The two categories of interventions that reduced all-cause readmissions and the composite outcome (home-visiting programs and MDS-clinic interventions) are multicomponent complex interventions. We could not separate out individual components from the overall bundle of interventions that showed efficacy; we found no single-component intervention that reduced all-cause readmissions. Few trials reported on whether transitional care interventions increased or decreased ER visits. Furthermore, few trials measured quality of life at the same timepoint with the same scale. No trial assessed whether transitional care interventions increased or decreased caregiver or self-care burden.

Whether certain interventions that reduce readmissions at 3 and 6 months would also be effective in reducing earlier readmissions remains uncertain. Data based on Medicare claims suggest that 35 percent of 30-day readmissions are for HF; the remainder are for diverse indications (e.g., renal disorders, pneumonia, arrhythmias, and septicemia or shock).[5] We found strong evidence for interventions that provided relatively frequent in-person monitoring following discharge—specifically, home-visiting programs and MDS-HF clinic interventions.

Interventions that did not show efficacy for all-cause readmissions tended to focus on HF self-care promotion alone (e.g., STS, primarily educational interventions). For reducing all-cause readmissions, focusing on HF disease management alone does not appear sufficient.

Current clinical practice in the care of adults with HF after hospitalization varies greatly; readmissions vary by geography and insurance coverage.[14] A recent telephone survey of 100 U.S. hospitals found wide variation in education, discharge processes, care transition, and quality improvement methods for patients hospitalized with HF.[15]

Our findings provide some guidance to quality improvement efforts, especially those that aim to reduce readmissions for people with HF. Specifically, systems or providers aiming to implement interventions to improve transitional care for patients with HF may be uncertain about what type of intervention to implement. Strong evidence supports the use of home-visiting programs and MDS-HF clinic interventions for reducing all-cause readmissions and mortality, and STS for reducing HF-specific readmissions and mortality. These interventions should receive the greatest consideration by systems or providers seeking to implement transitional care interventions for people with HF.

Applicability

Most trials included adults with moderate to severe HF. The mean age of subjects was generally in the 70s; very few trials enrolled patients who were, on average, either younger or older. We did not find evidence to confirm or refute whether transitional care interventions are more or less efficacious for many other subgroups, including groups defined by sex, racial or ethnic minorities, people with higher severity of HF, and those with certain coexisting conditions. Included trials commonly excluded patients who had end-stage renal disease or severe or unstable cardiovascular disease (e.g., recent myocardial infarction). The interventions included are applicable only to patients who are discharged to home; whether interventions would benefit patients who are discharged to another institution (e.g., assisted living facility) remains unclear. Most included trials did not use a readmission risk-prediction tool to determine inclusion eligibility.

All included trials enrolled patients with HF, but some degree of population heterogeneity across intervention categories would affect our findings (e.g., variation in HF severity, etiology, or number of coexisting conditions). The majority of trials included patients with moderate to severe HF based on the New York Heart Association classification and enrolled patients with both preserved and reduced ejection fraction.

One of three trials assessing MDS-HF clinics was conducted in the United States; the other two were conducted in Taiwan and Canada. Whether results reflect differences in populations or health care systems is unclear. Approximately one-half of the home-visiting programs were conducted in the United States; the others were conducted in Australia, the United Kingdom, and various European countries. Across most included trials, the majority of patients were prescribed an ACEI or ARB (when information was reported); however, the percentages of patients across trials who were prescribed beta-blockers at discharge varied widely across trials.

Whether "usual care" in trials published during the early 1990s is comparable to current practice is questionable. In general, trials did not report on details of usual care, including whether followup was scheduled soon after discharge or whether patients were receiving additional services such as home health care. However, rates of readmission in the usual-care arms of included trials are similar to recent rates of readmission in Medicare populations.[2]

Included trials were conducted in a mix of settings; these settings included academic medical centers, VA hospital settings, and community hospitals.

We did not prespecify a magnitude of effect (i.e., a specific reduction in RR) that should be considered a meaningful change in readmission rates from a clinical or policy perspective. The percentage of readmissions that are preventable may differ across settings and patient populations.

Limitations of the Comparative Effectiveness Review Process

The interventions in the included trials were quite diverse; they probably could be categorized using a variety of classification schemes or conceptual models. As explained previously, we classified them in a manner that we believe is both descriptive and informative; it accords with how numerous experts conceptualize these highly varied programs. Nonetheless, we acknowledge that other approaches to categorization could lead analysts to different conclusions. Other reviews have highlighted the difficulty in classifying trials into distinct categories. For example, we classified one trial by Rainville et al.[40] as STS, as did a 2011 Cochrane review,[41] but a 2012 Cochrane review classified the same trial as case management, grouping it with trials that assessed home-visiting programs.[42]

We use the term "transitional care" broadly; generally we were guided by Coleman's definition of "a set of actions designed to ensure the coordination and continuity of health care as patients transfer between different locations or different levels of care within the same location" (p. 30).[22] The included interventions are diverse in terms of whether they aimed to coordinate care at the provider level or focused more on strategies to transfer care back to the patient (e.g., through self-care promotion for managing HF). We did not include or exclude trials based on any specific set of components; for that reason, included trials assess diverse interventions. We chose to cast a broad net to be able to examine a comprehensive set of strategies to reduce readmissions, lower mortality, improve quality of life, or influence other patient-centered outcomes, on the grounds that doing so would be useful to stakeholders in different settings (hospitals, outpatient clinics, or others).

Our inclusion and exclusion criteria specified that included trials had to enroll patients during or soon after a hospitalization for HF and also had to measure a readmission rate at or before 6 months. We did not include readmission rates or mortality rates measured beyond 6 months; interventions that we did not find efficacious may or may not be beneficial in long-term disease management in patients with HF (e.g., perhaps for reducing 12-month readmission rates).

Finally, publication bias and selective reporting are potential limitations. Although we searched for unpublished trials and unpublished outcomes, we did not find direct evidence of either of these biases. Many of the included trials were published before trial registries (e.g., clinicaltrials.gov) became available; had we been able to consult such registries, we would have had greater certainty about the potential for either type of bias.

Limitations of the Evidence Base

The evidence base was inadequate to draw conclusions for some of our questions or subquestions of interest. In particular, as described above, direct evidence was insufficient to permit us to draw conclusions on comparative effectiveness of transitional care interventions. In addition, evidence was quite limited for some outcomes (e.g., readmissions within 30 days, other utilization outcomes such as ER visits, and quality of life). Evidence was insufficient to draw any definitive conclusions about whether any transitional care interventions are more or less efficacious in reducing readmissions or mortality based on patient subgroups defined by age, sex, race, ethnicity, socioeconomic status, disease severity, or coexisting conditions. Only two eligible trials reported information on different subgroups. We identified little evidence on the potential harms of transitional care interventions. No trial measured caregiver burden.

Many trials had methodological limitations introducing some risk of bias. Some trials did not clearly describe methods used for assessing utilization outcomes (e.g., readmissions, ER visits). Methods of handling missing data varied; some trials did nothing to address missing data (i.e., analyzed only completers). However, many trials conducted true ITT analyses and used appropriate methods of handling missing data.

Limitations also included inadequate sample size and heterogeneity of outcome measures across trials (specifically, types of readmission rates). Reporting use of health services other than for the primary outcomes, such as ER visits, was variable across the included trials.

Sometimes usual care and certain aspects of treatment interventions were not adequately described. Specifically, descriptions of whether (and how) interventions addressed medication management were often unsatisfactory. Categories of interventions that showed efficacy (e.g., MDS-HF clinic interventions and home-visiting programs) often included frequent visits with clinicians. Separating out individual components that are necessary from the overall type of interventions that showed efficacy was not possible. Moreover, some confounding components that were not described may be associated with efficacy as well (e.g., addressing social needs, optimizing HF pharmacotherapy).

Research Gaps

We identified important gaps in the evidence that future research could address; many are highlighted above. Of note, these gaps relate only to the KQs this report addresses, and they should not eliminate a wide range of potentially important research that falls outside the specified scope of this review. Table D summarizes the gaps and offers examples of potential future research that could address the gaps.

Table D. Evidence gaps for future research, by Key Question

KQ	Evidence Gap	Potential Future Research and Improved Methods
1	Few trials measured 30-day all-cause readmission outcomes (including those rated as high or unclear risk of bias); we found low SOE for home-visiting programs in reducing all-cause readmission and the composite outcome (all-cause readmission or death). Evidence was insufficient to determine the efficacy of other intervention categories in reducing 30-day readmission rates.	If 30-day readmission rates remain an important metric for policy, reimbursement, and quality, then future studies should evaluate whether interventions that show efficacy in reducing 3- and 6-month readmission rates (e.g., care in an MDS-HF clinic following discharge) are also effective in reducing 30-day readmission rates. Future trials should ensure that the sample sizes and methods of ascertaining readmission outcomes are adequate to determine the effect of transitional care interventions on 30-day readmission rates. Future research could also include methods such as meta-analysis of individual patient data to ascertain whether other intervention categories reduce 30-day readmission rates.

Table D. Evidence gaps for future research, by Key Question (continued)

KQ	Evidence Gap	Potential Future Research and Improved Methods
1, 2	Only one trial evaluated one intervention that was based in a primary care clinic; this intervention primarily aimed to increase access. Evidence was insufficient to determine the efficacy of this intervention in reducing readmissions or mortality.	Given that many patients do not have access to specialty care (e.g., in rural settings) or may prefer to receive care following an HF admission in primary care clinics, future studies should evaluate the efficacy of transitional care interventions based in primary care clinics. Such experimental programs could include features such as home visits or a series of clinic-based visits following discharge. In addition, future research could examine the features of patients receiving services in primary care clinics versus those of patients in cardiology-run HF clinics; these variables might include severity of HF or coexisting conditions.
1, 3, 4	Key intervention components (content and process) were inconsistently described across trials. Some trials provided great detail, others very little. Researchers who aim to assess whether interventions reduce readmissions for the included timepoints (30 days to 6 months) do not use a common conceptual framework.	Future research of transitional care interventions could rely on guidance from the AHA statement offering a taxonomy for disease management for investigators to categorize and compare such programs.[43] Alternatively, the AHA or others might amend this taxonomy to include more specific guidance on categorizing transitional care–type interventions; for instance, incorporating subdomains in the "environment" domain that are more specific to the transition period might be helpful.
1	Evidence was insufficient to determine the comparative effectiveness of transitional care interventions. Nearly all trials examined a particular program against "usual care" of various sorts. No trial tested a single complex intervention with and without a particular component thought to be critical to the intervention.	Future RCTs should address whether certain types of interventions are more efficacious than others. Examples of head-to-head trials include: (1) home-visiting programs that are higher vs. lower intensity or that differ in specific components; and (2) MDS-HF clinic followup compared with home visits that provide similar periodicity of followup and content (e.g., education on self-care and medication reconciliation).
1	Telemonitoring interventions did not reduce readmissions over 6 months; whether this can be attributed to lack of care coordination or other factors remains unclear.	Future RCTs of telemonitoring interventions should include additional components that appear to be necessary for efficacy (based on our results for KQs 1-3). For example, conventional telemonitoring might be combined with one (or more) of three key components: (1) starts immediately after discharge, (2) is combined with initial in-person visits (in the clinic or in the home), and (3) is integrated with the patient's established outpatient care.
2	Evidence was insufficient to determine whether transitional care interventions can reduce 30-day mortality.	Future trials and observational studies should evaluate whether interventions that reduce 30-day readmission rates increase or decrease mortality rates over the same period. There remains a concern about the relationship between reductions in 30-day readmission rates and mortality, especially for vulnerable populations.
2	The literature did not adequately address the effect of interventions on burdens placed on either patients themselves or their caregivers. It also did not adequately examine the effect of interventions on health-related quality of life or physical functioning, beyond measuring changes in disease-specific outcomes (with the MLWHFQ).	Future research should include validated measures of caregiver burden, patient-reported measures of the self-care burden, or both.

Table D. Evidence gaps for future research, by Key Question (continued)

KQ	Evidence Gap	Potential Future Research and Improved Methods
2	The literature did not adequately examine the effect of interventions on health-related quality of life or physical functioning, beyond measuring changes in disease-specific outcomes (with the MLWHFQ).	Health-related quality of life (in the form of PROs) is a crucial variable for many patients, families, professional societies, and research groups. Investigators could continue to use an HF-specific instrument (such as the MLWHFQ, the Kansas City Cardiomyopathy Questionnaire, or the Chronic Heart Failure Assessment tool). For broader quality of life outcomes, researchers should also consider use of reliable and valid PRO instruments; widely administered ones include the Medical Outcomes Study Short Forms and the EURO-QOL.
5	Evidence was insufficient to determine whether certain subgroups of patients benefit from transitional care interventions.	Future research should assess whether readmission rates or other key outcomes differ by sex, racial or ethnic minority status, disease severity, literacy level, income, or socioeconomic status.

AHA = American Heart Association; EURO-QOL = European Quality of Life questionnaire; HF = heart failure; KQ = Key Question; MDS-HF = multidisciplinary heart failure; MLWHFQ = Minnesota Living With Heart Failure Questionnaire; PRO = patient-reported outcome; RCT = randomized controlled trial; SOE = strength of evidence.

We also identified several methodological issues that increased the risk of bias for trials measuring readmission rates; these issues should be addressed in future research. Often trials inadequately described the method of ascertaining use of health care services (e.g., readmissions, ER visits)—specifically, whether measurements were based on patient report, chart review, or some combination of measurements. Masking outcome assessments also raised concerns; for example, in some trials personnel delivering the intervention also appeared to be primarily responsible for measuring health care use. Future studies should consider methods (such as blinded outcome assessments) that guard against measurement bias.

Conclusions

Few trials evaluating transitional care interventions for adults with HF reported 30-day readmission rates; we identified one home-visiting trial that reduced all-cause readmission and the composite endpoint (low SOE). For outcomes measured over 3 to 6 months, home-visiting programs and MDS-HF clinic interventions reduced all-cause readmissions and mortality; STS reduced HF-specific readmissions and mortality. The SOE for these conclusions was high for the readmission measures and moderate for mortality. Based on current evidence, telemonitoring interventions and primarily educational interventions are not efficacious for reducing readmissions or mortality. Direct evidence was insufficient to conclude whether one type of intervention was more efficacious than any other type. Evidence was generally insufficient to determine whether the efficacy of interventions differed for subgroups of patients. We found no evidence on potential harms of transitional care interventions, such as caregiver burden.

References

1. Centers for Medicare & Medicaid Services, Office of Information Services (OIS). Medicare Ranking for All Short-Stay Hospitals by Discharges. Fiscal Year 2005 Versus 2004. 2006. www.cms.hhs.gov/MedicareFeeforSvcParts AB/Downloads/SSDischarges0405.pdf. Accessed December 18, 2012.

2. Jencks SF, Williams MV, Coleman EA. Rehospitalizations among patients in the Medicare fee-for-service program. N Engl J Med. 2009 Apr 2;360(14):1418-28. Epub: 2009/04/03. PMID: 19339721.

3. Bernheim SM, Grady JN, Lin Z, et al. National patterns of risk-standardized mortality and readmission for acute myocardial infarction and heart failure. Update on publicly reported outcomes measures based on the 2010 release. Circ Cardiovasc Qual Outcomes. 2010 Sep;3(5):459-67. Epub: 2010/08/26. PMID: 20736442.

4. Bueno H, Ross JS, Wang Y, et al. Trends in length of stay and short-term outcomes among Medicare patients hospitalized for heart failure, 1993-2006. JAMA. 2010 Jun 2;303(21):2141-7. Epub: 2010/06/03. PMID: 20516414.

5. Dharmarajan K, Hsieh AF, Lin Z, et al. Diagnoses and timing of 30-day readmissions after hospitalization for heart failure, acute myocardial infarction, or pneumonia. JAMA. 2013 Jan 23;309(4):355-63. Epub: 2013/01/24. PMID: 23340637.

6. Centers for Medicare & Medicaid Services. Readmissions Reduction Program. August 2, 2013. www.cms.gov/Medicare/Medicare-Fee-for-Service-Payment/AcuteInpatientPPS/Readmissions-Reduction-Program.html. Accessed September 6, 2013.

7. Roger VL, Go AS, Lloyd-Jones DM, et al. Heart disease and stroke statistics--2012 update: a report from the American Heart Association. Circulation. 2012 Jan 3;125(1):e2-e220. Epub: 2011/12/20. PMID: 22179539.

8. Heidenreich PA, Trogdon JG, Khavjou OA, et al. Forecasting the future of cardiovascular disease in the United States: a policy statement from the American Heart Association. Circulation. 2011 Mar 1;123(8):933-44. Epub: 2011/01/26. PMID: 21262990.

9. Lloyd-Jones DM, Larson MG, Leip EP, et al. Lifetime risk for developing congestive heart failure: the Framingham Heart Study. Circulation. 2002 Dec 10;106(24):3068-72. Epub: 2002/12/11. PMID: 12473553.

10. Kalogeropoulos A, Georgiopoulou V, Kritchevsky SB, et al. Epidemiology of incident heart failure in a contemporary elderly cohort: the health, aging, and body composition study. Arch Intern Med. 2009 Apr 13;169(7):708-15. Epub: 2009/04/15. PMID: 19365001.

11. Roger VL, Weston SA, Redfield MM, et al. Trends in heart failure incidence and survival in a community-based population. JAMA. 2004 Jul 21;292(3):344-50. Epub: 2004/07/22. PMID: 15265849.

12. Levy D, Kenchaiah S, Larson MG, et al. Long-term trends in the incidence of and survival with heart failure. N Engl J Med. 2002 Oct 31;347(18):1397-402. Epub: 2002/11/01. PMID: 12409541.

13. Chen J, Normand SL, Wang Y, et al. National and regional trends in heart failure hospitalization and mortality rates for Medicare beneficiaries, 1998-2008. JAMA. 2011 Oct 19;306(15):1669-78. Epub: 2011/10/20. PMID: 22009099.

14. Allen LA, Tomic KE, Smith DM, et al. Rates and predictors of 30-day readmission among commercially insured and Medicaid-enrolled patients hospitalized with systolic heart failure. Circ Heart Fail. 2012 Nov 1;5(6):672-9. Epub: 2012/10/18. PMID: 23072736.

15. Kociol RD, Peterson ED, Hammill BG, et al. National survey of hospital strategies to reduce heart failure readmissions: findings from the Get With the Guidelines-Heart Failure registry. Circ Heart Fail. 2012 Nov 1;5(6):680-7. Epub: 2012/08/31. PMID: 22933525.

16. Medicare Payment Advisory Committee (MedPAC). Report to the Congress: Promoting Greater Efficiency in Medicare. June 2007. www.medpac.gov/documents/Jun07_Entire Report.pdf.

17. Konstam MA. Home monitoring should be the central element in an effective program of heart failure disease management. Circulation. 2012 Feb 14;125(6):820-7. Epub: 2012/02/15. PMID: 22331919.

18. Krumholz HM, Lin Z, Keenan PS, et al. Relationship between hospital readmission and mortality rates for patients hospitalized with acute myocardial infarction, heart failure, or pneumonia. JAMA. 2013;309(6):587-93. PMID: 23403683.

19. Naylor MD, Kurtzman ET, Grabowski DC, et al. Unintended consequences of steps to cut readmissions and reform payment may threaten care of vulnerable older adults. Health Aff (Millwood). 2012 July 1;31(7):1623-32. PMID: 22722702.

20. Naylor MD, Aiken LH, Kurtzman ET, et al. The care span: the importance of transitional care in achieving health reform. Health Aff (Millwood). 2011 Apr;30(4):746-54. Epub: 2011/04/08. PMID: 21471497.

21. Stauffer BD, Fullerton C, Fleming N, et al. Effectiveness and cost of a transitional care program for heart failure: a prospective study with concurrent controls. Arch Intern Med. 2011 Jul 25;171(14):1238-43. Epub: 2011/07/27. PMID: 21788541.

22. Coleman EA, Boult C. Improving the quality of transitional care for persons with complex care needs. J Am Geriatr Soc. 2003 Apr;51(4):556-7. Epub: 2003/03/27. PMID: 12657079.

23. Jessup M, Abraham WT, Casey DE, et al. 2009 focused update: ACCF/AHA Guidelines for the Diagnosis and Management of Heart Failure in Adults: a report of the American College of Cardiology Foundation/American Heart Association Task Force on Practice Guidelines: developed in collaboration with the International Society for Heart and Lung Transplantation. Circulation. 2009 Apr 14;119(14):1977-2016. Epub: 2009/03/28. PMID: 19324967.

24. Agvall B, Alehagen U, Dahlstrom U. The benefits of using a heart failure management programme in Swedish primary healthcare. Eur J Heart Fail. 2013 Feb;15(2):228-36. Epub: 2012/10/31. PMID: 23109650.

25. Lindenfeld J, Albert NM, Boehmer JP, et al. Executive Summary: HFSA 2010 Comprehensive Heart Failure Practice Guideline. J Card Fail. 2010 Jun;16(6):475-539.

26. Heart Failure Society of America. Executive summary: HFSA 2006 Comprehensive Heart Failure Practice Guideline. J Card Fail. 2006 Feb;12(1):10-38. Epub: 2006/02/28. PMID: 16500578.

27. The Joint Commission. A Comprehensive Review of Development and Testing for National Implementation of Hospital Core Measures. Oak Brook Terrace, IL; 2010 November. www.jointcommission.org/accreditation/acc reditation_main.aspx. Accessed February 14, 2014.

28. Bonow RO, Ganiats TG, Beam CT, et al. ACCF/AHA/AMA-PCPI 2011 performance measures for adults with heart failure: a report of the American College of Cardiology Foundation/American Heart Association Task Force on Performance Measures and the American Medical Association-Physician Consortium for Performance Improvement. Circulation. 2012 May 15;125(19):2382-401. Epub: 2012/04/25. PMID: 22528524.

29. Raman G, DeVine D, Lau J. Non-pharmacological interventions for post-discharge care in heart failure. Technology Assessment. Prepared by the Tufts-New England Medical Center Evidence-based Practice Center (EPC). Contract No. 290-02-0022. Rockville, MD: Agency for Healthcare Research and Quality; February 29, 2008.

30. Kimmelstiel C, Levine D, Perry K, et al. Randomized, controlled evaluation of short- and long-term benefits of heart failure disease management within a diverse provider network: the SPAN-CHF trial. Circulation. 2004 Sep 14;110(11):1450-5. Epub: 2004/08/18. PMID: 15313938.

31. Viswanathan M, Ansari MT, Berkman ND, et al. Assessing the Risk of Bias of Individual Studies in Systematic Reviews of Health Care Interventions. Agency for Healthcare Research and Quality Methods Guide for Comparative Effectiveness Reviews AHRQ Publication No. 12-EHC047-EF. Rockville, MD: March 2012. www.effectivehealthcare.ahrq.gov.

32. Cohen J. Statistical Power Analysis for the Behavioral Sciences. 2nd ed., Hillsdale, NJ: Erlbaum; 1988.

33. Higgins JP, Thompson SG. Quantifying heterogeneity in a meta-analysis. Stat Med. 2002 Jun 15;21(11):1539-58. Epub: 2002/07/12. PMID: 12111919.

34. Higgins JP, Thompson SG, Deeks JJ, et al. Measuring inconsistency in meta-analyses. BMJ. 2003 Sep 6;327(7414):557-60. Epub: 2003/09/06. PMID: 12958120.

35. Schünemann HJ, Oxman AD, Vist GE, et al. Chapter 12: Interpreting results and drawing conclusions. In: Higgins JPT, Green ST, eds. Cochrane Handbook for Systematic Reviews of Interventions Version 5.1.0 [updated March 2011]. The Cochrane Collaboration; 2011.

36. Owens DK, Lohr KN, Atkins D, et al. AHRQ series paper 5: grading the strength of a body of evidence when comparing medical interventions--Agency for Healthcare Research and Quality and the Effective Health Care Program. J Clin Epidemiol. 2010 May;63(5):513-23. Epub: 2009/07/15. PMID: 19595577.

37. Atkins D, Chang S, Gartlehner G, et al. Chapter 6: Assessing the Applicability of Studies When Comparing Medical Interventions. AHRQ Publication No. 11-EHC019-EF. Agency for Healthcare Research and Quality; January 11 2011. www.effectivehealthcare.ahrq.gov.

38. Naylor MD, Brooten DA, Campbell RL, et al. Transitional care of older adults hospitalized with heart failure: a randomized, controlled trial. J Am Geriatr Soc. 2004 May;52(5):675-84. Epub: 2004/04/17. PMID: 15086645.

39. Jaarsma T, Halfens R, Huijer Abu-Saad H, et al. Effects of education and support on self-care and resource utilization in patients with heart failure. Eur Heart J. 1999 May;20(9):673-82. Epub: 1999/04/20. PMID: 10208788.

40. Rainville EC. Impact of pharmacist interventions on hospital readmissions for heart failure. Am J Health Syst Pharm. 1999 Jul 1;56(13):1339-42. Epub: 2000/02/22. PMID: 10683133.

41. Inglis SC, Clark RA, Cleland JG. Telemonitoring in patients with heart failure. N Engl J Med. 2011 Mar 17;364(11):1078-9. PMID: 21410377.

42. Takeda A, Taylor SJ, Taylor RS, et al. Clinical service organisation for heart failure. Cochrane Database Syst Rev. 2012(9):CD002752. Epub: 2012/09/14. PMID: 22972058.

43. Krumholz HM, Currie PM, Riegel B, et al. A taxonomy for disease management: a scientific statement from the American Heart Association Disease Management Taxonomy Writing Group. Circulation. 2006 Sep 26;114(13):1432-45. Epub: 2006/09/06. PMID: 16952985.

Introduction

Background

Heart failure (HF) is a major clinical and public health problem and a leading cause of hospitalization and health care costs in the United States. It is the most common principal discharge diagnosis among Medicare beneficiaries and the third highest for hospital reimbursements, according to 2005 data from the Centers for Medicare & Medicaid Services (CMS).[1] Up to 25 percent of patients hospitalized with HF are readmitted within 30 days.[2-5] These numbers vary by geographic area and insurance coverage.[6]

Interventions aimed specifically at preventing early readmission among patients with HF have been developed; they are often referred to as "transitional care interventions."[7,8] To reduce the frequency of rehospitalization of Medicare patients, in October 2012 CMS began lowering reimbursements to hospitals with excessive risk-standardized readmission rates as part of the Hospital Readmissions Reduction Program authorized by the Affordable Care Act.[9] These measures apply to patients readmitted to any hospital within 30 days of discharge for applicable conditions (HF, acute myocardial infarction, and pneumonia). These policies may promote hospitals to develop effective transition programs to reduce readmission rates for people with HF.

An assessment of the effectiveness and harms of transitional care interventions is needed to support evidence-based policy and clinical decisionmaking. Despite advances in the quality of acute and chronic HF disease management, gaps remain in knowledge about effective interventions to support the transition of care for patients with HF.

Epidemiology of Heart Failure in the United States

In 2010, nearly 7 million Americans 18 years of age and older had a diagnosis of HF; by 2030, an additional 3 million Americans will have the condition.[10,11] The incidence of HF increases with age; it affects 1 of every 100 people after 65 years of age.[12] Coronary disease and uncontrolled hypertension are the highest population-attributable risks for HF.[13] Three-quarters of HF patients have antecedent hypertension.

Survival after HF diagnosis has improved over time, as shown by data from the Framingham Heart Study.[14,15] However, the death rate remains high: 50 percent of people diagnosed with HF die within 5 years after diagnosis.[14,15] Among Medicare beneficiaries, more than 30 percent of patients with HF die within 1 year after hospitalization.[16]

HF hospitalizations in the United States have declined by almost 30 percent during the past decade. However, national data show no evidence that readmission rates for HF patients have fallen during the past 2 decades.[17]

Heart Failure and Preventable Readmissions

Goldfield and colleagues defined a preventable readmission as one clinically related to the prior admission if there was a reasonable expectation that it could have been prevented by provision of quality care in the initial hospitalization, adequate discharge planning, adequate postdischarge followup, or improved coordination between inpatient and outpatient health care teams.[18] Although hospital readmission within 30 days of discharge is a crude measure, it has long been used as a quality metric.

In 2007, the Medicare Payment Advisory Commission called for hospital-specific public reporting of readmission rates, identifying HF as a priority condition. The Commission stated that readmissions for HF were common, costly, and often preventable.[19] An estimated 12.5 percent of admissions for HF were potentially preventable; this number is based on claims data analysis that identifies "red flags" in readmission diagnoses that are likely to represent conditions associated with a prior admission (and, therefore, likely preventable).[20]

Readmissions following an index hospitalization for HF appear to be related to various conditions. An analysis of 2007 to 2009 Medicare claims data showed that 24.8 percent of beneficiaries admitted with HF were readmitted within 30 days; 35.2 percent of those readmissions were for HF, and the remainder of readmissions were for diverse indications (e.g., renal disorders, pneumonia, arrhythmias, and septicemia/shock).[5] The broad range of conditions responsible for readmissions may reflect a "posthospitalization syndrome"—a generalized vulnerability to illness among recently discharged patients.[5,21]

The relationship between readmission rates and other important outcomes (e.g., mortality, emergency room visits) is unclear. Some data suggest that hospitals with the lowest mortality rate among patients with HF tend to have higher readmission rates.[22] Some predict that interventions aimed at reducing readmissions may increase use of other health care services, such as emergency room observational visits.[23]

Transitional Care for People With Heart Failure

Poorly executed care transitions can lead to inappropriate use of hospital, emergency care, and other services. Recently, experts have used the phrase *transitional care interventions* to describe disease-management interventions targeted toward populations transitioning from one care setting to another.[7,24] Naylor and colleagues defined transitional care as "a broad range of time-limited services designed to ensure health care continuity, avoid preventable poor outcomes among at-risk populations, and promote the safe and timely transfer of patients from one level of care to another or from one type of setting to another" (p.747).[7,24]

Transitional care interventions overlap with other forms of care (primary care, care coordination, discharge planning, disease management and case management). However, they aim specifically to avoid poor clinical outcomes arising from uncoordinated care.[24]

Similarly, the American Geriatrics Society defines transitional care as "a set of actions designed to ensure the coordination and continuity of health care as patients transfer between different locations or different levels of care within the same location" (p. 30).[24] Interventions include logistical arrangements, education of the patient and family, and coordination among the health professionals involved in the transition. In general, the intended mechanism of action of these interventions is to prevent complications that can occur during the transition from one care setting to another (e.g., medication errors or misunderstanding of self-care instructions) and thus avoid unnecessary readmissions that result from those complications.

No clear consensus exists about when the transition period ends. Although evaluating 30-day readmissions is important for certain stakeholders (hospitals, payers, quality improvement organizations, health care providers), outcomes beyond this period are clinically important and may benefit from overall improvements in care. Outcomes far away from the index hospitalization probably reflect the natural history of HF or an unrelated illness, whereas a higher proportion of early readmissions are thought to be preventable. No clear recipe or set of intervention components defines transitional care interventions; interventions occurring at the patient, health care provider, facility, and system levels are emphasized throughout the care transition. Transitional care interventions tend to focus on the following: patient or caregiver education (including education on self-care, e.g., self-titrating diuretics), medication reconciliation, coordination with outpatient providers, arrangements for future care (e.g., home health, outpatient followup), and symptom monitoring or reinforcement of education during the transition (e.g., home visits, telephone support, or additional outpatient visits).

Existing Guidelines and Current Practice

Existing Guidelines

The 2013 American Heart Association/American College of Cardiology (AHA/ACC) Heart Failure guidelines addressed postdischarge HF interventions.[25] These guidelines focus on the importance of optimizing HF pharmacotherapy before discharge, providing HF education before discharge (including self-care management), and addressing barriers to care among other factors. Specifically, the following components were noted as reasonable care options: a follow-up visit within 7 to 14 days of disease or a telephone followup within 3 days of discharge (or both).[26] The AHA/ACC guidelines also recommend initiating multidisciplinary (MDS)-HF disease management programs for patients at high risk for readmission.

The 2010 Heart Failure Society of America guidelines are similar; their guidance emphasizes particular components of discharge planning.[27] The Society does not provide specific guidance on the optimal components of transitional care interventions aimed at preventing readmissions for patients with HF.

Current Practice

Several national performance measures pertain to the standard of care for hospital discharge of HF patients. The Joint Commission performance measures mandate that all patients with HF should receive comprehensive written discharge instructions or other educational materials that address activity level, diet, discharge medications, follow-up appointment, weight monitoring, and planned actions to take should symptoms worsen.[28] Hospitals publicly report these measures. In 2011, the ACC/AHA/AMA (American Medical Association) Performance Consortium added a documented postdischarge appointment to the list of recommended HF performance measures.[29] Required documentation includes location, date, and time for a follow-up office visit or home health care visit.

Current clinical practice in the care of adults with HF after hospitalization is quite diverse. A recent telephone survey of 100 U.S. hospitals found wide variation in education, discharge processes, care transition, and quality-improvement methods for patients hospitalized with HF.[17] Readmission rates vary by both geographic location and insurance coverage.[6]

Rationale for Evidence Review

Targeting preventable readmissions is an important goal in reducing overall health care costs from both societal and payer perspectives. The cost of care for HF patients is growing as the population ages; the predominant cost driver is hospitalization. Readmissions account for an estimated $15 billion in annual Medicare spending.[30] For hospitals, reducing 30-day risk-stratified readmission rates may prevent decreases in Medicare reimbursement. From a patient perspective, addressing preventable readmissions may improve quality of life or function, reduce personal costs, and lower caregiver burden.

3

Uncertainty remains about effective strategies to reduce early readmission rates among adults with HF. Recent systematic reviews that have addressed HF disease management or transitional care programs have tended to focus on outcomes at 6 to 12 months after an index hospitalization,[31] include a narrow range of interventions,[32] or exclude interventions that are disease specific (i.e., specific to HF patients).[33] Potential harms or unintended consequences of interventions do not appear to have been widely considered in previous reviews. For example, HF may place a tremendous burden on patients and families. Effective self-care involves adhering to medication regimens, observing dietary restrictions, managing symptom (e.g., adjusting diuretic dosing), and notifying providers when problems arise.[34,35] Interventions aimed to promote self-care among HF patients may increase (or decrease) patient and caregiver burden.

Scope and Key Questions

A community hospital administrator nominated this topic; the nominator wanted to know how to prevent readmissions for patients with HF. The primary interest involved the Hospital Readmissions Reduction Program and penalties assigned by CMS for excess risk-stratified readmissions. The nominator commented that reducing mortality and improving quality of life were also important outcomes.

To address these issues, we conducted a systematic review and meta-analysis of the effectiveness of transitional care interventions for adults with HF. Our report focuses mainly on transitional care interventions that aim to reduce "early" readmissions and mortality for patients hospitalized with HF. We consider early to include these events occurring at any time up to 6 months following an index hospitalization. We also examine several related issues, including use of other health care services (e.g., emergency room visits), quality of life, and potential harms such as increased caregiver burden. We include these outcomes because they provide information on the potential implications on other health and utilization outcomes of strategies aimed at preventing readmissions. Specifically, we address the following five Key Questions (KQs):

Key Question 1. Among adults who have been admitted for heart failure, do transitional care interventions increase or decrease the following health care utilization rates?

a. Readmission rates

b. Emergency room visits

c. Acute care visits

d. Hospital days (of subsequent readmissions)

Key Question 2. Among adults who have been admitted for heart failure, do transitional care interventions increase or decrease the following health and social outcomes?

a. Mortality rate

b. Functional status

4

c. Quality of life

d. Caregiver burden

e. Self-care burden

Key Question 3. This question has three parts:

a. What are the components of effective interventions?

b. Among effective interventions, are particular components necessary?

c. Among multicomponent interventions, do particular components add benefit?

Key Question 4. This question has three parts:

a. Does the effectiveness of interventions differ based on intensity (e.g., duration, frequency or periodicity) of the interventions?

b. Does the effectiveness of interventions differ based on delivery personnel (e.g., nurse, pharmacist)?

c. Does the effectiveness of interventions differ based on method of communication (e.g., face-to-face, telephone, Internet)?

Key Question 5. Do transitional care interventions differ in effectiveness or harms for subgroups of patients based on age, sex, race, ethnicity, disease severity (left ventricular ejection fraction or New York Heart Association classification), coexisting conditions, or socioeconomic status?

Analytic Framework

We developed an analytic framework to guide the systematic review process (Figure 1). It notes all five KQs. Both KQ 1 and KQ 2 address the potential benefits and harms of transitional care interventions. The two overarching boxes (components; the effectiveness variables) address KQ 3 and KQ 4, respectively.

Figure 1. Analytic framework for transitional care interventions to prevent readmissions in people with heart failure

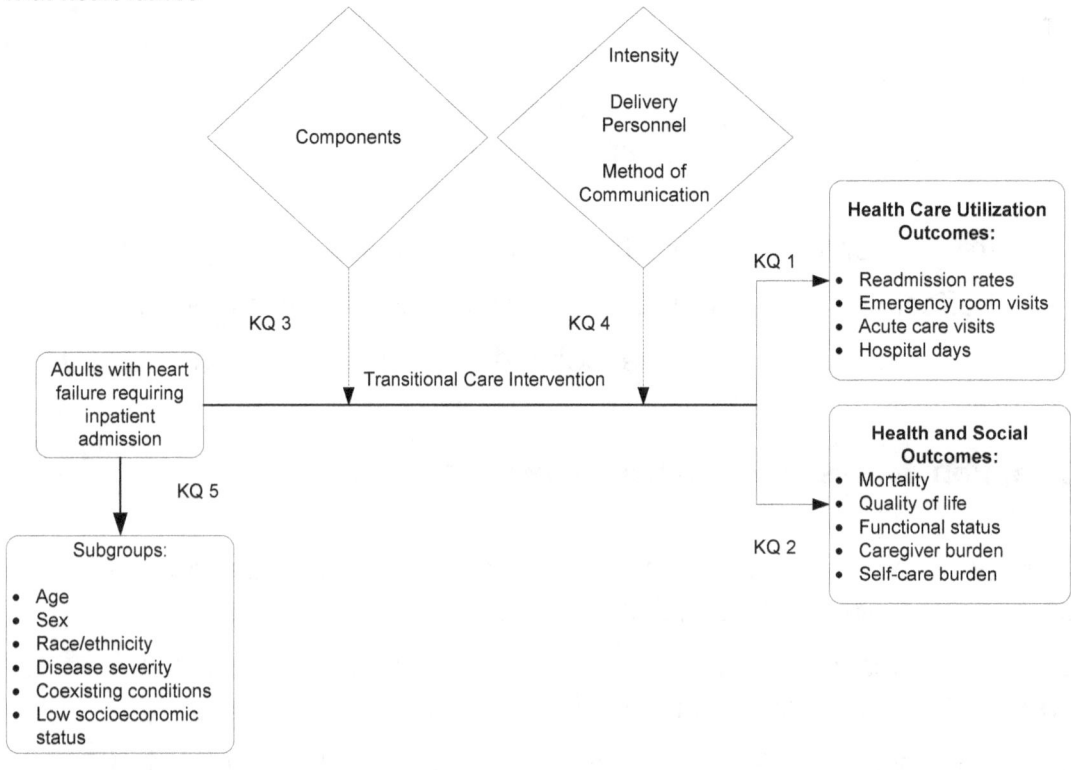

KQ = key question

Organization of This Report

The remainder of the review describes our methods in detail and presents the results of our synthesis of the literature with summary tables and the strength-of-evidence grades for major comparisons and outcomes. The discussion section offers our conclusions, summarizes our findings, and provides other information relevant to the interpretation of this work for clinical practice and future research. References, a list of acronyms and abbreviations, and a glossary of terms follow the discussion section.

Appendix A contains the exact search strings we used in our literature searches. Studies excluded at the stage of reviewing full-text articles with reasons for exclusion are listed in Appendix B. Detailed tables of intervention components appear in Appendix C. Appendix D provides the specific questions used for evaluating the risk of bias of all included trials, documents risk-of-bias ratings for each study, and explains the rational for high or unclear ratings. Appendices E and F document various meta-analyses (Appendix E gives forest plots to summarize results of individual trials and pooled analyses; Appendix F presents sensitivity analyses). Appendix G presents information about our grading of the strength of the various bodies of evidence (tables for individual domain assessments and overall strength-of-evidence grades for each KQ, organized by intervention category).

Methods

The methods for this review of transition care for heart failure (HF) patients follow those specified for the Agency for Healthcare Research and Quality (AHRQ) Evidence-based Practice Center (EPC) program. This guidance is codified in the "Methods Guide for Effectiveness and Comparative Effectiveness Reviews" (hereafter, Methods Guide, available at http://www.effectivehealthcare.ahrq.gov/methodsguide.cfm).

Topic Refinement and Review Protocol

During the topic development and refinement processes, we engaged in a public process to develop a draft and final protocol for the systematic review process. We generated an analytic framework, preliminary Key Questions (KQs), and preliminary inclusion/exclusion criteria in the form of PICOTS (populations, interventions, comparators, outcomes, timing, settings). The processes were guided by the information provided by the topic nominator, a scan of the literature, methods and content experts, and Key Informants. We worked with six Key Informants during the topic refinement; three were subsequently members of our Technical Expert Panel (TEP) for this report. Key Informants and a total of eight TEP members participated in conference calls and discussions through email to review the analytic framework, KQs, and PICOTS, discuss the preliminary assessment of the literature, provide input on the information and categories included in evidence tables, and comment on the data analysis plan.

Our KQs were posted for public comment on AHRQ's Effective Health Care Web site from February 22, 2013, through March 21, 2013; we revised them as needed after review of the comments and discussion with AHRQ and the TEP, primarily for clarity and readability. We then drafted a protocol, which was also posted on the Effective Health Care Web site on June 10, 2013.

Literature Search Strategy

Search Strategy

We searched MEDLINE®, the Cochrane Library, and the Cumulative Index to Nursing and Allied Health Literature (CINAHL)® from July 1, 2007 to May 9, 2013. We also used a previous AHRQ Technology Assessment on a similar topic to identify randomized controlled trials (RCTs) published before 2007.[36] Appendix A presents the full search strategy.

We used either Medical Subject Headings (MeSH) or major headings as search terms when available or key words when appropriate, focusing on terms to describe the relevant population and interventions of interest. We reviewed our search strategy with the TEP and incorporated their input into our search strategy. An experienced information scientist (an EPC librarian) conducted the searches; another information scientist at the EPC peer-reviewed them. We conducted quality checks to ensure that our searches identified known studies (i.e., studies identified during topic nomination and refinement).

Using the previously published AHRQ Technology Assessment on Non-Pharmacological Interventions for Postdischarge Care in Heart Failure, we identified relevant studies published from 1990 through July 1, 2007.[36] Its start date (1990) reflects the timing of advances in the medical management of HF, including the increased use of beta-blockers. We applied our current inclusion and exclusion criteria to RCTs in this earlier publication; our criteria are similar but narrower in scope—that is, limited to outcomes (readmissions, deaths, or other outcomes) timings occurring no more than 6 months from the index hospitalization.

We also searched MEDLINE, the Cochrane Library, and CINAHL for nonrandomized trials or prospective cohort studies of transitional care interventions that measured caregiver or self-care burden from 1990 to May 5, 2013. The previous review did not include these outcomes. We considered observational studies to ensure that we captured relevant literature addressing these potential consequences of transitional care interventions that RCTs may be less likely to report.

We searched for unpublished studies relevant to this review using ClinicalTrials.gov and the World Health Organization's International Clinical Trials Registry Platform.

We manually searched reference lists of pertinent reviews, included trials, and background articles on this topic to look for any relevant citations that our searches might have missed. We imported all citations into an EndNote® X4 electronic database.

We updated the database searches through October 29, 2013 (of the same databases), while the report was undergoing peer review. We investigated any literature suggested by peer reviewers or public comment respondents and, if found appropriate, incorporated the publications into the final review. We determined appropriateness of the publications by the same inclusion and exclusion criteria as we applied to the original searches.

Inclusion and Exclusion Criteria

We developed eligibility (inclusion and exclusion) criteria with respect to PICOTS, study designs, and study durations for each KQ (Table 1). The focus of this review is on the primary outcomes of readmission rates and mortality. Specifically, we included the following primary outcomes: all-cause readmission, HF-specific readmission, composite all-cause readmission or death, and all-cause mortality. We also evaluated the following outcomes when studies assessing readmission rates or mortality reported them: emergency room visits, acute care visits, hospital days (of subsequent readmissions), quality of life, functional status, caregiver or self-care burden. We were specifically interested in validated measures of caregiver outcomes and outcomes specific to patient self-care burden; however, we also sought evidence on burden of treatment in general (experienced by patients or caregivers) associated with transitional care interventions (e.g., confusion regarding medical information, stress or difficulty related to frequent outpatient appointments). We cast a broad net and initially included any outcomes that might be relevant in both RCTs and observational studies. During full-text review, we specifically excluded outcomes that measured patient satisfaction and self-care knowledge.

Study Selection

Two members of the research team independently reviewed all titles and abstracts (identified through searches) for eligibility against our inclusion/exclusion criteria (Table 1); we retrieved any publications marked for inclusion by either reviewer for evaluation of the full text. For titles and abstracts that lacked adequate information to determine inclusion or exclusion, we retrieved the full text for review. Then two investigators independently reviewed the full texts to determine final inclusion or exclusion. The reviewers resolved any disagreements by discussion and consensus or by consulting a third member of the review team.

All results in both review stages were tracked in an EndNote® database. We recorded the principal reason that each excluded full-text publication did not satisfy the eligibility criteria (Appendix B).

Table 1. Inclusion/exclusion criteria for studies of transitional care interventions for patients hospitalized for heart failure

Category	Criteria	
	Inclusion	**Exclusion**
Population	• Adults (ages 18 years or older) with HF requiring inpatient admission • Recruited during or immediately following an index hospitalization for HF[a]	Children and adolescents under 18
Interventions	Any transitional care interventions aimed at reducing readmissions, including one or more of the following components: • Education to patient or caregiver (or both), delivered pre- or postdischarge (or both) • Discharge planning • Appointment scheduling before discharge • Increased planned or scheduled outpatient clinic visits (primary care, multidisciplinary HF) • Home visits • Telemonitoring (including remote clinical visits) • Telephone support • Transition coach or case management • Interventions to increase provider continuity (same provider-continuity between inpatient and outpatient care)	• proBNP guided therapy • Pharmacotherapy (e.g., randomized trials of using a medication compared with placebo) • Physician training (e.g., continuing medical education on evidence-based treatment for HF patient management) • Surgical interventions or invasive procedures (e.g., left ventricular assist device, ultrafiltration, dialysis) • Technology aimed at guiding evaluation of patient volume status (e.g., pulmonary artery pressure sensor, segmental multifrequency bioelectrical impedance analysis) • Hospital-at-home interventions
Comparators	• Usual care, routine care, or standard care (as defined by the primary studies) • Comparison of one intervention with another eligible intervention	Comparison of one intervention with an excluded intervention.
Outcomes[b]	KQ 1: Readmission rates or the composite outcome (all-cause readmission or death), emergency room visits, acute care visits, all-cause hospital days (of subsequent readmissions) KQ 2: Mortality, quality of life, functional status[c] caregiver or self-care burden KQ 3: All-cause readmissions, mortality, and the composite outcome (all-cause readmission or death) KQ 4: All-cause readmission and mortality KQ 5. Subgroups: any outcome eligible for KQ 1 or KQ 2	Trials that reported only an eligible quality-of-life or functional status outcome (and no readmission or mortality rate) were excluded from the analysis unless they were a companion to a trial that measured readmission rates. Other composite endpoints (e.g., all-cause readmission or emergency room visits) were excluded.
Timing of outcome measurement Length of followup	• Outcomes (readmissions, deaths, or other outcomes) occurring no more than 6 months from the index hospitalization • Followup must be at least 30 days	• Outcomes measured at any time after 6 months • Followup is less than 30 days
Time period	Studies published from 1990 to October 29, 2013	Studies published earlier than 1990
Settings	• Interventions occurring during the index hospitalization, before discharge • Interventions initiated as an outpatient following the index hospitalization • Interventions bridging the transition from inpatient to outpatient care	All other settings (e.g., discharge to a skilled nursing facility or rehabilitation center)
Publication language	English	All other languages

Table 1. Inclusion/exclusion criteria for studies of transitional care interventions for patients hospitalized for heart failure (continued)

Category	Criteria	
	Inclusion	Exclusion

Admissible evidence (study design and other criteria)	• Original research
	• Eligible study designs include the following:
	  – For all KQs, randomized controlled trials
	  – For caregiver burden and self-care burden, nonrandomized controlled trials or prospective cohort studies with an eligible comparison group
		• Case series
		• Case reports
		• Nonsystematic reviews
		• Systematic reviews
		• Editorials
		• Letters to the editor
		• Case-control studies
		• Retrospective cohort studies
		• Studies with historical, rather than concurrent, control groups

[a] During data abstraction we required that populations had been recruited during or within 1 week of an index hospitalization. If the study authors did not reported this clearly, we contacted them to obtain additional information. When we could not verify whether the majority of the population had been recruited during this time period, we excluded the study.

[b] We did not consider results presented only in figures (e.g., Kaplan-Meier curves) as eligible for inclusion when the investigators did not clearly report results for an eligible outcome timing (readmission rate no more than 6 months from the index hospitalization).

[c] Eligible quality of life and functional status measures included the Minnesota Living With Heart Failure Questionnaire (MLWHFQ), the Quality of Life Index – Cardiac Version, Kansas City Heart Failure Questionnaire, 6-minute walk test, change in the New York Heart Association (NYHA) classification from baseline, Medical Outcomes Study Short Form with 36 items (SF-36), 12-Item Short form Health Survey (SF-12) and EuroQoL (or EQ-5D).

HF = heart failure; KQ = Key Question; proBNP = probrain natriuretic peptide; PICOTS = populations, interventions, comparators, outcomes, timing, and setting.

Data Extraction

For studies that met our inclusion criteria, we designed and used structured data extraction forms to gather pertinent information from each article, including characteristics of study populations, settings, interventions, comparators, study designs, methods, and results. One investigator extracted the relevant data from each included article; all data abstractions were reviewed for completeness and accuracy by a second member of the team. We recorded intention-to-treat (ITT) results if available. All data abstraction was performed using Microsoft Excel® software.

Risk-of-Bias Assessment of Individual Studies

To assess the risk of bias (internal validity) of studies, we used predefined criteria based on the AHRQ Methods Guide. These criteria included questions to assess selection bias, confounding, performance bias, detection bias, and attrition bias (i.e., those about adequacy of randomization, allocation concealment, similarity of groups at baseline, masking, attrition, use of ITT analysis, method of handling dropouts and missing data, reliability and validity of outcome measures, and treatment fidelity).[37] Appendix D provides the specific questions used for evaluating the risk of bias of all included studies. It also includes a table showing the responses to these questions and risk-of-bias ratings for each study and explains the rationale for all ratings that were either high or unclear.

In general terms, results from a low risk-of-bias study are considered to be valid. A study with moderate risk of bias is susceptible to some risk of bias but probably not enough to invalidate its results. A study assessed as high risk of bias has significant risk of bias (e.g., stemming from serious errors in design, conduct, or analysis) that may invalidate its results. To assess publication bias, we looked for evidence of unpublished literature through searches of gray literature (clinicaltrials.gov). We also reviewed (when available) the original protocols for included trials to assess for selective outcome reporting.

We determined the risk-of-bias rating using the responses to all questions assessing the various types of bias listed above. To receive a low risk-of-bias rating, we required favorable responses to most questions, and any unfavorable responses had to be relatively minor (e.g., lack of provider masking in home-visiting programs, which is generally not considered possible). We gave medium risk-of-bias ratings to studies that did not meet criteria for low or high risk of bias. We rated studies as medium risk of bias that we determined to have more than one unfavorable response and that were not considered to have major methodological shortcomings, but had shortcomings which may introduce some bias. We gave high risk-of-bias ratings to studies that we determined to have a major methodological shortcoming in one or more categories based on our qualitative assessment. Common methodological shortcomings contributing to high risk-of-bias ratings were high rates of attrition or differential attrition, inadequate methods used to handle missing data, lack of ITT analysis, and unclear or invalid measures of readmission or mortality rates. When assessing measurement bias related to readmission ascertainment, we considered whether a study had access to all potential readmission data (versus readmissions collected from only a single institution's database). When investigators used data from only a single institution to measure readmission rates (without at least collecting additional data on admissions to other institutions from patients or caregivers), we considered this a major methodological shortcoming (e.g., high risk of measurement bias). We rated studies as unclear risk of bias when information provided was inadequate for judging the validity of outcome measures (primarily readmission rates and mortality).

Two independent reviewers assessed the risk of bias for each study. Disagreements between reviewers were resolved by discussion and consensus or by consulting a third member of the team.

We did not use studies deemed high or unclear risk of bias in our main analyses; we included them only in sensitivity analyses. These studies are represented in the counts of included studies.

Categorization of Interventions

We grouped studies of similar interventions for our evidence synthesis. We categorized interventions into six types defined in Table 2 based primarily on the mode and environment of delivery. In our judgment, this method of categorization would best address the needs of multiple stakeholders that may be interested in interventions that could be implemented in specific health care settings. One investigator categorized the intervention, and a second team member reviewed the categorization. Disagreements were resolved by consensus.

Most studies included components delivered both during hospitalization and after discharge. Most studies included components delivered both during hospitalization and after discharge. We did not use timing of intervention delivery as a primary categorization scheme, but we did abstract detailed information regarding the timing of intervention components in relationship to the index hospitalization. Appendix C provides more information on components of interventions.

Table 2. Categories and definitions of transitional care interventions

Category	Definition
Home-visiting programs	Home visits by clinicians such as nurses or pharmacists, who deliver education, reinforce self-care instructions, perform physical examination, or provide other care (e.g., physical therapy, medication reconciliation). These interventions are often referred to as nurse case management interventions but they also can include home visits by a pharmacist or multidisciplinary team.
Structured telephone support	Monitoring, education, or self-care management (or various combinations) using simple telephone technology after discharge in a structured format (e.g., series of scheduled calls with a specific goal, structured questioning, or use of decision support software).
Telemonitoring	Remote monitoring of physiological data (e.g., electrocardiogram, blood pressure, weight, pulse oximetry, respiratory rate) with digital, broadband, satellite, wireless, or Bluetooth transmission to a monitoring center, with or without remote clinical visits (e.g., video monitoring).
Outpatient clinic-based interventions	Services provided in one of several different types of outpatient clinics—multidisciplinary HF, nurse-led HF, or primary care clinic. The clinic-based intervention can be managed by a nurse or other provider and may also offer unstructured telephone support (e.g., patient hotline) outside clinic hours.
Primarily educational interventions	Patient education (and self-care training) delivered before discharge or upon discharge by various delivery personnel or modes of delivery: in-person, interactive CD-ROM, video education. Interventions in this category do not feature home visiting, or structured telephone support. They are not delivered primarily through a clinic-based intervention (described above). Follow-up telephone calls may occur to ascertain outcomes (e.g., readmission rates) but not to monitor patients' physiological data.
Other	Unique interventions or interventions that did not fit into any of the other categories (e.g., individual peer support for HF patients).

CD-ROM = compact disc read-only memory; HF = heart failure.

Data Synthesis

We conducted meta-analyses of outcomes reported by multiple studies that were homogeneous enough to justify combining their results. To determine whether meta-analyses were appropriate, we assessed the clinical and methodological heterogeneity of the studies under consideration following established guidance.[38] We did this by qualitatively assessing the PICOTS of the included studies, looking for similarities and differences. When quantitative synthesis was not appropriate (e.g., because of clinical heterogeneity, insufficient numbers of similar studies, or insufficiency or variation in outcome reporting), we synthesized the data qualitatively.

For analyses of the efficacy of transitional care interventions, our main analyses include trials comparing an intervention with usual care (or treatment as usual) control groups. In some cases, "usual care" refers to usual home health care (e.g., home-visiting program); when this was a cointervention, we included it along with usual care in our analysis. For readmission and mortality outcomes, we stratified analyses for each intervention category by outcome timing, separating rates reported at 30 days from those beyond 30 days (i.e., rates reported over 3 to 6 months were combined).

For all readmission rates, we distinguished measures of the numbers of people readmitted versus measures of the total readmissions per group. We ran meta-analyses of trials that reported the number of people readmitted in each group. When the only information available was on the total number of readmissions (and not the total number of people readmitted), we contacted authors requesting additional data. When we could not obtain information on the number of people readmitted, we did not include these trials in meta-analyses for number of people readmitted; instead, we included these results in a qualitative synthesis.

We used random-effects models (DerSimonian and Laird) to estimate pooled effects.[39] For binary outcomes (e.g., readmission rates, mortality), we calculated the relative risk (RR) and

95% confidence interval (CI). When necessary, we calculated rates using the number of all randomized patients as the denominator to reflect a true ITT analysis. For continuous outcomes (e.g., scales of quality of life or function) measured with the same scale (e.g., Minnesota Living With Heart Failure Questionnaire [MLWHF]), we report the weighted mean difference between intervention and control subjects. When we had to combine multiple scales in one meta-analysis, we used the standardized mean difference (SMD), Cohen's d. A Cohen's d of zero means that the intervention and control groups have equivalent effects; a small effect size is 0.20, medium effect size is 0.50, and large effect size is 0.80.[40] Forest plots graphically summarize results of individual trials and of the pooled analyses (Appendix E).

For KQ 4, we assessed whether the efficacy of interventions differed based on intensity, delivery personnel, and method of communication both across intervention categories and within categories of interventions. When appropriate, we conducted meta-analyses stratified by intensity, delivery personnel, and method of communication within each intervention category.

Given the heterogeneity of included interventions, we were unable to develop a single measure of intensity that could be applied to all interventions. For most interventions, we defined intensity as the duration, frequency, or periodicity of patient contact, categorizing each intervention as low, medium, or high intensity. We also considered resource use as a dimension of intensity. For example, we included factors such as the total number of intervention components in the determination of intensity. We reserved the low-intensity category for interventions that included one episode of patient contact or that required few resources (e.g., no additional components, such as time spent coordinating care). We considered the majority of interventions to be medium or high intensity; most were multicomponent and included repeated patient contacts.

Few trials reported readmission rates separately by patient subgroups. For that reason, we were unable to conduct any meta-analysis. We present this information qualitatively.

For each meta-analysis in KQ 1 and KQ 2, we conducted sensitivity analyses by adding trials excluded for having high or unclear risk of bias and calculated a pooled effect to determine whether including them would have changed conclusions. Appendix F documents these sensitivity analyses; we mention them in the results section only when they changed our overall findings. We did not conduct sensitivity analyses for the subgroup comparisons in KQ 4 (intensity, delivery personnel and method of communication).

We calculated the chi-squared statistic and the I^2 statistic (the proportion of variation in study estimates attributable to heterogeneity) to assess statistical heterogeneity in effects between studies.[41,42] An I^2 from 0 to 40 percent might not be important, 30 percent to 60 percent may represent moderate heterogeneity, 50 percent to 90 percent may represent substantial heterogeneity, and ≥75 percent represents considerable heterogeneity.[41] The importance of the observed value of I^2 depends on the magnitude and direction of effects and on the strength of evidence (SOE) for heterogeneity (e.g., p value from the chi-squared test, or a confidence interval for I^2). Whenever we include a meta-analysis with considerable statistical heterogeneity in this report, we explain our reasoning considering the magnitude and direction of effects.[41]

In addition, we calculated the number needed to treat (NNT) for readmission and mortality outcomes when interventions were efficacious. We derived the NNTs from the RR and median usual care event rates using the methods described in the Cochrane Handbook.[43] Meta-analyses were conducted using Stata® version 11.1 (StataCorp LP, College Station, TX).

KQ 3 asks primarily "What are the components of effective interventions?" and "Are particular components necessary?" The aim of KQ 3 was to describe the components of effective interventions; it is intended as a descriptive question to provide information about the interventions that work for providers, health systems, etc. who may want to implement transitional care interventions. We considered "necessary" to mean that a particular component (e.g., inpatient education) was included in every effective intervention but was not necessarily sufficient (i.e., the component could be included in some interventions that were not efficacious). To address the first issue, we extracted detailed information on intervention components. We focused on content (e.g., specific educational content) and process (e.g., timing of first home visit following discharge), based on previous literature suggesting important components in HF treatment and transitional care.[24,33,36] We describe common components and combinations of components for all interventions that were efficacious in reducing all-cause readmissions, mortality, or the composite endpoint (all-cause readmission or death).

For KQ 3, we defined effective interventions as: (1) intervention categories (defined in Table 2) that reduced either all-cause readmissions or the composite endpoint (from our meta-analyses for KQ 1); (2) intervention categories that reduced mortality rates as shown in our meta-analyses; and (3) individual trials in other categories that reduced all-cause readmission, mortality, or the composite endpoint. Few trials reported outcomes at 30 days; for KQ 3 we describe the components of interventions that showed efficacy at any eligible time point up to 6 months following an index hospitalization for HF. For KQ 3, we focused on all-cause readmissions (rather than HF-specific readmission rates) for two reasons: (1) this outcome is relevant to stakeholders who are seeking to develop programs that reduce readmission rates in the context of CMS's decision to reduce reimbursement for excessive risk-standardized readmission rates;[9] (2) the majority of early readmissions in HF patients are for diverse indications (e.g., renal disorders, pneumonia, arrhythmias, and septicemia/shock).[5] We also included mortality as an outcome for two reasons: (1) addressing current uncertainty about the proportion of readmissions that are preventable is critical to the broad issue; (2) considering lower mortality as an outcome acknowledges the fact that some readmissions are warranted.

Strength of the Body of Evidence

We graded the SOE of the accumulated evidence on a given issue to answer the specific KQs on the benefits and harms of the interventions in this review; we used the guidance established for the EPC program.[44] Developed to grade the overall strength of a body of evidence, this approach incorporates four key domains: risk of bias (includes study design and aggregate quality), consistency, directness, and precision of the evidence. It also considers other optional domains that may be relevant for some scenarios, such as a dose-response association, plausible confounding that would decrease the observed effect, strength of association (magnitude of effect), and publication bias. Table 3 defines the grades of evidence that we assigned.

Table 3. Definitions of the grades of overall strength of evidence

Grade	Definition
High	**High confidence that the evidence reflects the true effect.** Further research is very unlikely to change our confidence in the estimate of effect.
Moderate	**Moderate confidence that the evidence reflects the true effect.** Further research may change our confidence in the estimate of the effect and may change the estimate.
Low	**Low confidence that the evidence reflects the true effect.** Further research is likely to change our confidence in the estimate of the effect and is likely to change the estimate.
Insufficient	**Evidence either is unavailable or does not permit estimation of an effect.**

Source: Owens et al.[44]

14

Two reviewers assessed each domain for each key outcome and resolved differences by consensus. For each assessment, one of the two reviewers was always an experienced EPC investigator. To give high SOE grades, we required consistent, direct, and precise evidence from studies with aggregate low risk of bias. An unfavorable assessment for any one of the four key domains (e.g., inconsistency, indirectness, imprecision, or medium aggregate risk of bias) typically resulted in downgrading to moderate SOE. Two unfavorable assessments typically resulted in downgrading to low SOE. We allowed reviewers to include the optional domains listed above (e.g., dose-response association, publication bias), if relevant, and to upgrade or downgrade the SOE for those domains if appropriate. When only one study reported an outcome of interest (with unknown consistency and imprecision), we usually graded the SOE as insufficient; when similar interventions had consistent results at other time points we graded the SOE as low.

We graded SOE for the following outcomes: all-cause readmissions rate, HF-specific readmission rates, composite endpoint, mortality, emergency room visits, length of hospital stay (of subsequent readmissions), and commonly reported measures of quality of life or functional status. We graded the SOE separately for each time point following an index hospitalization. For readmission rates, we graded the evidence for rates that were specific to the number of people readmitted (not total number of readmissions per group); however, we considered outcome measures of total readmission per group when assessing the consistency of evidence. We did not grade the SOE for results specific to KQ 3 (components of effective interventions), KQ 4 (intensity, delivery personnel, method of communication), or KQ 5 (subgroups). Appendix G presents tables showing our assessments for each domain and the resulting SOE grades KQs 1 and 2, organized by intervention category.

Applicability

We assessed applicability of the evidence following guidance from the Methods Guide.[45] We used the PICOTS framework to explore factors that affect applicability. Some factors identified a priori that may limit the applicability of evidence include the following: age of enrolled populations; sex of enrolled populations; race or ethnicity of enrolled populations; few studies enrolling subjects who are uninsured or lack social support; and setting (e.g., trials conducted outside the United States).

Peer Review and Public Commentary

This report received extensive external peer review and was posted for public comment October 29, 2013, to November 26, 2013. We addressed all comments in the final report, making revisions as needed; a disposition of comments report will be publicly posted 3 months after release of the final report.

Results

This chapter begins with the results of our literature search and a general description of the included studies. We then present our findings by Key Question (KQ), grouped by transitional care intervention, in the categories defined in Table 2 (in Methods). Appendix C presents a table of intervention components organized by intervention.

After describing included studies, we present results by KQ. For each KQ, we give the key points, including the strength-of-evidence (SOE) grades. We then present a detailed synthesis of the literature. Appendix D includes the risk-of-bias assessment for all included studies, organized by intervention category.

In the remainder of this chapter, we present the results of interventions compared with usual care first, followed by trials comparing one transitional care intervention with another type of intervention (generally in a subsection labeled "comparative effectiveness"). In the text, we usually report results as relative risks (RRs) with 95% confidence intervals (CIs); this is specifically the case when trials reported the number of people in each group who were readmitted. When investigators reported the total number or readmissions per group (or gave hazard ratios or some other metric), we present the results as they had been presented in the trial. We mention statistical significance in text only for significant findings; no mention means that differences between groups are not significant.

Tables describing studies (Tables 4–9) are organized first in chronological order by year of publication and, when necessary for more than one study in a year, alphabetically by author. Generally, we present figures with meta-analyses and RR calculations for our primary outcomes (readmission rates and mortality). We document other meta-analyses in Appendix E (e.g., hospital days, quality of life) or Appendix F (sensitivity analyses).

Literature Search and Screening

Searches of all sources identified a total of 2,419 potentially relevant citations. We included 47 studies described in 53 publications. Figure 2 describes the flow of literature through the screening process according to PRISMA (Preferred Reporting Items for Systematic Reviews and Meta-Analyses) categories.[46] Appendix B provides a complete list of articles excluded at the full-text screening stage, with reasons for exclusion. Only randomized controlled trials (RCTs) met the inclusion/exclusion criteria specified in Table 1 (Methods).

Figure 2. Disposition of articles about transitional care interventions for patients hospitalized for heart failure

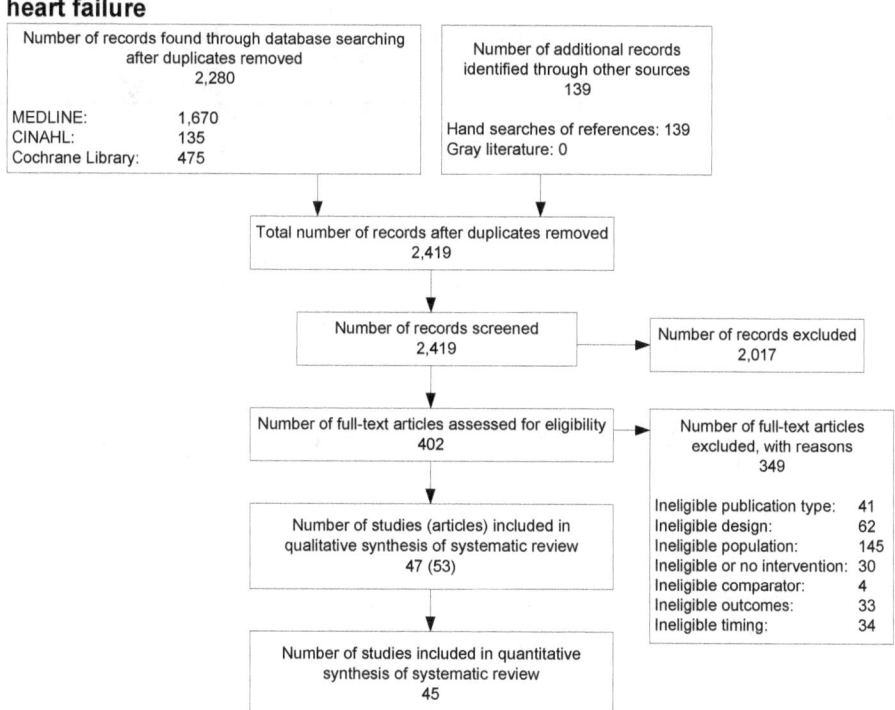

Characteristics of Included Studies

We grouped trials of similar interventions based primarily on the mode and environment of delivery as described in Methods (Table 2). These included only RCTs: home-visiting programs (15 RCTs), structured telephone support (STS, 13 trials), telemonitoring (8 trials), outpatient clinic-based interventions (7 trials), and primarily educational interventions (4 trials). We also included two unique interventions in an "other" category; one featured individual peer support and one emphasized cognitive training for patients with coexisting mild cognitive impairment.

Most trials compared a transitional care intervention with usual care; only two directly compared more than one transitional care intervention. Usual care was somewhat heterogeneous across trials and often was not well described. In all tables, the timing for outcome measurement(s)—readmissions, deaths, or other outcomes—reflects a period of 6 months or less (i.e., meeting our inclusion criteria noted in Table 1 in Methods). Below we describe the characteristics of included trials by intervention category.

Home-Visiting Programs

Characteristics of Trials

Fourteen RCTs compared a home-visiting program with usual care,[47-60] and one trial comparing a home-visiting program with telemonitoring (Table 4).[61] Sample sizes ranged from 58 to 339. Only one trial reported a readmission rate at 30 days.[47]

We rated all but five trials as medium or low risk of bias. We rated three trials as high risk of bias and two as unclear risk of bias;[48,49,52,61] the primary problems were high risk of selection bias, measurement bias (readmission rates), and inadequate handling of missing data.

Table 4. Characteristics of trials assessing home-visiting programs

Author, Year Setting	Intervention Category (N), Comparator (N)	Timing (m)[a]	Baseline NYHA Class; Mean EF	Age (y)	Female (%)	Non-White (%)	Taking BB or ACEI at Discharge (%)	Co-occurring Condition(s) (%)	Risk of Bias
Rich et al., 1993[58] US; single institution	Home-visiting program (63), Usual care (35)	3	NYHA mean: 2.8	79	59	50	NR	DM: 31 MI: 23	Med
Rich et al., 1995[57] US; single institution	Home-visiting program (142), Usual care (140)	3	NYHA mean: 2.4 EF: 43%	79	63	55	ACEI: 59 BB: 12	DM: 28 MI: 43	Med
Stewart et al., 1998[51] Australia; single institution	Home-visiting program (49), Usual care (48)	6	NYHA class III or IV: 48%	75	52	NR	ACEI: 81 BB: NR	DM: 22 IHD: 67 MI: 42 AF: 31	Med
Jaarsma et al., 1999[47] Netherlands; single institution	Home-visiting program (84), Usual care (95)	1, 3	NYHA III or IV: 100% LVEF: 34%	73	42	NR	ACEI or ARB: 70 BB: NR	DM: 30	Med
Stewart et al., 1999[50] Australia; single institution	Home-visiting program (100), Usual care (100)	6	NYHAIII or IV: 56% EF: 37%	76	38	NR	ACEI or ARB: 71 BB: 28	DM: 34 IHD: 78 AF: 35	Med
Pugh et al., 2001[52] US; multicenter	Home-visiting program (27), Usual care (31)	6	NYHA III or IV: 51%	74	57	NR	NR	NR	High
Benatar et al., 2003[61] US; multicenter	Home-visiting program (108), Telemonitoring (108)	6	NYHA mean class: 3.1 EF: 38%	63	63	93	ACEI or ARB: 76 BB: 53	DM: 23 CAD or other cardiac disorders: 61	Unc.
Kimmelstiel et al., 2004[53] US; multicenter	Home-visiting program (97), Usual care (103)	3	NYHA II or III: 97%	72	42	NR	ACEI or ARB: 92 BB: 57	DM: 48	Med
Naylor et al., 2004[55] US; multicenter	Home-visiting program (118), Usual care (121)	1, 3, 6	EF<30%: 57%	76	57	36	NR	DM: 38 CAD: 49 Pulmonary disease: 30	Low

Table 4. Characteristics of trials assessing home-visiting programs (continued)

Author, Year Setting	Intervention Category(N), Comparator (N)	Timing (m)[a]	Baseline NYHA Class; Mean EF	Age (y)	Fe-male (%)	Non-White (%)	Taking BB or ACEI at Discharge (%)	Co-occurring Con-dition(s) (%)	Risk of Bias
Sethares et al., 2004[48] US; single institution	Home-visiting program (33), Usual care (37)	3	NYHA mean class: 3 EF: 40%	76	53	8.5	ACEI or ARB: 61 BB: 49	NR	High
Thompson et al., 2005[60] UK; multicenter	Home-visiting program (58), Usual care (48)	6	NYHA III or IV: 40% EF: 30%	73	28	NR	ACEI or ARB: 69 BB: 18	DM: 21 MI: 52 AF: 30 chronic airways limitation: 24	High
Aldamiz-Echevarría Iraúrgui et al., 2007[56] Spain; single institution	Home-visiting program (137), Usual care (142)	6	EF: 50%	76	61	NR	ACEI or ARB: 84 BB: 12	DM: 36 IHD: 30.5 AF: 49.6	Med
Holland et al., 2007[59] UK; multicenter	Home-visiting program (148), Usual care (143)	6	NYHA III or IV: 67%	77	36	NR	ACEI or ARB: 77 BB: 39	NR	Med
Kwok et al., 2007[54] Hong Kong; multicenter	Home-visiting program (44), Usual care (46)	6	EF <40%: 24%	78	55	100	ACEI or ARB: 57 BB: 22	DM: 33 IHD: 47 MI: 23 AF: 30 COPD: 10	Med
Triller et al., 2008[49] US; multicenter	Home-visiting program (77), Usual care[b] (77)	6	NR	80	72	7	ACEI or ARB: 47 BB: 62	NR	Unc

[a] Timing of readmission outcome.

[b] Triller et al. compared pharmacist home visits among a population of patients receiving home nursing visits.[49]

ACEI = ACE inhibitor; AF = atrial fibrillation; ARB = angiotensin II receptor blocker; BB = beta-blocker; CAD = coronary artery disease; COPD = chronic obstructive pulmonary disease; DM = diabetes mellitus; EF = ejection fraction; HF = heart failure; IHD = ischemic heart disease; LVEF = left ventricular ejection fraction; m = months; Med = medium; MI = myocardial infarction; N = number (group size); NR = not reported; NYHA = New York Heart Association functional classification; QoL = quality of life; UK = United Kingdom; Unc. = unclear; US = United States; y = years.

Population

The mean age of participants was similar across trials, ranging from 63 to 80 years. All trials enrolled both women and men; the percentage of women ranged from 28 to 72. The percentage of nonwhite participants ranged from 0 percent to 93 percent in the six trials that described patient race or ethnicity;[48,52,55,57,58,61] one trial did not comment on race but was conducted among Hong Kong residents.[54]

Seven trials reported the percentage of patients who had moderate or severe heart failure (HF) (New York Heart Association [NYHA] class III or IV); 40 percent to 67 percent of patients

19

had moderate or severe HF.[47,50-53,59,60] Four trials reported the mean NYHA classification for patients: 2.8,[58] 3.0,[48,61] and 2.4[57] (scores range from 1 to 4). One trial did not describe the HF severity among patients.[49]

Two trials commented on the percentage of patients with a reduced ejection fraction (EF): 57 percent of patients had an EF less than 35 percent in one trial,[55] and 24 percent of patients had an EF less than 40 percent in another.[54] One trial gave the mean EF for the population (50 percent) but no information on NYHA classifications or the percentage of patients with a reduced EF.[56]

Five trials did not describe the percentage of patients receiving a beta-blocker at discharge,[47,51,52,55,58] 12 percent to 62 percent of patients in other trials were prescribed a beta-blocker at discharge. Three of these trials did not report on the percentage of patients taking an angiotensin-converting-enzyme inhibitor (ACEI) or angiotensin receptor blocker (ARB) medication at discharge[52,55,58]; 47 percent to 92 percent of patients in other trials were on an ACEI or ARB at discharge.

In nine trials, 30 percent to 78 percent of patients had ischemic heart disease or coronary artery disease.[51-57,60,61] In all other trials, 20 percent to 48 percent of patients had diabetes.

Interventions

Most trials delivered a series of home visits immediately following discharge. Five trials involved one comprehensive home visit following an index hospitalization;[47,50,51,53,60] of these five trials, two specified that additional home visits would be provided if a person experienced more than two unplanned hospitalizations within 6 months.[50,51] In most trials, nurses conducted the home visits; one trial evaluated home visits led by pharmacists;[59] and one evaluated whether additional home visits by a pharmacist among patients already receiving home-nursing visits was associated with improved outcomes.[49] In one trial, a physician accompanied the nurse on the first home visit.[56] Most home visits began within 7 days of discharge; three trials included visits within 24 to 48 hours of discharge;[55,57,58] and three trials specified that visits occurred within 14 days of discharge.[48,52,59]

All trials included education or training (or both) focused on self-care, diet, HF medications, and early recognition of symptoms. About half the trials delivered educational components both before discharge and during home visits. Two trials included planned, structured telephone calls in addition to home visits.[47,52] Most interventions offered a "patient hotline" for questions or advice throughout the intervention.

In one trial, usual care referred to usual "home health" that included nursing home visits in both groups.[49] Among other trials, descriptions of usual care tended to include "normal discharge planning," "followup as usual," or "care directed by inpatient team" with little other description provided.

Setting

One trial was conducted in Hong Kong,[54] two in the United Kingdom,[59,60] one in the Netherlands,[47] one in Spain,[56] and two by the same group of investigators in Australia.[50,51] The remaining trials were conducted in the United States. Eight trials were multicenter; seven were single center.[47,48,50,51,56-58]

Structured Telephone Support

Characteristics of Trials

Thirteen RCTs described in 15 publications compared STS with usual care (Table 5).[62-74] One three-arm trial compared two modes of delivering STS (standard telephone versus videophone) with usual care.[69,75] Trial sample size ranged from 32 to 715. Only one trial reported a readmission rate at 30 days.[64]

We rated all but three trials as medium risk of bias. We rated three trials as high risk of bias primarily for high risk of selection bias and measurement bias.

Table 5. Characteristics of trials assessing structured telephone support

Author, Year, Setting	Intervention Category (N), Comparator (N)	Timing (m)[a]	Baseline NYHA Class; Mean EF	Age (y)	Female (%)	Non-White (%)	Taking BB or ACEI at Discharge (%)	Co-occurring Con-dition(s) (%)	Risk of Bias
Rainville et al., 1999[71] US; single institution	STS (17), Usual care (17)	6	NYHA III or IV: 85%	70	50	NR	ACEI or ARB: 88 BB: 44	NR	Med
Barth et al., 2001[62] US; single institution	STS (17), Usual care (17)	2	NR	75	53	NR	NR	DM: 33 Any other cardiac disease: 68	High
Jerant et al., 2001[70] Jerant et al., 2003[76] US; single institution	STS (12), Usual care (12), Telemonitoring (13)	6	NYHA III or IV: 35%	70	54	51	ACEI or ARB: 68 BB: 38	IHD: 27	High
Riegel et al., 2002[63] US; multicenter	STS (130), Usual care (228)	3, 6	NYHA III or IV: 97% EF: 43%	72	51	NR	ACEI or ARB: 54 BB: 17	DM: 42 CAD: 65 AF: 24 COPD: 36	Med
Laramee et al., 2003[65] US; single institution	STS (141), Usual care (146)	2	NYHA III or IV: 35%	70	46	NR	ACEI or ARB: 82 BB: 63	DM: 43 Prior MI: 42 IHD: 71	Med
Tsuyuki et al., 2004[72] Canada; multicenter	STS (140), Usual care (136)	6	NYHA III or IV: 37%: EF: 31.5%	72	20	NR	ACEI or ARB: 85 BB: 43	NR	Med
Dunagan et al., 2005[68] US: single institution	STS (76), Usual care (75)	6	NYHA III or IV: 80% EF <40%: 58%	70	56	56	ACEI or ARB: 71 BB: NR	NR	Med

Table 5. Characteristics of trials assessing structured telephone support (continued)

Author, Year, Setting	Intervention Category (N), Comparator (N)	Timing (m)[a]	Baseline NYHA Class; Mean EF	Age (y)	Female (%)	Non-White (%)	Taking BB or ACEI at Discharge (%)	Co-occurring Con-dition(s) (%)	Risk of Bias
Cabezas et al., 2006[73] Spain; multicenter	STS (70), Usual care (64)	2, 6	NYHA III or IV: 10% EF: 51%	75	56	NR	ACEI or ARB: 72 BB: 7	DM: 34 MI: 20	Med
Riegel et al., 2006[64] US; multicenter	STS (69), Usual care (65)	1, 3, 6	NYHA III or IV: 81% EF <40%; 55%	72	54	100	ACEI or ARB: 75 BB: 54	DM: 59 IHD: 44 MI: 28 AF: 17	Med
Wakefield et al., 2008[69] Wakefield et al., 2009[75] US; single center (VAMC)	STS (47), Videophone (52), Usual care (49)	6	NYHA class III or IV: 72% EF: 41%	69	1	6	NR	NR	Med
Duffy et al., 2010[74] US; multicenter	STS (15), Usual care (17)[b]	6	NR	81	59	35 [b]	NR	NR	High
Domingues et al., 2011[67] Brazil; single institution	STS (48), Usual care (63)	3	LVEF: 29%	63	32	19	NR	NR	Med
Angermann et al., 2012[66] Germany; multicenter	STS (352), Usual care (363)	6	NYHA III or IV: 40% EF: 30%	69	29	NR	ACEI or ARB: 88 BB: 80	DM: 36 CAD: 58 AF: 29 COPD: 19	Med

[a] Both groups in Duffy et al.[74] also received home health care co-intervention that included nursing home visits.

[b] Duffy et al.[74] reported in text that >35 percent of participants were minorities but did not provide exact numbers.

ACEI = ACE inhibitor; AF = atrial fibrillation; ARB = angiotensin II receptor blocker; BB = beta-blockers; CAD = coronary artery disease; COPD = chronic obstructive pulmonary disease; DM = diabetes mellitus; EF = ejection fraction; HF = heart failure; IHD = ischemic heart disease; LVEF = left ventricular ejection fraction; m = months; MI = myocardial infarction; N = number (group size); NR = not reported; NYHA = New York Heart Association functional classification; STS = structured telephone support; US = United States; VAMC = Veterans Affairs Medical Center; Y = years

Population

The mean age of patients ranged from 63 to 81. One trial, conducted at a Veterans Affairs Medical Center (VAMC), enrolled primarily males (99 percent);[69] all other trials included 20 percent to 59 percent women. One trial was conducted in a completely Hispanic population.[64] Seven trials did not report the race or ethnicity of participants;[62,63,65,66,71-73] all other trials enrolled 6 percent to 56 percent nonwhite participants.

Most trials included a majority of patients with moderate to severe HF; five trials included a minority of patients with moderate to severe HF.[65,66,70,72,73] Two trials did not report HF disease severity.[62,74] Four trials did not report the percentage of patients receiving HF pharmacotherapy (ACEI or ARB; beta-blocker) at discharge.[62,67,69,74,75] All other trials included 54 percent to 86 percent of patients who were prescribed an ACEI or ARB and 7 percent to 63 percent of patients who were prescribed a beta-blocker. Most trials included patients with coexisting coronary artery disease or ischemic heart disease (20 percent to 79 percent); four trials did not describe the prevalence of coexisting heart disease among included patients.[62,70,71,74] Approximately half of the trials reported information on coexisting diabetes; the prevalence of coexisting diabetes ranged from 32 percent to 59 percent.[62-66,73]

Interventions and Comparators

All trials involved a series of scheduled, structured telephone calls to patients following discharge. Most trials averaged one or two calls during the intervention period. In most trials, the first telephone contact was within 7 days of discharge; in one, the first call occurred at 2 weeks after discharge;[72] and two trials did not describe the timing of the first call.[70,74] Most calls were delivered by nurses; two trials focused on STS delivered by a pharmacist.[71,73]

All trials included patient education. In most trials, education or self-care training began as an inpatient and was reinforced after discharge during telephone followup, but five trials did not include an educational component before discharge.[53,62-64,68,74] Most trials included a patient-initiated hotline for questions or additional support.[62,65,66,68,69,71,73]

The types of other components delivered (in addition to STS) varied across trials. One intervention involved nurse case management at the time of discharge; care coordination with primary care and individualized discharge planning was part of the intervention (e.g., obtaining needed services for patients such as physical therapy, and facilitating communication in the hospital among the family and providers).[65] Two trials included an inpatient intervention that focused on optimizing evidence-based HF pharmacotherapy before discharge.[71,72] Six trials included coordination between intervention personnel and the patient's outpatient care providers during the course of telephone support.[62-66,69]

Usual care was described as planned outpatient followup in four trials.[65-67,69,75] One other trial was conducted among patients receiving home health following discharge: "usual care" included in-home nursing visits administered by the home-health agency without additional details.[74]

Setting

Most trials were conducted in the United States: three in multicenter settings[63,64,74] and all others at a single center. Three trials were conducted in multicenter settings in Europe and Canada;[66,72,73] one trial was conducted at a single center in Brazil.[67]

Telemonitoring

Characteristics of Trials

Eight RCTs described in nine publications (Table 6) dealt with telemonitoring. Seven RCTs compared remote monitoring of clinical data (e.g., weight, vital signs) with usual care;[70,76-82] one compared remote monitoring of clinical data with home nurse visits.[61] Sample sizes ranged from 37 to 280 patients. Only one trial reported a readmission rate at 30 days.[82]

Table 6. Characteristics of trials assessing telemonitoring

Author, Year, Setting	Intervention Category(N), Comparator (N)	Timing (m)[a]	Baseline NYHA Class; Mean EF	Age (y)	% Fe-male	Non-White (%)	Taking BB or ACEI at Discharge (%)	Co-occurring Con-dition(s) (%)	Risk of Bias
Jerant et al., 2001[70] Jerant et al., 2003[76] US; single institution	Telemonitoring (13), Usual care (12), STS (12)	6	NYHA III or IV: 35%	70	54	51	ACEI or ARB: 68 BB: 38	IHD: 27	High
Benatar et al., 2003[61] US; multicenter	Telemonitoring (108), Home-visiting program (108)	6	NYHA mean class: 3.1 EF: 38%	63	63	93	ACEI or ARB: 76 BB: 53	DM: 23 CAD or other cardiac disorders: 61	Unc
Goldberg et al., 2003[79] US; multicenter	Telemonitoring (138), Usual care (142)	6	NYHA III-IV: 100%	59	32	36	ACEI: 74 ARB: 16 BB: 38	DM: 41 MI: 39 AF: 35	Med
Schwarz et al., 2008[78] US; single institution	Telemonitoring (51), Usual care (51)	3	NYHA class III or IV: 79%	78	52	19	NR	DM: 50 MI: 51 AF: 30 COPD: 29	Med
Woodend et al., 2008[81] Canada; single institution	Telemonitoring (62), Usual care (59)	3	NYHA III or IV: 62%	67	28	NR	NR	Prior MI: 57	High
Dar et al., 2009[80] UK; multicenter	Telemonitoring (91), Usual care (91)	6	EF ≥40%: 39%[b]	72	34	20 (South Asian)	ACEI or ARB: 88 BB: 56	DM: 36 CAD: 55 Prior MI: 48 COPD: 91	Med
Dendale et al., 2012[77] Belgium; multicenter	Telemonitoring (80), Usual care (80)	6	NYHA mean class: 3.0 LVEF: 35%	76	35	NR	NR	NR	Unc
Pekmezaris et al., 2012[82] US; multicenter	Telemonitoring (83), Usual care (85)[c]	1, 3	NR	82	62	9	NR	NR	Med

[a] Timing of readmission outcome.

[b] EF data reported in Dar et al. are based on data from 168 patients (92 percent of total sample).[80]

[c] In Pekmezaris et al., both groups received home health care, including nursing home visits.[82]

ACEI = ACE inhibitor; AF = atrial fibrillation; ARB = angiotensin II receptor blocker; BB = beta-blocker; CAD = coronary artery disease; COPD = chronic obstructive pulmonary disease; DM = diabetes mellitus; EF = ejection fraction; HF = heart failure; IHD = ischemic heart disease; LVEF = left ventricular ejection fraction; m = months; Med. = medium; MI = myocardial infarction; N = group size; NR = not reported; NYHA = New York Heart Association functional classification; UK = United Kingdom; Unc = unclear; US = United States; Y = years

We rated four trials as medium risk of bias. We rated two trials as high risk of bias and two others as unclear risk of bias; the primary problems were inadequate handling of missing data and unclear fidelity to the protocol.

Population

The mean age of patients ranged from 59 to 82 years. Half of the trials enrolled fewer women than men (range, 28 percent to 35 percent women);[77,79-81] the remainder included 52 percent to 63 percent women.[61,70,76,78,82] One trial was conducted primarily in nonwhite patients (86 percent African American, 6 percent Hispanic, 1 percent Asian);[61] the other trials included 9 percent to 51 percent nonwhite patients[70,76,78-80,82] or did not report information on race.[77,81]

Most trials enrolled a majority of patients with moderate to severe HF based on NYHA classification (class III or IV). In one trial, a majority of patients had less severe HF (65 percent with NYHA class II HF);[70,76] two trials did not report baseline disease severity based on NYHA classification.[80,82]

Four trials described the percentage of patients on an ACEI or ARB at discharge (68 percent to 88 percent of patients) and the percentage of patients on a beta-blocker at discharge (38 percent to 56 percent of patients).[61,70,79,80] Three trials did not report information on pharmacotherapy at discharge,[77,81,82] and one trial reported the mean number of "heart medications" at discharge (5.5 medications) without defining which medications were counted.[78]

The proportion of patients with coronary artery disease or prior myocardial infarction (MI) ranged from 27 percent to 61 percent in most trials.[61,70,76,78-81] The proportion of patients with diabetes ranged from 23 percent to 50 percent in four RCTs.[61,78-80]

Interventions and Comparators: Remote Monitoring of Clinical Data

Five RCTs evaluated remote clinical data monitoring using equipment installed in patients' homes that transmitted clinical data to a central site.[61,77-80] Remote monitoring equipment was generally either sent home with a patient from the hospital or delivered within 1 to 3 weeks of discharge. In four of these RCTs, nurses or physicians (or both) contacted patients when weights or vital signs were outside protocol-defined parameters.[61,78-80] In three RCTs, patients also answered questions about symptoms (e.g., shortness of breath, edema) through the remote monitoring system.[78-80] In one RCT, alerts about abnormal clinical data were sent directly to the primary care clinician and HF clinic.[77]

Four RCTs compared remote monitoring of clinical data with usual care.[77-80] Usual care was defined as standard care from primary care clinicians or cardiologists (or both) in three trials;[77-79] in one trial, usual care included an initial home visit to deliver education about HF self-monitoring, telephone support, and care from a specialized HF clinician.[80] One trial randomized patients to either home nursing visits or nurse remote monitoring.[61]

Interventions and Comparators: Remote Monitoring With Video Clinical Visits

Three trials used specialized equipment to allow for video assessments and interactions with patients.[70,76,81,82] The equipment could also check clinical data such as blood pressure or included stethoscopes to allow remote heart and lung auscultation. The specialized equipment was generally delivered to patients' homes within 48 hours to 7 days of discharge from the hospital.

In one trial, the intervention group was instructed to monitor weight and blood pressure daily; this information was then transmitted to a central site and monitored by a nurse who also completed video conferences with the patients. Outcomes for this group were compared with those for usual care.[81] Another RCT had three arms and compared (1) video nursing visits including video interaction and a remote stethoscope with (2) telephone nursing visits and with (3) usual care; both intervention groups also had access to a nurse hotline for questions or concerns.[70,76] In both of these trials, usual care was defined as directed by a primary care physician or cardiologist. In one usual-care group, patients also had a telephone number with which to reach an advanced practice nurse with questions about their care;[81] patients in the other usual-care group received two nurse home visits (after discharge and at 60 days), during which standard education and clinical assessment were conducted.[70,76]

One trial evaluated adding video nursing visits to home nursing visits through a home health care agency; the comparison was usual home nursing visits without additional video visits.[82] The equipment in this trial allowed for blood pressure checks and stethoscope examination during the video visits.[82] In both groups, a nurse determined the frequency of home visits; in addition, all nurses followed standardized disease management guidelines to manage patients.

Interventions and Comparators: Educational Components

All trials included an educational component; most delivered education after discharge. One trial delivered education before discharge about general self-care, weight monitoring, and low-sodium diets.[79] In five trials, nurses delivered general HF self-care education after discharge by telephone, video, or in person.[70,76,77,80 ,81,82] Educational content included weight monitoring in four trials,[70,76-79] low-sodium diets in five trials,[61,70,76,77,79,82] medication education and adherence promotion in four trials,[61,70,76,77,82] and exercise promotion in one trial.[77]

Setting

Five trials were conducted in the United States; two were at a single center,[70,76,78] and the remainder were multicenter.[61,79,82] Three trials were conducted outside the United States: one at a single institution in Canada,[81] one in a multicenter setting in Belgium,[77] and one in a multicenter setting in the United Kingdom.[80]

Clinic-Based Interventions

Characteristics of Trials

Seven RCTs described in nine publications (Table 7) tested interventions in three main types of outpatient clinics. Six trials compared interventions in HF specialty clinics;[83-90] four were in multidisciplinary (MDS) clinics (denoted MDS-HF) and two were in nurse-led clinics. A single trial compared enhanced access (increased access) to primary care with usual care.[91] Sample sizes ranged from 98 to 443. One trial reported a readmission rate at 30 days.[84]

Of these seven trials, we rated six as low or medium risk of bias; we rated one trial as unclear, primarily because the investigators did not describe the validity of their measures of health care use well.

Table 7. Characteristics of trials assessing outpatient clinic-based interventions

Author, Year, Setting	Intervention Category (N), Comparator (N)	Timing (m)[a]	Baseline NYHA Class; Mean EF	Age (y)	Female (%)	Non-White (%)	Taking BB or ACEI at Discharge (%)	Co-occurring Condition(s) (%)	Risk of Bias
Ekman et al., 1998[83] Sweden; single institution	Nurse-led clinic (79), Usual care (79)	6	NYHA mean class: 3.2 EF: 41%[c]	80	42	NR	ACEI or ARB: 37 BB: 30	DM: 28 AF: 41 Prior MI: 45	Med
Oddone et al., 1999[91] US; multicenter	Primary care clinic (222), Usual care (221)	6	NYHA III or IV: 53%	65	1	34	ACEI or ARB: 74 BB: 12	NR	Med
McDonald et al., 2001[84] McDonald et al., 2002[85] Ledwidge et al., 2003[86] Ireland; single institution	At 3 months[b]: MDS-HF clinic (51), Usual care (47) At 30 days: MDS-HF clinic (35), Usual care (35)	1, 3[b]	EF<45%: 63%[b]	71[b]	34[b]	NR	ACEI or ARB: 61[b] BB: NR	NR	Unc
Kasper et al., 2002[87] US; multicenter	MDS-HF clinic (102), Usual care (98)	6	NYHA III: 59% (no patients with class IV) EF <45%: 88%	64	40	35	ACEI or ARB: 86 BB: 39	DM: 40	Low
Stromberg et al., 2003[88] Sweden; multicenter	Nurse-led clinic (52), Usual care (54)	3	NYHA III or IV: 82%	78	39	NR	ACEI or ARB: 82 BB: 58	DM: 24 IHD: 68	Low
Ducharme et al., 2005[89] Canada; single institution	MDS-HF clinic (115), Usual care (115)	6	NYHA III or IV: 91% EF: 35%	69	28	NR	ACEI or ARB: 80 BB: 43	DM: 30 CAD: 66 Prior MI: 50	Low
Liu et al., 2012[90] Taiwan; single institution	MDS-HF clinic (53), Usual care (53)	6	NYHA III or IV: 62% EF: 28%	61	35	100	ACEI or ARB: 40 BB: 65	DM: 46	Low

[a] Timing of readmission outcome.

[b] Data come from the McDonald et al., 2002, publication;[85] the percentages from companion studies differ slightly.[84,86]

[c] EF values reported in Ekman et al. are based on data from 99 patients (63 percent of total sample).[83]

ACEI = ACE inhibitor; AF = atrial fibrillation; ARB = angiotensin II receptor blocker; BB = beta-blocker; CAD = coronary artery disease; DM = diabetes mellitus; EF = ejection fraction; HF = heart failure; IHD = ischemic heart disease; m = months; MDS-HF = multidisciplinary heart failure clinic; Med. = medium; MI = myocardial infarction; N = group size; NR = not reported; NYHA = New York Heart Association functional classification; Unc. = unclear; US = United States; Y = years

Population

The mean age of patients ranged from 61 to 80 years. The percentage of female patients ranged from 39 percent to 42 percent in most trials; one trial focused on increased primary care access for HF patients was conducted in a VAMC setting (1 percent were women). Four trials did not include information on race or ethnicity. One trial was conducted only among Taiwanese patients;[90] the percentage of nonwhite subjects in two U.S. trials was approximately 34 percent.[87,91] Most trials enrolled a majority of subjects with moderate to severe HF based on NYHA classification. The percentage of patients on pharmacotherapy at discharge ranged from 37 percent to 86 percent for an ACEI or ARB and 12 percent to 65 percent for beta-blockers. Most trials included populations with a variety of coexisting chronic conditions: 24 percent to 46 percent of patients had diabetes, and 46 percent to 71 percent of patients had a prior history of MI. Two trials reported no information on coexisting diabetes, cardiac disease, or respiratory disorders.[84-86,91]

Interventions and Comparators

All trials involved a series of scheduled outpatient clinic visits following discharge, regular structured telephone calls to patients beginning within 7 days after the hospital discharge or enrollment, and individualized care planning. These interventions did not include regularly scheduled home visits as a primary component; none included telemonitoring. All trials provided a brief description of usual care that included "management in accordance with current clinical practice" or stated that patients received conventional followup in primary health care.

Among the six trials evaluating HF clinic interventions, four were described as MDS-HF clinic interventions;[84-87,89,90] they involved more emphasis on physician contact and access to a multidisciplinary care team (cardiology, nurses, dieticians, pharmacists) than nurse-led clinics. The two trials described as nurse-led focused more on patient education delivered by nurses during scheduled clinic appointments than on multidisciplinary management.[83,88]

In general, most trials included an educational component. Two trials included education on self-care delivered before discharge and education reinforcement during telephone followup.[85,91]

One trial focused on enhanced access to primary care.[91] Three services coordinated care with a patient's primary care physician by scheduling appointments for acute needs or alerting physicians to changes in symptoms.[83,85,90]

Setting

Three trials were conducted in North America,[87,89,91] three in Europe,[83-86,88] and one in Asia.[90] Four trials were at a single center[83,84,89,90] and three were conducted in a multicenter setting.[87,88,91]

Primarily Educational Interventions

Characteristics of Trials

Four RCTs compared primarily educational interventions with usual care (Table 8).[92-95] Sample sizes ranged from 76 to 230. No trial reported a 30-day readmission rate. We rated one trial as low risk of bias and one as medium risk of bias. We rated one trial as high risk of bias and one as unclear risk of bias, primarily because of potential for measurement bias and inadequate handling of missing data, respectively.

Table 8. Characteristics of trials assessing primarily educational interventions

Author, Year, Setting	Intervention Category(N), Comparator (N)	Timing (m)[a]	Baseline NYHA Class; Mean EF	Age (y)	Female (%)	Non-White (%)	Taking BB or ACEI at Discharge (%)	Co-occurring Con-dition(s) (%)	Risk of Bias
Koelling et al., 2005[95] US; single institution	Primarily educational (107), Usual care (116)	6	EF: 27%	65	42	22	ACEI or alternative: 61 BB: 55	CAD: 64	Low
Linne et al., 2006[94] Sweden; multicenter	Primarily educational (122), Usual care (108)	6	EF < 40%: 100%	70	29	NR	ACEI or ARB: 80 BB: 49	NR	Unc
Nucifora et al., 2006[93] Italy; single institution	Primarily educational (99), Usual care (101)	6	NYHA III or IV: 65%	73	38	NR	ACEI or ARB: 80 BB: 13	DM: 26 IHD: 46 COPD: 27	Med
Albert et al., 2007[92] US; single institution	Primarily educational (37), Usual care (39)	3	EF <40%: 100%	60	23	17	ACEI or ARB: 88 BB: 56	DM: 33 CAD: 66 MI: 45 AF: 37	High

[a] Timing of readmission outcome.

ACEI = ACE inhibitor; AF = atrial fibrillation; ARB = angiotensin II receptor blocker; BB = beta-blocker; CAD = coronary artery disease; COPD = chronic obstructive pulmonary disease; DM = diabetes mellitus; EF = ejection fraction; HF = heart failure; IHD = ischemic heart disease; LVEF = left ventricular ejection fraction; m = months; Med. = medium; MI = myocardial infarction; N = group size; NR = not reported; NYHA = New York Heart Association functional classification; Unc = unclear; US = United States; VAMC = Veterans Affairs Medical Center; Y = years

Population

Mean age ranged from 60 to 73 years. Trials included 23 percent to 42 percent women. Two trials described the race or ethnicity of patients (17 percent and 22 percent nonwhite).[92,95] Three trials included patients with an EF of <40 percent,[92,94,95] and one trial included a majority of patients with moderate to severe HF.[93] The majority of patients were on an ACEI or ARB at discharge (60 percent to 88 percent). Approximately half of patients in three trials were on a beta-blocker at discharge.[92,94,95]

One trial did not describe the prevalence of coexisting conditions among patients.[94] Two trials reported prevalence rates of diabetes of 26 percent and 33 percent.[92,93] Three trials included populations among whom 46 percent to 66 percent of patients had coronary artery disease.[92,93,95]

Interventions and Comparator

All trials involved primarily educational interventions aimed at preventing HF readmission; however, they differed in the mode of delivery and timing of education in relationship to the index HF hospitalization. One trial compared the effects of a 1-hour in-person patient education program with usual discharge care; no other components were delivered after discharge.[95] Another trial featured intensive education about HF symptoms and treatment administered by a nurse ahead of discharge. In addition, one telephone call was conducted 3 to 5 days after discharge with the goal of reinforcing education, a nurse hotline was available for questions, and education was reinforced at scheduled outpatient visits (15 days, 1 and 6 months).[93]

Two trials investigated the effects of HF education delivered via technology.[92,94] One study included education before discharge focused on HF symptoms and treatment that was delivered via CD; the same educational CD was repeated 2 weeks after discharge (patients returned to the hospital to view the CD).[94] Another study evaluated the effects of a 60-minute, six-chapter video on HF that was intended to be viewed at home.[92]

Setting

Two single-center trials were conducted in the United States[92,95] and one in Italy.[93] One multicenter study was conducted in Sweden.[94]

Other Interventions

Characteristics of Trials

Two RCTs evaluated unique interventions that did not fit into any other category (Table 9). One used peer support for patients with HF following discharge,[96] and the other examined the effect of cognitive training on patients with HF and coexisting cognitive dysfunction.[97] Sample sizes were 88 and 125, respectively. Both trials reported a 30-day readmission rate. We rated one trial as medium risk of bias and the other as high risk of bias, primarily because of a high risk of selection bias and inadequate handling of missing data.

Table 9. Characteristics of trials assessing other interventions

Author, Year, Setting	Intervention Category(N), Comparator (N)	Timing (m)[a]	Baseline NYHA Class; Mean EF	Age (y)	Female (%)	Non-White (%)	Taking BB or ACEI at Discharge (%)	Co-occurring Con-dition(s) (%)	Risk of Bias
Riegel et al., 2004[96] US; multi-center	Peer support (45), Usual care (43)	1, 3	NYHA III or IV: 64% EF: 45%	73	58	NR	NR	DM: 46 History of MI: 35 COPD: 25	High
Davis et al., 2012[97] US; single institution	Self-care teaching and cognitive training (63), Usual care (62)	1	NYHA III or IV: 53% EF: 34%	59	53	69	NR	DM: 39 AF: 26 COPD: 22 MCI: 100	Med.

[a] Timing of readmission outcome.

ACEI = ACE inhibitor; AF = atrial fibrillation; ARB = angiotensin II receptor blocker; BB = beta-blocker; COPD = chronic obstructive pulmonary disease; DM = diabetes mellitus; EF = ejection fraction; HF = heart failure; m = months; MCI = mild cognitive impairment; Med. = medium; MI = myocardial infarction; N = group size; NR = not reported; NYHA = New York Heart Association functional classification; US = United States; Y = years

Population

Mean age was 73 years (peer support) and 59 years (cognitive training). Approximately one-half the patients in both trials were women. Only the trial assessing cognitive training described patient race or ethnicity (69 percent nonwhite).[97] Both trials enrolled a majority of patients with moderate to severe HF. Neither study reported on the percentage of patients taking an ACEI or beta-blocker at discharge. Patients with coexisting diabetes made up 46 percent or 39 percent of the study populations. The trial assessing cognitive training screened patients for inclusion with the Montreal Cognitive Assessment;[98] patients were included if they had a score suggesting mild cognitive impairment (score between 17 and 25 out of 30; scores less than 17 suggest dementia).

Interventions and Comparators

One trial focused on peer monitoring as a means of social support and mentoring on self-care management for patients with HF.[96] The investigators recruited nine patients with HF and trained them as mentors; mentors were described as elderly men and women with mild to moderate HF. Patients randomized to peer support chose the gender and geographic location of their mentor. Contact began during the index hospitalization (in person) or immediately after discharge via telephone contact. Mentoring occurred during home visits, telephone calls, and joint outings; weekly contact was encouraged for the 30 days following discharge and then at least monthly for 3 months. Usual care was described as inpatient education on HF.

The other trial focused on dealing with impairments in memory and executive function through environmental manipulations and training strategies and on improving self-confidence related to the ability to handle self-care.[97] Specifically, during the hospitalization, each patient was given a spiral workbook with pictograms and space to personalize a self-care schedule focused on their medication schedule and future appointments. Patients were provided with typical HF self-care problems and a case manager helped them to solve problems; an audiotape of the sessions was given to patients at discharge. One telephone call was conducted after discharge (24 to 72 hours) for a teach-back session.[97] Usual care was described as "standard discharge teaching for HF, including verbal review of a HF patient education booklet."

Setting

Both trials occurred in the United States. The study assessing peer support was conducted in a multicenter setting,[96] and the trial assessing cognitive training was conducted at a single center.[97]

KQ 1. Transitional Care Interventions and Health Care Utilization Outcomes

Key Points: All-Cause Readmissions

- A high-intensity home-visiting program (e.g., first visit within 24 hours and multiple planned home visits) reduced all-cause readmission at 30 days (low SOE). A lower-intensity home-visiting program did not reduce all-cause readmission at 30 days (low SOE).
- Home-visiting programs and MDS-HF clinic interventions reduced all-cause readmission over 3 to 6 months (high SOE for both).
- The following intervention categories did not reduce all-cause readmission over 3 to 6 months: STS (moderate SOE), telemonitoring (moderate SOE), and nurse-led clinic interventions (low SOE).

- Evidence was insufficient to determine the efficacy of the following intervention categories at any time point: the primary care clinic intervention, primarily educational interventions, and cognitive training.

Key Points: Heart Failure–Specific Readmissions

- Two intervention categories reduced HF-specific readmission over 3 to 6 months: Home-visiting programs (moderate SOE) and STS (high SOE).
- Telemonitoring interventions did not reduce HF-specific readmission over 3 to 6 months (moderate SOE).
- Evidence was insufficient to determine the efficacy of the following interventions in reducing HF-specific readmission either at 30 or at any time point: MDS-HF clinic interventions, nurse-led clinic interventions, and primarily educational interventions.

Key Points: Composite All-Cause Readmission or Death

- Home-visiting programs reduced the composite outcome (all-cause readmission or death) at 30 days (low SOE) and over 3 to 6 months (moderate SOE).
- The following intervention categories did not reduce the composite outcome: STS (low SOE), MDS-HF (moderate SOE), and primarily educational interventions (low SOE).
- Evidence was insufficient to determine the efficacy of nurse-led clinic interventions in reducing the composite outcome.

Key Points: Emergency Room Visits, Acute Care Visits, Hospital Days

- Few trials reported rates of emergency room (ER) or acute care visits.
- STS interventions did not increase or decrease ER visits over 3 to 6 months (low SOE).
- Evidence was insufficient to determine whether other intervention categories increased or decreased ER or acute care visits at any time point.
- The following interventions showed efficacy in reducing the number of hospital days of subsequent readmissions over 3 to 6 months: home-visiting programs (low SOE) and STS (moderate SOE).

Key Points: Comparative Effectiveness

- Direct evidence was insufficient to determine whether one type of transitional care intervention was more or less efficacious than any other type of intervention for any health care utilization outcome.

Detailed Synthesis: Transitional Care Interventions Compared With Usual Care

All-Cause Readmissions: Transitional Care Interventions Compared With Usual Care

Figure 3 presents our meta-analysis and forest plot of trials reporting all-cause readmission (number of people readmitted) stratified by intervention category and outcome timing. We present detailed results by intervention category and outcome timing below.

Figure 3. All-cause readmission for transitional care interventions compared with usual care, by intervention category and outcome timing: Meta-analysis and forest plot of individual trials

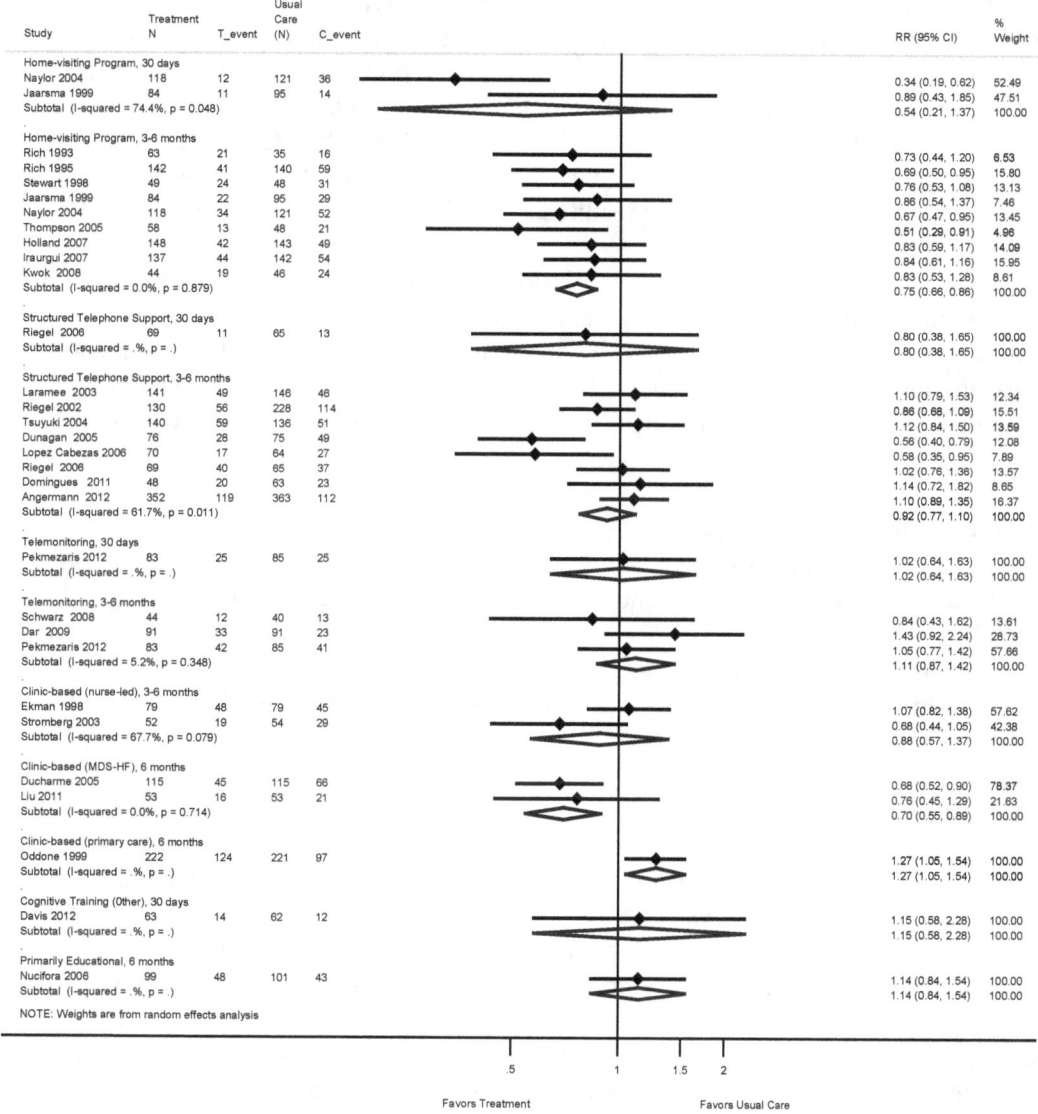

C_event = number of people readmitted in the control (usual care) group; N = sample size; T event = number of people readmitted in the intervention group.

Home-Visiting Programs

At 30 days, our meta-analysis (two trials) found no difference in the risk of all-cause readmission between the patients receiving home visits and those receiving usual care (RR, 0.54; 95% CI, 0.21 to 1.37).[47,55] However, the statistical heterogeneity between these two trials was considerable (I^2 =74.4 %), and they also had important clinical differences in the intervention delivered. Although both trials included comprehensive inpatient education and individualized discharge planning, the interventions differed in the timing of the first home visit and total number of planned home visits.

In the trial by Naylor et al., an advanced practice nurse visited patients at home within 24 hours of discharge, and a total of eight home visits were planned. In the trial by Jaarsma et al., patients were called within 7 days following discharge to schedule a home visit; most visits were scheduled within 10 days of discharge and no additional visits were planned. The trial by Naylor et al., which evaluated a more intensive intervention, found a lower risk of readmission for patients receiving home visits than for patients in the control group (RR, 0.34; 95% CI, 0.19 to 0.62).[55] The trial by Jaarsma et al. found no difference in all-cause readmission between patients receiving the home visit and patients in the control group (RR, 0.89; 95% CI 0.43 to 1.85).[47]

Over 3 to 6 months, our meta-analysis (nine trials) found that patients receiving home visits had a significantly reduced risk of all-cause readmission (RR, 0.75; 95% CI, 0.66 to 0.86).[47,51,54-60]

Two trials reported the number of total readmissions per group (rather than people readmitted) at 6 months. In one trial (N=200), patients receiving home visits had significantly fewer unplanned readmissions (68) than those receiving usual care (118) (p=0.031).[50] In another trial (N=200), all-cause readmissions did not differ between patients receiving home visits and those receiving usual care (measured as mean readmissions per patient-year alive: RR, 0.89; p=0.61).[53]

Structured Telephone Support

One trial (N= 134) reported all-cause readmission at 30 days; the readmission rate did not differ between patients receiving STS and those receiving usual care (RR, 0.80; 95% CI, 0.38 to 1.65).[64]

Over 3 to 6 months, our meta-analysis (eight trials) found no difference in the relative risk of all-cause readmission between patients receiving STS and those receiving usual care (RR, 0.92; 95% CI, 0.77 to 1.10).[63-65,67,68,72,73]

Telemonitoring

One trial (N=168) reported all-cause readmissions at 30 days; the risk of all-cause readmission among patients receiving telemonitoring and those receiving usual care did not differ (RR, 1.02; 95% CI, 0.64 to 1.63).[82]

Over 3 to 6 months, our meta-analysis (three trials) found no difference in the risk of readmission between patients receiving telemonitoring and those receiving usual care (RR, 1.11; 95% CI, 0.87 to 1.42).[78,80,82]

Four telemonitoring trials reported the total number of readmissions per group (rather than the number of people readmitted). All-cause readmissions did not differ between patients receiving telemonitoring and those receiving usual care at 30 days,[76] 3 months,[81] or 6 months.[76,77,79]

34

Clinic-Based Interventions

Given the diversity in interventions among the clinic-based interventions, we pooled data separately by clinic setting: MDS-HF clinic, nurse-led HF clinic, and primary care clinic. Among the MDS-HF interventions, our meta-analysis (two trials) found that patients receiving the intervention had a significantly lower risk of all-cause readmission than patients receiving usual care (RR, 0.70; 95% CI, 0.55 to 0.89).

Over 3 to 6 months, our meta-analysis (two trials) found that patients receiving a nurse-led clinic intervention and those receiving usual care had a similar risk of all-cause readmission (RR, 0.88; 95% CI, 0.57 to 1.37).[83,88]

One trial (N=443) found that HF patients with better access to primary care following discharge through a VAMC setting had a significantly higher risk of all-cause readmission than patients in the control group (RR, 1.27; 95% CI, 1.05 to 1.54).[91]

Primarily Educational Interventions

One trial (N= 200) found no difference in the risk of all-cause readmission at 6 months between patients receiving intensive predischarge education and controls (RR 1.14; 95% CI, 0.84 to 1.54).[93]

Other Interventions

One trial (N=125) of cognitive training among patients with HF and coexisting cognitive dysfunction found no difference in the risk of 30-day readmission between patients receiving the intervention and controls (RR, 1.15; 95% CI, 0.58 to 2.28).[97]

Heart Failure-Specific Readmissions: Transitional Care Interventions Compared With Usual Care

Our meta-analysis of trials reporting HF-specific readmissions (number of people readmitted) is shown in Figure 4. We present detailed results by intervention category and outcome timing below.

Home-Visiting Program

At 3 months, one trial (N=282) found that patients receiving home visits had a significantly lower risk of HF-specific readmissions than controls (RR, 0.51; 95% CI, 0.31 to 0.82).[57] Another trial (N=200) reported the total number of readmissions per group (rather than the number of patients readmitted) at 3 months; patients receiving home visits had significantly fewer total HF-specific readmissions than did patients receiving usual care (measured as readmissions per patient-year alive, RR, 0.54; p<0.001).[53]

Structured Telephone Support

One trial (N=134) found no difference in the risk of HF-specific readmission between patients receiving STS and those receiving usual care at 30 days (RR, 0.63; 95% CI, 0.84 to 1.54).[64] Over 3 to 6 months, our meta-analysis (nine trials) found that people receiving STS had a significantly lower risk of HF readmission than controls (RR, 0.74; 95% CI, 0.61 to 0.90).[63-68,71-73]

Telemonitoring

At 6 months, one trial (N=182) found no difference in the risk of HF-specific readmission between patients receiving telemonitoring and controls (RR, 1.70; 95% CI, 0.82 to 3.51).[80] Two trials reported the total number of readmissions per group (rather than patients readmitted); neither study found a difference between these two groups.[77,79]

Figure 4. HF-specific readmission for transitional care interventions compared with usual care, by intervention category and outcome timing: Meta-analysis and forest plot of individual trials

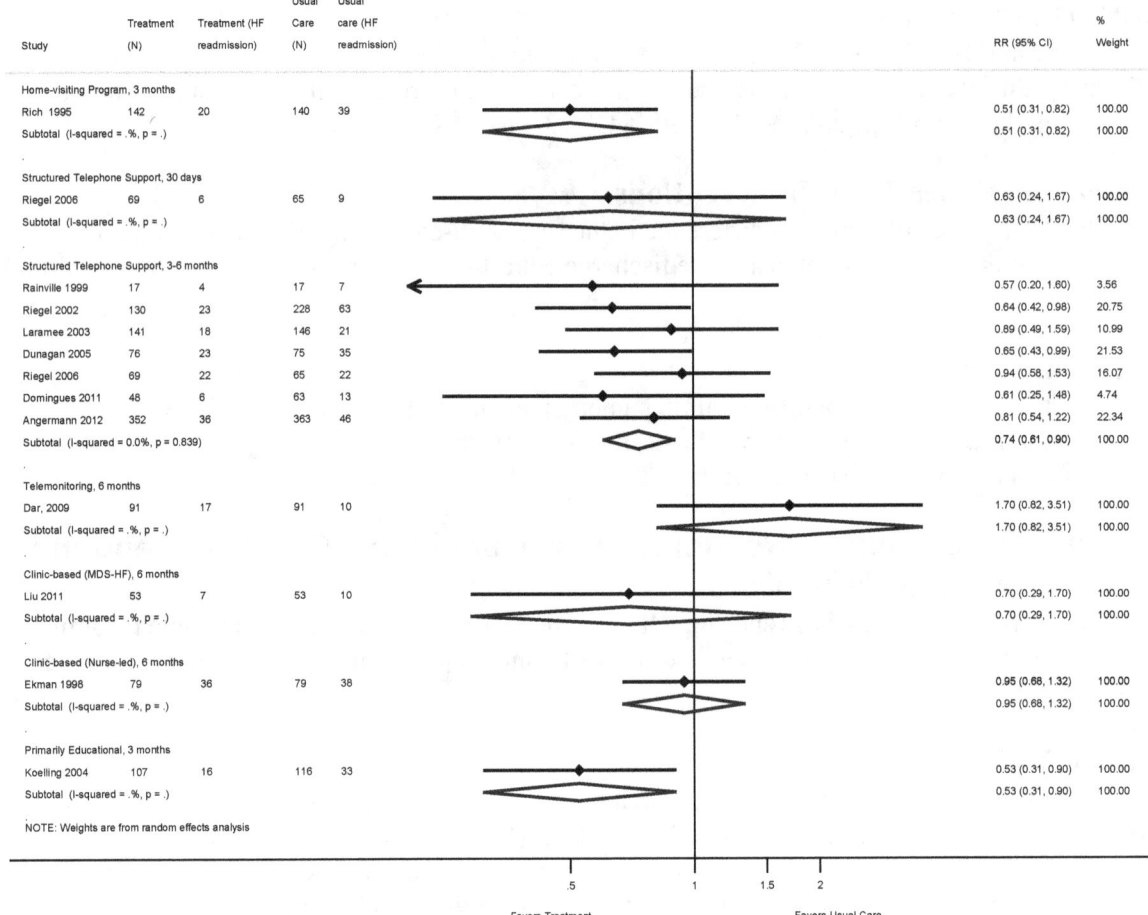

N= sample size; Treatment (HF readmissions) = number of people in the intervention group who were readmitted; Usual care (HF readmissions) = number of people in the usual care group who were readmitted

Clinic-Based Interventions

Two clinic-based interventions reported HF-specific readmissions at 6 months—one in an MDS-HF clinic and the other in a nurse-led clinic. The MDS-HF trial (N=106) found no difference in the risk of HF-specific readmission between patients receiving the intervention and those receiving usual care (RR, 0.70; 95% CI, 0.29 to 1.70).[90] The nurse-led clinic trial (N=158) also found no difference in the risk of HF-specific readmission between the intervention and control groups (RR, 0.95; 95% CI, 0.68 to 1.32).[83]

Primarily Educational Interventions

One trial (N=123) found a significantly lower risk of HF-specific readmission among patients receiving face-to-face intensive HF education before discharge compared with those receiving usual care at 3 months (RR, 0.53; 95% CI, 0.31 to 0.90).[95] A sensitivity analysis, for which we added a second educational intervention trial rated as high risk of bias, showed attenuated effect in the risk of HF-specific readmission between patients receiving an educational intervention and those receiving usual care that was no longer statistically significant (RR, 0.76; 95% CI, 0.36 to 1.63; Appendix F).[92,95]

Other Interventions

One trial (N=88) assessing peer support among patients recently discharged for HF (rated high risk of bias) found a higher risk of HF-specific readmission among the intervention group than among the control group at 30 days and 3 months; the authors stated that the differences were not statistically significant (p-value or CIs not reported).[96]

Composite All-Cause Readmission or Death: Transitional Care Interventions Compared With Usual Care

Our meta-analysis of trials reporting the composite outcome is shown in Figure 5. We present detailed results by intervention category and outcome timing below.

Figure 5. Composite all-cause readmission or death for transitional care interventions compared with usual care, by intervention category and outcome timing: Meta-analysis and forest plot of individual trials

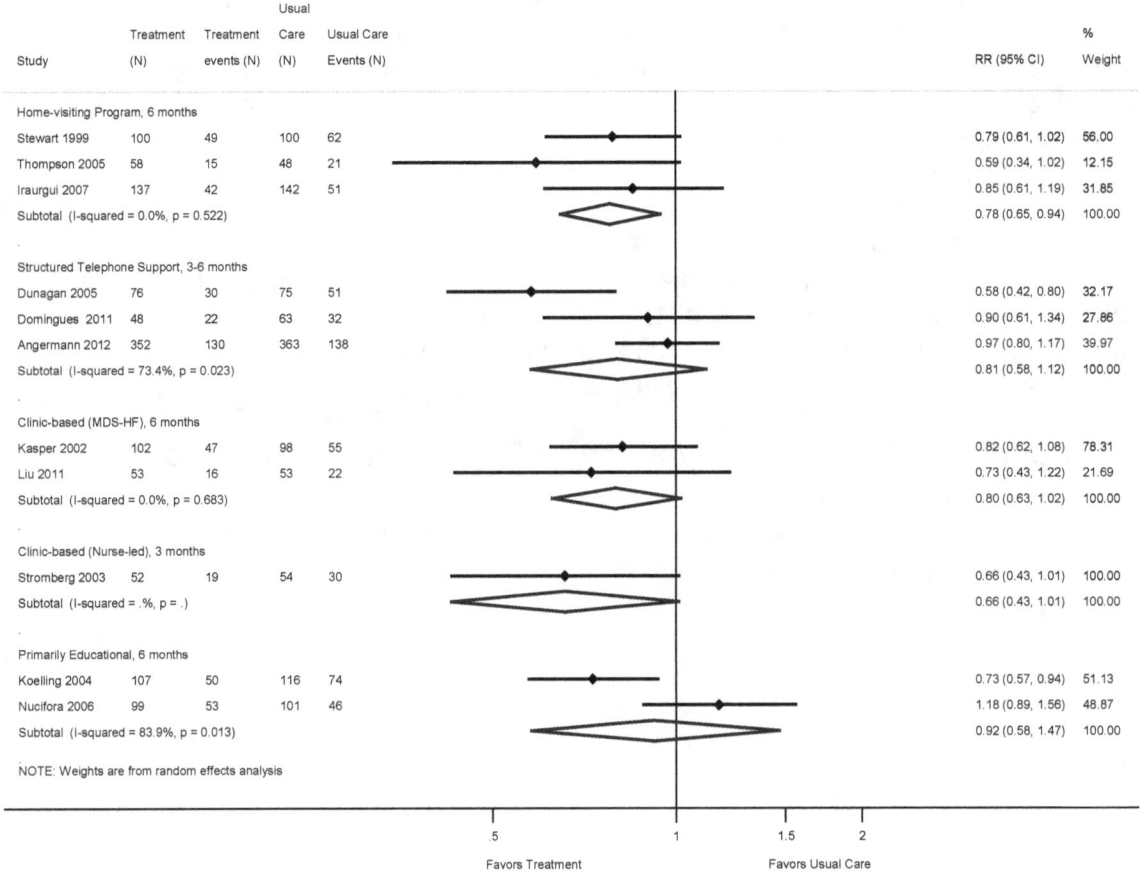

N= sample size; Treatment events= number of people readmitted in the intervention group; Usual Care Events= number of people readmitted in the usual care group.

Home-Visiting Programs

Our meta-analyses (three RCTs) found a significantly lower risk of the composite outcome among patients receiving home visits than among controls (RR, 0.78; 95% CI, 0.65 to 0.94).[50,56,60] One other trial (N=239) presented the estimated proportion of patients alive and with no hospital readmissions at various points after the intervention.[55] Patients in the intervention group were more likely to be alive with no hospitalizations than those receiving usual care at 30 days (hazard ratios 0.869 [standard error 0.033] versus 0.737 [0.041]), 3 months (0.071 [0.045] versus 0.558 [0.047]), and 6 months (0.600 [0.047] versus 0.444 [0.047]); p-values were not reported.

Structured Telephone Support

Over 3 to 6 months, our meta-analysis (three trials) found no difference in the risk of the composite outcome between patients receiving STS and controls (RR, 0.81; 95% CI, 0.58 to 1.12).[66-68]

Clinic-Based Interventions

Our meta-analysis (two trials) showed no difference in the risk of the composite outcome between patients receiving MDS-HF clinic care and controls (RR, 0.80; 95% CI, 0.63 to 1.02).[87,90] One trial (N=106) assessing a nurse-led clinic intervention found a lower risk of readmission in patients receiving the intervention compared with controls (RR, 0.66; 95% CI, 0.43 to 1.01).[88]

Primarily Educational Interventions

Our meta-analysis (two trials) found no difference in the risk of the composite outcome between patients receiving an educational intervention and patients receiving usual care (RR, 0.92; 95% CI, 0.58 to 1.47, I^2 83.9).[93,95] Despite the heterogeneity, we considered the interventions similar enough in terms of included population and intervention components to justify combining in a meta-analysis. The trial by Koelling et al. included a 1-hour individual teaching session with a nurse educator before discharge and focused on self-care behaviors, with no additional followup after discharge; patients receiving this intervention experienced a lower risk of the composite outcome than controls.[95] The trial by Nucifora et.al included a similar predischarge educational intervention and one nurse telephone followup after discharge with the goal of reinforcing education.[93] Baseline population characteristics between patients in these two trials did not differ in any obvious way. The trials were conducted in different settings (Italy; the United States), and differences in usual care (not reported in detail) may explain the inconsistent results.

Emergency Room or Acute Care Visits: Transitional Care Interventions Compared With Uual Care

Few trials reported on the number of patients seeking emergency care or acute care visits. All trials categorized these visits as "emergency department" or ER visits. We found no trials reporting acute care visits separately.

Home-Visiting Program

Three home-visiting trials reported on ER visits; all reported on different lengths of followup and used different methods to calculate the rate of ER visits. One of these trials (N=179) found that the number of patients who had an ER visit did not differ between those receiving home visits and those receiving usual care at 30 days (5 percent versus 4 percent, p-value NR) or at 3 months (17 percent versus 22 percent, p-value NR).[47] At 6 months, another trial (N=97) found significantly fewer total ER visits per group among patients receiving home visits than among those receiving usual care (48 versus 87 visits, p=0.05).[51] Finally, one trial (N=58), rated high risk of bias, found no difference in mean ER visits per patient over 6 months between patients in the intervention and control groups.[52]

Structured Telephone Support

Six STS trials provided data on ER visits at different time points and using different methods. At 3 months, one trial (N=111) found no difference in the total number of ER visits among patients receiving STS and patients receiving usual care (RR, 0.66; 95% CI, 0.21 to 2.05; p=0.67).[67] Two trials reported on the number of ER visits at 6 months; neither found a difference between patients receiving STS and those receiving usual care. In one trial (N=276), 22.1 percent of patients receiving STS and 27.9 percent of patients receiving usual care had at least one ER visit (p=0.266).[72] Another trial (N= 358) reported the mean number of ER visits per person in each group; those receiving STS had 0.14 visits (standard deviation [SD], 0.45) and those receiving usual care had 0.11 visits (SD, 0.34) (p=0.58).[63] One trial (N=37), rated high risk of bias, found that patients receiving STS had fewer ER visits related to HF over 6 months than controls; however, the number of all-cause ER visits did not differ between the intervention and control groups.[70]

Telemonitoring

No trial assessing a telemonitoring intervention found either an increase or a decrease in ER visits in patients receiving the intervention compared with those receiving usual care. At 3 months in one trial (N=102), the average number of ER visits per patient did not differ between the telemonitoring group (0.34) and the control group (0.38) (p=0.73).[78] Two trials, rated high risk of bias, did not find a difference in total ER visits at 3 months between patients receiving telemonitoring and those receiving usual care.[70,81]

At 6 months, one trial (N=182) found that the total number of ER visits was lower in the intervention group (20) than in the control group (32); the authors stated that the difference was not significant.[80] The authors of one trial (N=280, rated high risk of bias) reported no difference in ER visits between intervention and control groups at 6 months (data not provided).[79] One trial (N=37), rated high risk of bias, found that patients receiving telemonitoring had fewer CHF-related ER visits over 6 months than controls; however, the number of all-cause ER visits did not differ between the intervention and control group.[70]

Clinic-Based Interventions

In one trial (N= 230), at 6 months, the percentage of patients seen in the ER did not differ between patients receiving MDS-HF clinic management and those receiving usual care (HR, 0.97; 95% CI, 0.70 to 1.36).[89]

Primarily Educational Interventions

One trial (N=76) found that the percentage of patients seen in the ER did not differ at 3 months between patients receiving video HF education and those receiving usual care (38 percent versus 33 percent; p=0.68).[92]

Hospital Days (of Subsequent Readmissions): Transitional Care Interventions Compared With Usual Care

Home-Visiting Programs

At 30 days, one trial (N=179) found no difference in the mean number of readmission hospital days between patients receiving home visits (2.2 days; SD, 7) and those receiving usual care (2.3 days; SD, 7).[47]

Our meta-analysis (four trials; see Appendix E) found no difference in the mean number of hospital days per person accumulated over 3 months between people receiving home visits and those receiving usual care (weighted mean difference [WMD], -1.17; 95% CI, -2.44 to 0.09).[47,53,57,58] At 6 months, three trials reported the total number of hospital days accumulated per group (along with a p-value).[50,51,60] All found that patients receiving home visits accumulated fewer readmission days than controls (Table 10).

Table 10. Hospital days accumulated over 6 months: Home visiting versus usual care

Author, Year	Sample Size	Home-Visiting Hospital Days	Usual Care Hospital Days	P-Value
Stewart et al., 1998[51]	Home visiting (49) Usual care (48)	261	452	0.05
Stewart et al., 1999[50]	Home visiting (100) Usual care (100)	875	1476	0.04[a]
Thompson et al., 2005[60]	Home visiting (58) Usual care (48)	108	459	<0.01[b]

[a] Excluding "planned" admissions (e.g., for surgical procedures, other planned admissions).

[b] Adjusted for the number of events per patient per month of followup.

Structured Telephone Support

At 30 days, one trial (N=134) found no difference in the mean hospital days accumulated between patients receiving STS and controls (WMD, -0.95; 95% CI, -2.43 to 0.53).[64]

Our meta-analysis (five trials; Appendix E) found that patients receiving STS accumulated significantly fewer total hospital days over 3 to 6 months than did patients receiving usual care (WMD, -2.49; 95% CI, -3.39 to -1.04).[63-65,72,73]

Telemonitoring

No RCT comparing telemonitoring with usual care found a reduction in length of hospital stay or total accumulated hospital days at any time point.

One trial (N=168) found no difference in mean length of hospital stay per patient readmitted both at 30 days (telemonitoring, 1.9 days [SD, 4.4]; control: 1.8 days [SD, 12.2]) and at 90 days (telemonitoring: 4.9 days [SD, 8.2]; usual care: 4.8 [SD, 10.2].[82] Another trial (N=121), rated high risk of bias, found no difference in mean length of hospital stay per person readmitted among patients receiving telemonitoring and controls (2.69 days versus 3.75 days; NS per authors).[81]

At 6 months, one trial (N=182) found no difference in median duration of readmission hospital stay between intervention and control groups (17 days versus 13 days; p=0.99).[80] Two trials, rated high[70] or unclear risk of bias,[77] each found no difference in mean length of hospital stay at 6 months between intervention and control arms.

Clinic-Based Interventions

One trial (N=230) found that patients receiving MDS-HF management had significantly fewer total hospital days at 6 months than did patients receiving usual care (HR, 0.61; 95% CI, 0.39 to 0.95).[89]

At 3 months, one trial (N=106) found that patients receiving care in a nurse-led HF clinic had significantly fewer hospital days per group than patients receiving usual care (350 days versus 592; p=0.045).[88] At 6 months, another nurse-led clinic trial (N=158) found no difference in mean hospital days per patient among patients receiving the intervention (26 days; SD, 31) and those receiving usual care (18 days; SD, 19) (p-value NS per investigators).[83]

One trial (N=443) evaluating increased access to primary care in a VA setting found that patients receiving the primary care intervention had a significantly higher mean hospital length of stay at 6 months than did patients receiving usual care (9.1 versus 7.3 days; p=0.04).[91]

Primarily Educational Interventions

One trial (N=200) found no difference in the mean length of hospital stay over 6 months for patients receiving intensive predischarge education and those receiving usual care (20 days versus 15 days; p=NS per authors).[93]

Other Interventions

The trial (N=88; rated high risk of bias) assessing the efficacy of peer support for HF patients found no difference in the mean number of all-cause hospital days per patient among those receiving peer support and patients receiving usual care at 30 days (0.87 days versus 1.2 days; p=NS per authors) and at 3 months (1.8 days versus 2.1 days, respectively; p=NS per authors).[96]

Detailed Synthesis: Comparative Effectiveness of Transitional Care Interventions

Telemonitoring Versus Home Visiting

A single trial (N= 216, rated unclear risk of bias) compared telemonitoring with a home-visiting program. At 3 months, the telemonitoring group had significantly fewer total HF readmissions than the group receiving home visits (13 versus 24 readmissions; $p \leq 0.001$).[61] Similarly, the telemonitoring group had significantly fewer HF readmissions at 6 months than the group receiving home visits (38 versus 63 readmissions; $p \leq 0.05$).[61] The group receiving telemonitoring also accumulated significantly fewer hospital days at 3 months than the group receiving home visits (49.5 versus 105.0 days; $p \leq 0.001$).[61]

Telemonitoring Versus Structured Telephone Support

One trial (N= 37, rated high risk of bias) had three arms: (1) telemonitoring (video nursing visits), (2) STS, and (3) usual care. Neither all-cause nor HF readmissions differed among groups over 6 months.[70] Mean ER visits and mean length of stay did not differ over 6 months between the telemonitoring and STS groups.[70]

KQ 2: Transitional Care Interventions and Health and Social Outcomes

Key Points: Mortality

- Home-visiting programs, STS, and MDS-HF clinic interventions were efficacious in reducing mortality over 3 to 6 months (moderate SOE for each category).
- Evidence was insufficient to determine whether home-visiting programs affected mortality at 30 days.
- Three categories of interventions did not reduce mortality rates over 3 to 6 months: telemonitoring, nurse-led clinic interventions, and primarily educational interventions (low SOE for each category).
- Evidence was insufficient to determine whether the following intervention categories affected mortality at any time point: the primary care clinic intervention and cognitive training.

Key Points: Quality of Life and Function

- Home-visiting programs improved HF-specific quality of life (measured by the Minnesota Living with Heart Failure Questionnaire [MLWHFQ]) at 3 months (low SOE). Evidence was insufficient to determine whether home-visiting programs improved HF-specific quality of life at 6 months (due to imprecision and inconsistent findings).
- STS did not improve HF-specific quality of life compared with usual care at 3 or 6 months (low SOE).
- Evidence was insufficient to determine whether telemonitoring, primarily educational interventions, and clinic-based interventions affected quality-of life outcomes at 3 or 6 months following an inpatient admission.
- Too few trials reported other quality-of-life outcomes or functional status outcomes using the same scales at similar time points to assess whether interventions improved these types of outcomes.

Key Points: Caregiver and Self-Care Burden

- No trial assessing the efficacy of a transitional care intervention reported outcomes on caregiver or self-care burden.

Key Points: Comparative Effectiveness

- Direct evidence was insufficient to determine whether one type of transitional care intervention was more or less efficacious than any other type of intervention for any health or social outcome.

Detailed Synthesis: Transitional Care Interventions Compared With Usual Care

Mortality: Transitional Care Interventions Versus Usual Care

Figure 6 presents our meta-analysis of trials reporting mortality stratified by intervention category and the outcomes measurement points. We present detailed results by intervention category and outcome timing below.

43

Figure 6. Mortality among patients receiving transitional care interventions compared with usual care, by intervention category and outcome timing: Meta-analysis and forest plot of individual trials

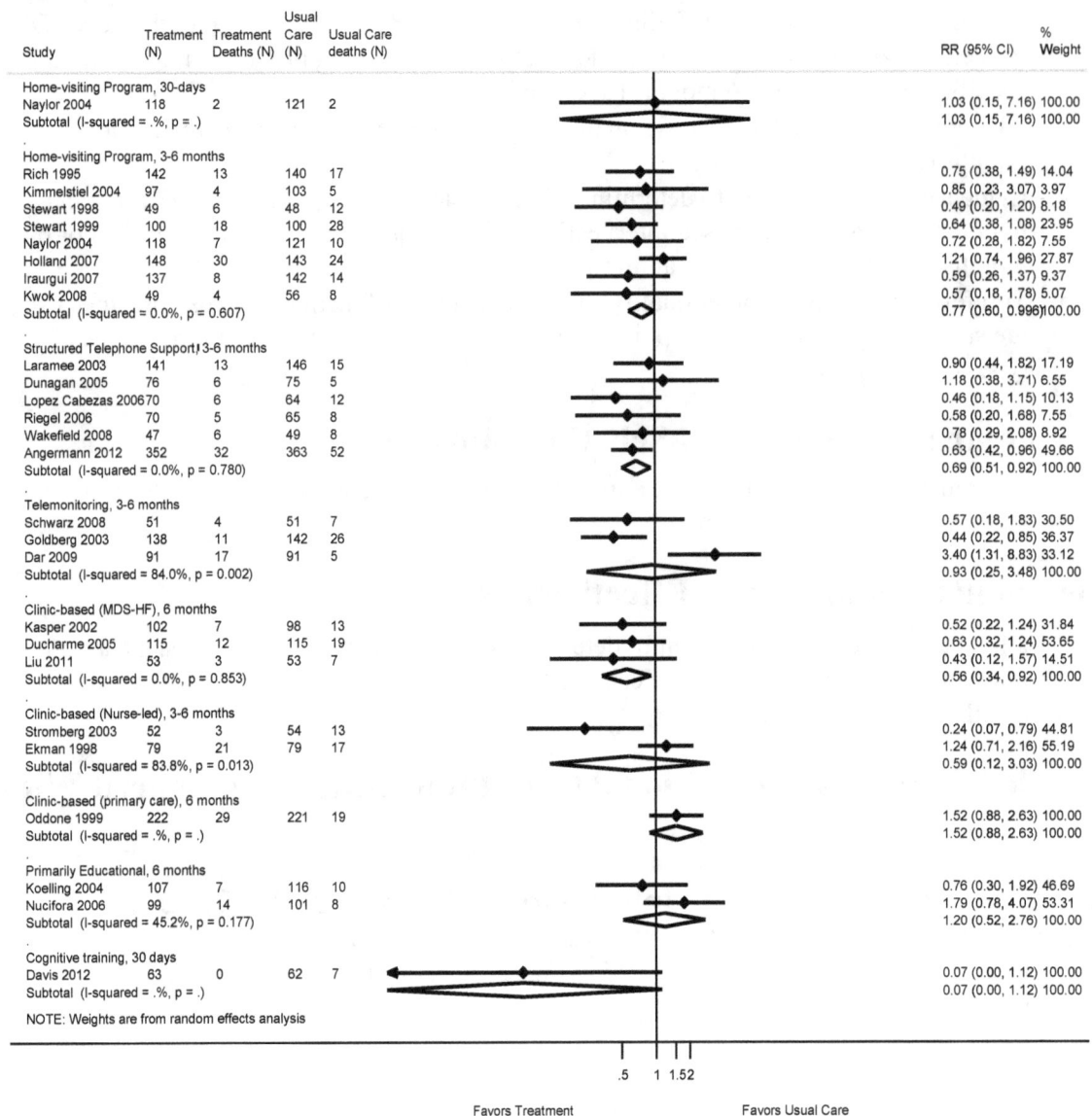

N = sample size; Treatment deaths = number of people who died in the intervention group; Usual Care deaths = number of people who died in the usual care group.

Home-Visiting Programs

One trial (N=239) reported mortality rates at 30 days; mortality did not differ between the intervention and control groups (RR, 1.03; 95% CI, 0.15 to 7.16).[55] Over 3 to 6 months, our meta-analysis (eight trials) found a significantly lower risk of mortality among patients receiving home visits than among those receiving usual care (RR, 0.77; 95% CI, 0.60 to 0.996).[50,51,53-57,59]

Structured Telephone Support

Our meta-analysis (six trials) found a significantly lower risk of mortality among patients receiving STS than among controls (RR, 0.69; 95% CI, 0.51 to 0.92).[64-66,68,69,73] Wakefield et al. evaluated the efficacy of two STS applications, one delivered by telephone and one by videophone, both compared with usual care.[69] In our meta-analysis, we included only the telephone arm (compared with usual care) as it is similar to other included trials assessing STS. The STS arm using videophone did not lower the risk of mortality compared with usual care.[69]

Telemonitoring

Our meta-analysis (three trials) found no difference in mortality over 3 to 6 months between patients receiving telemonitoring and those receiving usual care (RR, 0.93; 95% CI, 0.25 to 3.48; I^2 84 percent).[78-80] These trials produced inconsistent findings. One found a significant improvement in mortality for patients receiving telemonitoring compared with patients receiving usual care;[79] another found a significant increase in mortality in the intervention group.[80] The third found no difference between the intervention and control group.[78] Studies used similar equipment in patient populations that appeared comparable; the UK study by Goldberg et al. (which produced a mortality benefit) also included one initial home visit when staff were setting up the telemonitoring equipment.[79] Patients may have benefited from the in-home assessment or usual care may have differed. A sensitivity analysis, which included two additional trials rated as unclear or high risk of bias, did not change the overall results (Appendix E).

Clinic-Based Interventions

Our meta-analysis (three trials) found that the MDS-HF clinic patients had a significantly lower risk of mortality over 3 to 6 months than control patients (RR, 0.56; 95% CI, 0.34 to 0.92).[87,89,90] Our meta-analysis (two trials) found no difference in mortality over 3 to 6 months between patients receiving nurse-led clinic interventions and patients receiving usual care (RR, 0.59; 95% CI, 0.12 to 3.03; I^2 83.8%).[83,88] Despite the significant heterogeneity, we judged these trials to be similar enough to combine in a meta-analysis. Both trials assessed similar, nurse-directed clinic interventions at a single institution in Sweden; the interventions featured similar components such as psychosocial support, individualized education, and coordination with a cardiologist.[83,88] The trial assessing increased access to primary care in a VAMC (N= 443) found no difference in mortality between the intervention and control groups (RR, 1.52; 95% CI, 0.88 to 2.63).[91]

Primarily Educational Interventions

Our meta-analysis (two trials) found no difference in mortality between patients receiving an educational intervention and those receiving usual care (RR, 1.20; 95% CI, 0.52 to 2.76).[93,95]

Other Interventions

One trial assessing cognitive training among patients with HF and coexisting mild cognitive dysfunction found that the group receiving the intervention experienced reduced mortality compared with patients receiving usual care (RR, 0.07; 95% CI, 0.00 to 1.12).[97]

Quality of Life or Functional Status

Table 11 describes the common quality of life and functional status measures used in this literature. Overall, the types of measure used varied considerably across categories of interventions and at each eligible point of measuring outcomes. Few trials reported on measurements of functional status; for each category of interventions, we present our data synthesis of quality of life and functional status measures together.

Table 11. Quality of life or function measures used in the included trials

Abbreviated Name	Complete Name	Range of Scores	Improvement Indicated By
MLWHFQ	Minnesota Living With Heart Failure Questionnaire	0-105	Decrease
NYHA	New York Heart Association Classification	II-IV	Decrease
6MWT	Six-Minute Walk Test	0-400+ meters[a]	Increase
EuroQoL or EQ-5D	European Quality of Life-5 Dimensions	0-100	Increase
SF-12	Medical Outcomes Study Short Form (12 items)	0-100	Increase
SF-36	Medical Outcomes Study Short Form (36 items)	0-100	Increase

[a] This is the distance a person can walk within 6 minutes on a flat surface. An improvement of 54 meters is considered clinically significant.[99]

Home-Visiting Programs

Seven trials reported on at least one quality of life or functional status measure. One trial (N=226) found that quality of life measured with the MLWHFQ did not differ between intervention and control groups at 2 weeks.[55] Our meta-analysis (two trials; Appendix E) found that patients receiving home visits had significantly better HF-specific quality of life than controls as measured by the MLWHFQ at 3 months (standardized mean difference [SMD], -0.26; 95% CI, -0.47 to -0.05) but not at 6 months (SMD, -0.04; 95% CI, -0.35 to 0.26).[55,59] At six months, these two trials found inconsistent results and there was moderate statistical heterogeneity. Although both of these trials measured MLWHFQ, one of them reported the results on a log scale,[55] placing scores into categories (from 1-5) and assigning "0" to patients who died. For this reason, we did not use a WMD in the meta-analysis but instead calculated an SMD. One additional trial (N=200) found significant improvement in MLWHFQ scores at 3 months in patients receiving home visits compared with those receiving usual care (change from baseline: -19 versus -1; p=0.04).[50]

Table 12 summarizes the results of other quality of life or functional status measures reported by trials assessing a home-visiting program. In one trial, patients receiving home visits had improved quality of life at 3 months as measured by the MLWHFQ and SF-36 physical health score.[50] Three additional trials found no improvement in any measure of quality of life or function at 3 or 6 months.

Two trials rated high risk of bias found no difference in function measured by the 6-minute walk test between patients receiving home visits and those receiving usual care; one measured function at 30 days[48] and the other at 6 months.[52]

Table 12. Results of quality of life and function: Home visiting versus usual care

Study	Arm (N)	Outcome Measures(s)	Baseline Value	Change From Baseline (or End of Treatment Mean)	P-Value[a]
Stewart et al., 1999[50]	HV (100)	MLWHFQ	HV: 65 (47 to 70) UC: 62 (49 to 73)	3 months (median change and IQR): HV: -19 (-41 to 1); UC: -1 (-29 to 10)	0.04
	UC (100)			6 months: HV: -17 (-35 to -8); UC: -12 (-35 to -8)	0.30
		SF-36 physical health score	HV: 26 (21 to 32) UC: 23 (18 to 28)	3 months: HV: 16 (5 to 2.7); UC: 3 (-8 to 14)	0.02
				6 months : HV: 17 (3 to 27); UC: 15 (3 to 31)	0.53
		SF-36 mental health score	HV: 58 (48 to 76) UC: 56 (37 to 68)	3 months : HV: 10 (-19 to 19); UC: 6 (-9 to 31)	0.48
				6 months: HV: 7 (-15 to 31); UC: 19 (10 to 31)	0.46
Thompson et al., 2005[60]	HV (58) UC (48)	MLWHFQ	NR	6 months (change from baseline): HV: -14.2; UC: -13.7	NS
		SF-36	NR	SF-36 (change from baseline for 8 sub-scores; authors presented data in figure only)	NS
Holland et al., 2007[59]	HV (148) UC (143)	EQ-5D	HV: 0.58 (SD 0.32) UC: 0.57 (SD 0.34)	3 months (mean score and SD): HV: 0.54 (0.33); UC: 0.51 (0.37)	NS
				6 months: HV: 0.58 (0.29); UC: 0.52 (0.34)	0.07
Kwok et al., 2008[54]	HV (44) UC (46)	6MWT	HV: 120.7 m (SD 62.0) UC: 118.5 m (SD 62.5)	6 months (changes in from baseline): HV: 44 (-15, 84) UC: 25 (-22, 69)	NS

[a] p-value is for result indicated—i.e., either change from baseline or difference in mean scores.

HV = home visiting; IQR = interquartile range; MLWHFQ = Minnesota Living with Heart Failure Questionnaire; 6MWT = 6-minute walk test; NR = not reported; NS = not significant; SD, standard deviation; SF-36= Medical Outcomes Study Short Form (36 items); UC = usual care.

Structured Telephone Support

Our meta-analysis (two trials; Appendix E) found no difference in MLWHFQ scores among patients receiving STS and those receiving usual care at either 3 months (WMD, -3.78; 95% CI, -10.39 to 2.83) or 6 months (WMD, -7.14; 95% CI, -21.07 to 6.78).[64,69] Wakefield and colleagues included STS delivered by standard telephone or by videophone (without telemonitoring);[69] we included only the comparison between telephone-based STS and usual care.

Three additional trials reported on quality of life at 6 months (Table 13). In one trial, patients receiving STS had significantly better NYHA classification and SF-36 physical functioning subscale and physical health summary measure scores at 3 months than patients receiving usual care.[66] Another reported on physical and emotional subscales of the MLWHFQ and on physical and mental health summary measures of the SF-12; patients receiving STS had significantly better scores on the SF-12 physical scale than controls at 6 months, but all other comparisons were not significant.[68]

Table 13. Results of quality of life and function: Structured telephone care versus usual care

Study	Arm (N)	Outcome Measures(s)	Baseline Value	Change From Baseline (or End of Treatment Mean)	P-Value[a]
Barth, 2001[62]	STS (17)	MLWHFQ	MLWHFQ total score:	Change from baseline (SD) at 2 months:	NS[c]
	UC (17)		STS: 50.9 (16.3); UC; 49.7 (15.7)	STS: 8.2 (4.3); UC: NR (NS per authors)	
Dunagan et al., 2005[68]	STS (64)	MLWHFQ	Mean (SD)	Change from baseline (SD) at 6 months	
	UC (66)	SF-12	MLWHFQ physical scale: STS: 23.6 (10.8); UC: 23.0 (11.3)	MLWHFQ physical scale: STS: 9.3 (8.9); UC: 5.2 (10.4)	0.33
			MLWHFQ emotional scale: STS: 46.2 (11.9); UC:46.6 (11.2)	MLWHFQ emotional scale: STS: 2.7 (6.0); UC:2.4 (6.8)	0.90
			SF-12 physical scale: STS: 24.1 (10.1); UC: 24.9 (11.3)	SF-12 physical scale: STS: 1.2 (9.9); UC: -2.7 (10.7)	0.028
			SF-12 mental scale: STS: 46.2 (11.9); UC: 46.6 (11.2)	SF12 mental scale: STS: 7.3 (12.7); UC: 5.5 (11.7)	0.20
Lopez Cabezas et al., 2006[73]	STS (70)	EuroQoL	NR	2 months: mean (SD) STS: 62.3 (17.3) UC: 65.0 (17.6)	NS[b]
	UC (64)			6 months: mean (SD) STS: 62.9 (14.9) UC: 62.8 (14.1)	NS[b]
Angermann et al., 2012[66]	STS (352)	NYHA class	% with NYHA III or IV: STS 40% UC 36%	NYHA class at 3 months Worsened: HV 17%; UC 10% Unchanged: HV 49%; UC 52% Improved: HV 33%; UC 38%	0.05[b]
	UC (363)	SF-36	STS: mean (SD) Physical function.: 48 (30) Physical health: 36 (11) Mental health: 44 (12)	Mean change (SD) at 3 months Physical function: STS: +2.8 (10.0); UC +1.3 (9.9)	0.03
			UC: mean (SD) Physical function.: 44 (29) Physical health: 36 (11) Mental health: 44 (12)	Physical health: STS: +5.9 (25.8); UC +1.8 (24.7)	0.03
				Mental health: STS: +2.3 (12.4); UC +2.3 (12)	0.57

[a] All p-values in this column are for the difference in change from baseline between groups unless noted otherwise.

[b] p-value for overall trend (improvement) is based on logistic regression.

[c] As reported by authors. The authors did not specifically report a p-value for the difference in mean change at 2 months between intervention and control groups. They did, however, report that the change from baseline to 2 months was p<0.00 for change from baseline (improvement) in STS group and "not significant" for the usual care group.

MLWHFQ = Minnesota Living with Heart Failure Questionnaire; NR = not reported; NS = not significant; NYHA = New York Heart Association Classification; SD = standard deviation; SF-12 = Medical Outcomes Study Short Form (12 items); STS = structured telephone support; UC = usual care.

Telemonitoring

In one trial (N=102), patients receiving telemonitoring and those receiving usual care did not differ in mean MLWHFQ scores at 3 months (27.4 versus 27.3, respectively, p=0.99 for difference in mean scores between groups).[78] Another trial (N=182) reported no difference in MLWHFQ or European Quality of Life-5 Dimensions outcomes at 6 months between intervention and control groups (authors did not provide data).[80]

Clinic-Based Interventions

At 6 months, one trial (N=200) found that patients receiving care through an MDS-HF clinic experienced significantly greater improvement on the total MLWHFQ score than patients receiving usual care (change from baseline -28.3 versus -15.7; p=0.01).[87] In the same trial, patients receiving care in the MDS-HF clinic also experienced significantly greater improvement in NYHA functional class than did controls (25 percent of intervention group and 43 percent of the usual care group had NYHA class III or IV at 6 months; p=0.03 [test for trend]).[87]

The one trial (N=443) assessing enhanced access to primary care found no difference between intervention and control groups in mean scores on the SF-36 mental and physical summary measures at 6 months (p=0.2 for both).[91]

Primarily Educational Interventions

Two trials evaluating a primarily educational intervention reported quality of life measured with the MLWHFQ at 6 months but produced inconsistent findings. In one trial (N=223), total MLWHFQ scores were significantly better among patients receiving predischarge, in-person education than among those receiving usual care (14 [SD, 20] versus 10 [SD, 16]; p<0.0001).[93] In another trial (N=149), patients receiving discharge education did not improve compared with patients receiving usual care (41 [SD, 22] versus 42 [SD, 25]; p-value not reported).[95]

Other Interventions

Neither trial in this category reported on a quality-of-life or functional status outcome.

Detailed Synthesis: Comparative Effectiveness of Transitional Care Interventions

Telemonitoring Compared With Home-Visiting Program

One trial (N=216, rated unclear risk of bias) compared a telemonitoring program with a home-visiting program. At 3 months, MLWHFQ scores did not differ between the groups (telemonitoring mean score: 51.64 [SD, 17.36]; home-visiting mean score: 57.72 [SD, 16.24]; p=0.47).[61]

KQ 3. Components of Effective Interventions

We defined effective interventions as: (1) intervention categories (defined in Table 2 in Methods) that reduced either all-cause readmission (from our meta-analyses for KQ 1) or the composite endpoint of all-cause readmission or death; (2) intervention categories that reduced mortality (from our meta-analyses for KQ 2); or (3) individual trials in other categories that were efficacious for reducing all-cause readmissions, mortality, or the composite endpoint. Few trials reported outcomes at 30 days. Below we describe the components of interventions that showed efficacy at any eligible time point (up to 6 months following an index hospitalization for HF).

For all included trials, we abstracted information about the intervention components as the authors had described them. We considered intervention "components" as any part of the intervention that could be separated out and that could influence efficacy. Across trials, authors provided varying levels of detail about interventions and components. Evidence tables (Appendix C) give the full data abstraction of intervention components of all included trials.

Here we focus on the content (e.g., education, exercise recommendations) and process (e.g., care coordination) components of interventions. We evaluate intensity, delivery personnel, and mode of delivery separately in KQ 4; we also mention mode of delivery (e.g., whether the intervention is delivered in person) in KQ 3 because we cannot separate mode of delivery from some intervention components (e.g., use of home visits or coordination of care with providers).

KQ 3a. Intervention Components

All-Cause Readmissions and Composite All-Cause Readmission or Death

Table 14 summarizes the components that we identified in the articles describing efficacious interventions that reduced all-cause readmission or the composite endpoint at either 30 days or over 3 to 6 months (or both). The main categories were home-visiting programs and MDS-HF clinic interventions. One education trial (a nursing education session) also was efficacious (for the composite endpoint at 6 months) and two trials of STS were efficacious in reducing all-cause readmission at 6 months.

Shared Components of Home-Visiting and MDS-HF Clinic Interventions

Both home-visiting programs and MDS-HF clinic interventions are multicomponent, complex interventions. No single-component intervention (including predischarge only) reduced all-cause readmission rates. As a whole, these two categories of interventions shared the following components:

- HF education, emphasizing self-care, recognition of symptoms, and weight monitoring.
- HF pharmacotherapy, emphasizing patient education about medications; promotion of adherence to medication regimens; promotion of evidence-based HF pharmacotherapy before discharge or during followup (or both).
- Face-to-face contact following discharge: via home-visiting personnel, MDS-HF clinic personnel, or both. In most cases, this contact occurred within 7 days of discharge.
- Streamlined mechanisms to contact care delivery personal (clinic personnel or visiting nurses or pharmacists) outside of scheduled visits (e.g., patient hotline).
- Mechanisms for medication adjustment after discharge. In most cases, home-visiting personnel either directly recommended medication adjustment or assisted with coordination of care (e.g., with primary care provider or cardiologist) to facilitate timely medication adjustment, based on a patient's needs (rather than advising patients to call for help themselves).

Components of Individual Studies in Other Categories That Were Effective

Two STS trials reduced all-cause readmissions (Lopez Cabezas et al., 2006[73] and Dunagan et al., 2005[68]); one other trial assessed a primarily nurse-based educational intervention that reduced the composite endpoint (Koelling et al., 2005).[95] Table 14 also includes components of these interventions.

Table 14. KQ 3, Components of effective interventions: All-cause readmissions or composite (all-cause readmission or death) outcome

Author, Year	Category	Primary Mode of Delivery	Self-Care Management Promotion	Weight-monitoring Education	Diet/Sodium Restriction Education	Promotion of Medication Adherence	Exercise Education or Promotion	Unspecified HF Education	Medication Reconciliation
Ducharme et al., 2005[89]	MDS-HF	Face-to-face	x	x	x	x	–	x	x
Liu et al., 2012[90]	MDS-HF	Face-to-face	x	–	–	x	–	–	x
Rich et al., 1993[58]	HV	Face-to-face	x	x	x	x	–	x	x
Rich et al., 1995[57]	HV	Face-to-face	x	x	x	x	–	x	x
Stewart et al., 1998[51]	HV	Face-to-face	x	–	–	x	–	–	–
Jaarsma et al., 1999[47]	HV	Face-to-face	x	–	x	x	–	x	–
Stewart et al., 1999[50]	HV	Face-to-face	x	x	–	x	x	–	–
Kimmelstiel et al., 2004[53]	HV	Face-to-face	x	x	x	x	–	x	–
Naylor et al., 2004[55]	HV	Face-to-face	x	x	x	x	–	–	x
Thompson et al., 2005[60]	HV	Face-to-face	x	x	x	x	x	x	x
Aldamiz-Echevarría Iraúrgui et al., 2007[56]	HV	Face-to-face	x	x	x	x	–	x	x
Holland et al., 2007[59]	HV	Face-to-face	x	x	x	x	x	x	x
Kwok et al., 2008[54]	HV	Face-to-face	x	–	x	x	x	–	x
Dunagan et al., 2005[68]	STS	Telephone	x	x	x	x	x	–	x
Lopez Cabezas et al., 2006[73]	STS	Telephone	–	–	x	x	–	x	–
Koelling et al., 2005[95]	Edu	Face-to-face	X	x	x	x	x	–	–

Table 14. KQ 3—Components of effective interventions: All-cause readmissions or composite (all-cause readmission or death) outcome (continued)

Author, Year	Category	Setting/ Timing of Education (Pre-d/c, Post-d/c or Both)	Transition Coach/ Case Management*	Coordination w/ Outpatient Provider While Inpatient	Individualized Discharge Plan	Planned Telephone Follow-up Post Discharge	Timing of First Telephone Follow-up (Days)	Series of Scheduled Calls	Patient Hotline	Timing of First Home Visit (Days)	Number of Scheduled Home Visits	Medication Reconciliation During Home Visit
Ducharme et al., 2005[89]	MDS-HF	Post-d/c	–	–	–	x	≤3	x	–	–	–	–
Liu et al., 2012[90]	MDS-HF	Both	x	–	x	x	≤7	x	x	–	–	–
Rich et al., 1993[58]	HV	Both	x	x	x	As needed	–	x	<7	>3	x	x
Rich et al., 1995[57]	HV	Both	x	x	x	As needed	–	x	<2	>3	x	x
Stewart et al., 1998[51]	HV	Both	x	–	–	–	–	–	–	<7	1	x
Jaarsma et al., 1999[47]	HV	Both	–	–	x	x	≤7	–	x	<7	1	–
Stewart et al., 1999[50]	HV	Post-d/c	x	–	–	–	–	–	–	>7	1	–
Kimmelstiel et al., 2004[53]	HV	Post-d/c	–	–	–	–	–	x	x	<7	1	x
Naylor et al., 2004[55]	HV	Both	x	x	x	–	–	–	x	<1	8	x
Thompson et al., 2005[60]	HV	Both	x	–	–	–	–	–	x	>7	1	–
Aldamiz-Echevarria Iraúrgui et al., 2007[56]	HV	Post-d/c	–	–	–	–	–	–	x	<2	2 to 3	x
Holland et al., 2007[59]	HV	Post-d/c	–	–	–	–	–	–	–	<14	2	x
Kwok et al., 2008[54]	HV	Both	x	–	–	–	–	–	x	<7	6	x
Dunagan et al., 2005[68]	STS	Post-d/c	–	–	–	x	≤7	x	x	–	–	–
Lopez Cabezas et al., 2006[73]	STS	Both	–	–	–	x	>7	x	x	–	–	–
Koelling et al., 2005[93]	Edu	Pre-d/c	–	–	–	–	–	–	–	–	–	–

Table 14. KQ 3—Components of effective interventions: All-cause readmissions or composite (all-cause readmission or death) outcome (continued)

Author, Year	Category	Unspecified HF Education/ Promotion During Home Visit	Symptom Checklist or Clinical Assessment During Home Visit (e.g. History, Symptoms)	Physical Exam During Home Visit	Home Visiting Personnel Coordinates Care or Collaborates With Outpatient Provider	Timing of First Clinic Visit Post Discharge (Days)	Consultation With a Dietician	Clinic Personnel on-Call/ Available for Acute Symptom Management (Outside of Scheduled Appt)	Clinical Pharmacist Visit/ Consultation	Medication Optimization; Predischarge or During Intervention
Ducharme et al., 2005[89]	MDS-HF	–	–	–	–	≤14	x	x	x	x
Liu et al., 2012[90]	MDS-HF	–	–	–	–	≤7	x	x	–	x
Rich et al., 1993[58]	HV	x	–	x	–	–	–	–	–	x
Rich et al., 1995[57]	HV	x	–	x	–	–	–	–	–	x
Stewart et al., 1998[51]	HV	x	–	–	x	–	–	–	–	–
Jaarsma et al., 1999[47]	HV	x	–	–	–	–	–	–	–	–
Stewart et al., 1999[50]	HV	x	x	x	x	–	–	–	–	–
Kimmelstiel et al., 2004[53]	HV	x	x	–	x	–	–	–	–	–
Naylor et al., 2004[55]	HV	x	x	–	x	–	–	–	–	–
Thompson et al., 2005[60]	HV	x	x	x	–	–	–	x	–	x
Aldamiz-Echevarría Iraúrgui et al., 2007[56]	HV	x	x	x	–	–	–	–	–	x
Holland et al., 2007[59]	HV	x	x	–	x	–	–	–	–	x
Kwok et al., 2008[54]	HV	–	x	x	x	Unclear	–	–	–	x
Dunagan et al., 2005[68]	STS	–	–	–	–	–	–	–	–	–
Lopez Cabezas et al., 2006[73]	STS	–	–	–	–	≥14	–	–	x	x
Koelling et al., 2005[95]	Edu	–	–	–	–	–	–	–	–	–

Note: x = this component was part of the study intervention. "–"= this component was not included in the intervention. appt = appointment; d/c = discharge; Edu = primarily educational; HV= home visits; MDS = multidisciplinary; MDS-HF = multidisciplinary heart failure; Med = medium; STS = structured telephone support; UC = usual care.

53

All three trials included a face-to-face inpatient education session before hospital discharge. Both STS trials had two additional components: promotion of medication adherence during scheduled calls and a patient hotline for questions or advice outside of scheduled calls. One STS trial also had the following components: nurse-directed diuretic adjustment during telephone followup; and flexibility of intervention based on patient need (e.g., 24 percent of patients received at least one home visit, and 24 percent were provided with a home bathroom scale).[73] The educational session trial included an hour-long visit with a nurse educator that focused on the following: mechanism of action of HF medications, specific guidance on sodium and water restriction, and comprehensive guidance on self-care management (e.g., daily weight monitoring, smoking cessation, actions to take if symptoms worsened).[95] In addition to the teaching session, patients receiving the intervention were given guidelines written in layman's terms.

Mortality

We found a wider range of intervention types that reduced mortality (as contrasted with the types of interventions that improved all-cause readmissions) within 6 months following an index hospital admission. Components of interventions that reduced mortality are summarized in Table 15.

Shared Components of Structured Telephone Support and MDS Clinic Interventions

As with all-cause readmission, STS and MDS clinic interventions are multicomponent. No single-component intervention reduced mortality. As a whole, these two categories of interventions shared the following components:

- HF education, emphasizing self-care, recognition of symptoms, and weight monitoring.
- A series of scheduled, structured visits (via telephone, home visits, or clinic followup) that reinforced education and monitored for HF symptoms.
- A mechanism to contact providers easily outside of scheduled visits (e.g., patient hotline).

Components of Individual Studies in Other Categories That Were Effective

Three trials from other categories showed efficacy in reducing mortality: one telemonitoring trial,[79] one study of cognitive training in HF patients with cognitive dysfunction,[97] and one nurse-led HF clinic intervention.[88] These intervention types involved different sets of components, but all focused on transitioning self-care management back to the patient. Components included giving inpatient education training on self-care;[97] implementing a series of nurse-led clinic visits featuring self-care education, training, and monitoring;[88] or encouraging daily weights and response to symptom questions via telemonitoring.[79] To some degree, all three interventions involved flexibility to individualize care (e.g., by coordinating with the patient's physician[79] or individualizing self-care training[88,97]). The telemonitoring trial specified that coordination of care with the patient's outpatient provider was a component of the intervention.[79]

Table 15. KQ 3—Components of effective interventions: Mortality

Author, Year	Category	Primary Mode of Delivery	Self-Care Management Education/Promotion	Weight-Monitoring Education or Promotion	Diet/Sodium Restriction Education or Promotion	Promotion of Medication Adherence	Exercise Education or Promotion	Other or Unspecified HF Education	Medication Reconciliation
Kasper et al., 2002[87]	MDS-HF	Face-to-face	x	–	–	–	–	x	–
Ducharme et al., 2005[89]	MDS-HF	Face-to-face	x	x	x	x	–	x	x
Liu et al., 2012[90]	MDS-HF	Face-to-face	x	–	–	x	–	–	x
Rich et al., 1993[58]	HV	Face-to-face	x	x	x	x	–	x	x
Rich et al., 1995[57]	HV	Face-to-face	x	x	x	x	–	x	x
Stewart et al., 1998[51]	HV	Face-to-face	x	–	–	x	–	–	–
Jaarsma et al., 1999[47]	HV	Face-to-face	x	–	x	x	–	x	–
Stewart et al., 1999[50]	HV	Face-to-face	x	x	–	x	x	–	–
Kimmelstiel et al., 2004[53]	HV	Face-to-face	x	x	x	x	–	x	–
Naylor et al., 2004[55]	HV	Face-to-face	x	x	x	x	–	–	x
Thompson et al., 2005[60]	HV	Face-to-face	x	x	x	x	x	x	x
Aldamiz-Echevarria Iraúrgui et al., 2007[56]	HV	Face-to-face	x	x	x	x	–	x	x
Holland et al., 2007[59]	HV	Face-to-face	x	x	x	x	x	x	x
Kwok et al., 2008[54]	HV	Face-to-face	x	–	x	x	x	–	x
Rainville et al., 1999[71]	STS	Telephone	–	x	–	x	–	x	–
Riegel et al., 2002[63]	STS	Telephone	x	–	x	x	–	x	x
Dunagan et al., 2005[68]	STS	Telephone	x	x	x	x	x	x	x
Lopez Cabezas et al., 2006[73]	STS	Telephone	–	–	x	x	–	x	–
Riegel et al., 2006[64]	STS	Telephone	x	x	x	x	–	x	–
Wakefield et al., 2008[69] 2009[75]	STS	Telephone	x	x	x	x	–	–	–
Wakefield et al., 2008[69] 2009[75]	STS	Video-phone	x	x	x	x	–	–	–
Angermann et al., 2012[66]	STS	Telephone	x	x	x	x	x	x	–
Davis et al., 2012	Other	Face-to-face	x	x	x	x	–	–	–
Stromberg et al., 2003[88]	Clinic (nurse)	Face-to-face	x	x	x	x	–	–	–
Goldberg et al., 2003[79]	TM	TM	x	x	x	–	–	–	–

Table 15. KQ 3—Components of effective interventions: Mortality (continued)

Author, Year	Category	Setting/Timing of Education (Pre-d/c, Post-d/c or Both)	Transition Coach or Coordination Between Inpatient/Outpatient Providers	Planned Telephone Followup After Discharge	Timing of First Phone or TM Follow up (Days)	Telephone Followup Conducted by Same Personnel Delivering Inpatient Intervention Component	Series of Structured Calls	Patient Hotline (e.g. Patients Can Call Anytime for Help)	Timing of First Clinic Visit After Discharge	Consult With Nutritionist	Clinic Personnel On-Call/Available for Outside of Clinic Hours	Outpatient Clinical Pharmacist Visit
Kasper et al., 2002[87]	MDS-HF	x	x	–	–	–	–	x	–	–	–	–
Ducharme et al., 2005[89]	MDS-HF	Post-d/c	–	x	≤3	–	x	–	≤14	x	x	x
Liu et al., 2012[90]	MDS-HF	Both	x	x	≤7	Unclear	x	x	≤7	x	x	–
Rich et al., 1993[58]	HV	Both	x	As needed	–	–	x	<7	–	–	–	–
Rich et al., 1995[57]	HV	Both	x	As needed	–	–	x	<2	–	–	–	–
Stewart et al., 1998[51]	HV	Both	x	–	–	–	–	–	–	–	–	–
Jaarsma et al., 1999[47]	HV	Both	–	x	≤7	–	–	x	–	–	–	–
Stewart et al., 1999[50]	HV	Post-d/c	x	–	–	–	–	x	–	–	–	–
Kimmelstiel et al., 2004[53]	HV	Post-d/c	–	–	–	–	x	x	–	–	–	–
Naylor et al., 2004[55]	HV	Both	x	–	–	–	–	x	–	–	–	–
Thompson et al., 2005[60]	HV	Both	x	–	–	–	–	x	–	–	x	–
Aldamiz-Echevarría Iraúrgui et al., 2007[56]	HV	Post-d/c	–	–	–	–	–	x	–	–	–	–
Holland et al., 2007[59]	HV	Post-d/c	–	–	–	–	–	–	–	–	–	–
Kwok et al., 2008[54]	HV	Both	x	–	–	–	–	x	Unclear	–	–	–
Rainville et al., 1999[71]	STS	Both	x	x	≤2	x	x	x	–	–	–	–
Riegel et al., 2002[63]	STS	Post-d/c	–	x	≤7	–	x	–	–	–	–	–
Dunagan et al., 2005[68]	STS	Post-d/c	–	x	≤7	–	x	x	–	–	–	–
Lopez Cabezas et al., 2006[73]	STS	Both	–	x	>7	x	x	x	–	–	–	x
Riegel et al., 2006[64]	STS	Post-d/c	–	x	≤7	–	x	–	–	–	–	–
Wakefield et al., 2008[69] Wakefield et al., 2009[75]	STS	Both	–	x	≤7	–	x	x	–	–	–	–
Wakefield et al., 2008[69] Wakefield et al., 2009[75]	STS	Both	–	–	–	–	–	–	–	–	–	–
Angermann et al., 2012[66]	STS	Both	x	x	≤7	x	x	x	–	–	–	–
Davis et al., 2012	STS	Both	–	x	≤7	x	–	–	–	–	–	–

56

Table 15. KQ 3—Components of effective interventions: Mortality (continued)

Author, Year	Category	Setting/ Timing of Education (Pre-d/c, Post-d/c or Both)	Transition Coach or Coordination Between Inpatient/Outpatient Providers	Planned Telephone Followup After Discharge	Timing of First Phone or TM Follow-up (Days)	Telephone Followup Conducted by Same Personnel Delivering Inpatient Intervention Component	Series of Structured Calls	Patient Hotline (e.g. Patients Can Call Anytime for Help)	Timing of First Clinic Visit After Discharge	Consult with Nutritionist	Clinic Personnel On-call/ Available for Outside of Clinic Hours	Outpatient Clinical Pharmacist Visit
Stromberg et al., 2003[88]	Clinic (nurse)	Post-d/c	—	—	—	—	—	—	>14	x	x	x
Goldberg et al., 2003[79] [a]	TM	Pre-d/c	—	—	—	—	—	—	—	—	—	—

[a] Telemonitoring components also included: first telehealth contact >7 days after discharge, telemonitoring device included an automated adherence reminder, transmitted vital signs and symptoms, and service coordinated care with outpatient provider(s).

Note: x = this component was part of the study intervention. "—"= this component was not included in the intervention.

d/c = discharge; HF = heart failure; MDS = multidisciplinary; MDS-HF = multidisciplinary heart failure; Med = Medium; Pharm = pharmacist; STS = structured telephone support; TM = telemonitoring.

57

KQ 3b. Necessity of Particular Components in Effective Interventions

Given the heterogeneity of interventions, we had insufficient detail across all interventions to determine whether certain components are necessary beyond what was addressed in KQ 3a. One intervention that reduced the composite outcome was delivered during the index hospitalization; no components were delivered after discharge.[95] In all other cases, efficacious interventions were delivered either both before and after discharge or in the postdischarge setting.

For all-cause readmissions (and the composite endpoint), four elements seem to be necessary. They are (1) education focused on self-care (delivered face-to-face); (2) early contact following discharge (e.g., home visit or outpatient followup); (3) a mechanism for patients to contact intervention personnel easily for problems or symptoms (e.g., availability of a patient hotline); and (4) flexibility in the intervention that allows tailoring the intervention to patient's needs (e.g., early adjustment of medications based on symptoms)

That these seem "necessary" for demonstrated utility in affecting key outcomes does not mean that they are "sufficient," certainly not as single components.

For mortality, including training or reinforcement on self-care (e.g., daily weights) and reinforcing these skills over time both seem necessary. Like interventions that reduced all-cause readmissions, interventions that reduced mortality rates included instructions (or a patient hotline) on who and when to call when symptoms worsen.

KQ 3c. Benefits of Particular Components in Multicomponent Interventions

We did not find any direct evidence to determine whether specific components add benefit. That is, no trials directly compared the delivery of an intervention having a specific component with the same intervention but lacking that specific component. When we attempted to use indirect evidence, the diversity of components in the interventions across categories (and within intervention categories) limited our ability to isolate specific factors that added benefit. Separating out individual components from the overall type (or "bundles") of interventions that showed efficacy (KQs 1 and 2) was not possible.

KQ 4. Intensity, Delivery Personnel, Method of Communication

To assess whether the efficacy of interventions varied based on intensity, delivery personnel, or method of communication, we assessed variation both across and within intervention categories (when variation was present). We did not pool trials in a meta-analysis from different intervention categories to assess the impact of these variables because many other factors (e.g., different intervention components) differed too much across categories.

For the KQ 4 analyses, we used trials in our main analyses for either of the two primary outcomes (all-cause readmission and mortality)—i.e., trials rated as medium or low risk of bias. Appendix C (Tables C1-C13) describes the subquestions of interest: intensity, primary delivery personnel, and method of communication for these trials. For some categories of interventions, variation was insufficient within categories or we had too few trials to conduct any meaningful stratified analyses. These limitations differed by subquestion; for each subquestion below, we address only the intervention categories with sufficient variation or sufficient number of trials to assess whether efficacy differed by these factors.

Key Points: Intensity

- In general, intervention categories that included higher-intensity interventions (i.e., home-visiting programs, STS, MDS-HF clinic interventions) reduced all-cause readmission or mortality. By contrast, categories with lower-intensity interventions (i.e., primarily educational interventions, nurse-led HF clinic interventions) did not affect these two outcomes in any meaningful way.
- Within categories, subgroup analyses found that higher intensity home-visiting programs reduced all-cause readmission at 30 days, whereas lower intensity programs did not (low SOE). STS interventions had no significant differences based on intensity. Subgroup analyses were not possible for other categories of interventions because of either lack of variation or too few trials reporting outcomes at similar time points.

Key Points: Delivery Personnel

- The two categories of interventions that reduced all-cause readmission and mortality— home-visiting programs and MDS-HF clinic interventions—were more likely to include teams of providers delivering the intervention (e.g., home visits conducted by a nurse and pharmacist together). STS interventions reduced mortality (but not all-cause readmission); primarily nurses or pharmacists delivered STS interventions (and not teams of providers).
- Within categories, evidence was insufficient to make definitive conclusions about whether specific delivery personnel had more (or less) impact in reducing all-cause readmissions or mortality.

Key Points: Method of Communication

- Across intervention categories, interventions were delivered primarily face-to-face or via technology (telephone, telemonitoring, video visits). The two categories of interventions delivered primarily face-to-face did reduce all-cause readmissions—namely, home-visiting programs and MDS-HF clinic interventions. For these two categories, method of delivery did not vary within each category. STS showed efficacy in reducing mortality; some of these interventions included a face-to-face component (e.g., predischarge educational intervention). In general, interventions delivered primarily remotely (i.e., telemonitoring, STS) did not reduce all-cause readmissions.
- Only STS interventions varied in their method of communication. Our subgroup analyses for reducing either all-cause readmission or mortality found no significant differences by method of communication at any time point.

Detailed Synthesis

KQ 4a. Intensity

For most interventions, we defined intensity as the duration, frequency, or periodicity of patient contact, and we categorized each intervention as low, medium, or high intensity. Given the heterogeneity of intensity across included interventions; however, we were unable to develop a single measure of intensity to apply to trials across all intervention categories.

We considered resource use as a dimension of intensity. For example, we included factors such as the total number of intervention components in the determination of intensity. We reserved the low-intensity category for interventions that included one episode of patient contact or that required few resources (e.g., no additional components, such as time spent coordinating care). We considered the majority of interventions to be of medium or high intensity; most were multicomponent and included repeated patient contacts.

Intensity Across Intervention Categories

Certain categories (as a whole) are higher intensity than others. The MDS-HF clinic interventions were all classified as high intensity. Two categories included no trials classified as high intensity: primarily educational interventions and trials in the "other" category. Trials involving home-visiting interventions and STS included a mix of medium- and high-intensity interventions. Overall, the home-visiting category included more trials classified as high intensity (five of six interventions) than the STS category (four of six).

Our meta-analysis (KQs 1 and 2) showed that trials involving higher-intensity interventions (i.e., home-visiting programs, STS, MDS-HF clinic interventions) reduced all-cause readmissions or mortality. By contrast, trials with lower-intensity interventions (i.e., primarily educational interventions, nurse-led HF clinic interventions) did not.

Intensity Within Intervention Categories

Home-Visiting Programs

Table 16 displays the intensity, delivery personnel, and method of communication for the 11 trials that we rated as either low or medium risk of bias (listed in chronological order). All were multicomponent, relatively complex interventions. We used the number of home visits (one visit or a series of visits) and the inclusion of other components (e.g., predischarge educational session, individualized discharge planning) to determine whether interventions were of medium or high intensity. We classified five as high intensity and six as medium intensity.

Table 16. Intensity, delivery personnel, and method of communication in trials assessing home-visiting programs compared with usual care

Author, Year	Intensity	Delivery Personnel	Method of Communication
Rich et al., 1993[58]	High	Multidisciplinary	Face-to-face
Rich et al., 1995[57]	High	Multidisciplinary	Face-to-face
Stewart et al., 1998[51]	Medium	Multidisciplinary	Face-to-face
Jaarsma et al., 1999[47]	Medium	Nurse	Face-to-face
Stewart et al., 1999[50]	Medium	Nurse	Face-to-face
Pugh et al., 2001[52]	Medium	Nurse	Face-to-face
Kimmelstiel et al., 2004[53]	Medium	Nurse	Face-to-face
Naylor et al., 2004[55]	High	Nurse	Face-to-face
Aldamiz-Echevarría Iraúrgui et al., 2007[56]	High	Multidisciplinary	Face-to-face
Holland et al., 2007[59]	Medium	Pharmacist	Face-to-face
Kwok et al., 2007[54]	High	Nurse	Face-to-face

All-Cause Readmissions

Eight trials reported all-cause readmission rates; among these, we rated five as high intensity[54-58] and three as medium intensity.[47,51,59] Higher-intensity home-visiting programs reduced all-cause readmissions at 30 days; lower-intensity interventions did not (Appendix E). This issue is also discussed in KQ 1. At measurements over 3 to 6 months, our analysis stratified by intensity found no significant difference between high-intensity and medium-intensity approaches (Appendix E). Our ability to draw definitive conclusions about impacts over 3 to 6 months is limited by lack of precision (wide and overlapping CIs); too few trials reported outcomes at the same time point to permit us to assess adequately whether efficacy of home-visiting programs differed by intensity.

Mortality

Eight trials reported mortality, among these, we rated four as high intensity[54-57] and four as medium intensity.[50,51,53,59] Intensity did not differ at any outcome time point (Appendix E). As with all-cause readmissions, however, lack of precision (wide and overlapping CIs) limited our ability to draw any definitive conclusions.

Structured Telephone Support

Table 17 displays the intensity, delivery personnel, and method of communication for 10 STS trials that we rated as low or medium risk of bias (chronological order). Determining whether trials varied sufficiently in the periodicity or frequency of telephone support was difficult. Trials included similar numbers of planned telephone calls at each time point (e.g., weekly for 1 month following hospitalization, then biweekly for 2 months or 3 months). Often, interventions specified that calls could occur more frequently based on need or the availability of a patient hotline for questions or concerning symptoms.

Table 17. Intensity, delivery personnel, and method of communication in trials assessing structured telephone support compared with usual care

Author, Year	Intensity	Delivery Personnel	Method of Communication
Rainville et al., 1999 [71]	Medium	Pharmacist	Telephone; Face-to-face
Riegel et al., 2002[63]	Medium	Nurse	Telephone
Laramee et al., 2003[65]	High	Non-nurse case manager	Telephone; Face-to-face
Tsuyuki et al., 2004[72]	High	Nurse	Telephone
Dunagan et al., 2005[68]	High	Nurse	Telephone
Cabezas et al., 2006[73]	Medium	Pharmacist	Telephone; Face-to-face
Riegel et al., 2006[64]	Medium	Nurse	Telephone
Wakefield et al., 2008[69] Wakefield et al., 2009[75]	Medium	Nurse	Group 1: Telephone Group 2: Videophone
Domingues et al., 2011[67]	Low	Nurse	Telephone
Angermann et al., 2012[66]	High	Nurse	Telephone; Face-to-face

Whether interventions included additional components other than STS also varied across these trials (e.g., intensive inpatient education). When interventions included STS and additional components that required face-to-face contact with patients or time spent coordination of care with a clinician in response to a patient's symptoms, we classified those interventions as high intensity (four trials).[65,66,68,72] We rated one trial as low intensity; it included a series of telephone calls (<8 per person over 3 months) with no other components (e.g., no care coordination or face-to-face contact).[67] The remaining interventions were considered medium intensity.

All-Cause Readmissions

As reported for KQ 1, STS interventions did not decrease all-cause readmission at any time point. Our analysis stratified by intensity found no significant difference between in high-intensity and medium-intensity trials at any point (Appendix E). Confidence intervals were wide and overlapped in all cases.

Mortality

Reductions in mortality rates did not differ between high-intensity and medium-intensity trials at any time point (Appendix E). Confidence intervals were wide and overlapped in all cases.

Telemonitoring

Table 18 displays the intensity, delivery personnel, and method of communication for four trials that we rated low or medium risk of bias. Intensity varied little across these trials; we considered two as high intensity and two as medium intensity. The two high-intensity trials involved components other than remote monitoring alone; one used both video visits and remote monitoring,[80] and one included an individualized weight goal along with direct communication with a clinician when the patient fell outside of his or her normal weight range.[79] Three trials reported all-cause readmissions (number of people readmitted);[78,80,82] three trials reported data on mortality.[78-80] Because of lack of precision and little variation in intensity, meaningful subgroup analyses were not possible.

Table 18. Intensity, delivery personnel, and method of communication in trials assessing telemonitoring compared with usual care

Author, Year	Intensity	Delivery Personnel	Method of Communication
Goldberg et al., 2003[79]	High	Nurse	Remote monitoring
Schwarz et al., 2008[78]	Medium	Nurse	Remote monitoring
Dar et al., 2009[80]	High	Nurse	Remote monitoring
Pekmezaris et al., 2012[82]	Medium	Nurse	Video visits

Outpatient Clinic-Based Interventions

Given heterogeneity among the clinic-based interventions, we pooled data separately in KQ 1 and KQ 2 for MDS-HF clinic interventions, nurse-led HF clinic interventions, and the primary care clinic intervention. These categories directly matched stratification by intensity, delivery personnel, and method of communication. Therefore, we did not conduct new analyses to stratify interventions by these factors.

In terms of intensity, we considered MDS-HF clinic interventions to be high intensity and the nurse-led and primary care interventions medium intensity. We determined intensity primarily on resource use (e.g., planned contact with multiple providers in a specialty clinic during each patient visit). The periodicity or frequency of clinic visits did not vary in any clear ways; most interventions increased clinic visit frequency based on a patient's need (i.e., they were tailored based on clinical status) in addition to planned visits.

All-Cause Readmissions

As described in KQ 1, high-intensity MDS-HF interventions reduced all-cause readmission at 6 months. The medium-intensity nurse-led HF clinic[83] and the primary care clinic intervention[91] did not.

Mortality

As described in KQ 2, both of the high-intensity MDS-HF interventions and one medium-intensity nurse-led HF intervention reduced mortality at 6 months. The primary care clinic based intervention did not.

Primarily Educational Interventions

Table 19 displays the intensity, delivery personnel, and method of communication for the two trials rated as low or medium risk of bias. Two primarily educational interventions reported mortality; we rated one as low intensity[95] and the other as medium intensity.[93] Both assessed inpatient educational interventions; the trial by Nucifora et al. included additional components (e.g., telephone contact following discharge to reinforce education).[93] One trial reported on all-cause readmissions; both reported mortality at 6 months.

Table 19. Intensity, delivery personnel, and method of communication in trials assessing primarily educational interventions compared with usual care

Author, Year	Intensity	Delivery Personnel	Method of Communication
Koelling et al., 2005[95]	Low	Nurse	Face-to-face
Nucifora et al., 2006[93]	Medium	Nurse	Face-to-face

Our meta-analysis of these two trials showed that neither intervention reduced mortality. Lack of precision (wide and overlapping CIs) and different lengths of followup limited our ability to draw definitive conclusions.

KQ 4b. Delivery Personnel

Delivery Personnel Across Intervention Categories

Nurses or MDS teams were the primary personnel for most interventions; pharmacists delivered a few home-visiting and STS interventions. The two categories of interventions that reduced all-cause readmissions (home-visiting; MDS-HF clinic) were more likely to use teams of clinicians to deliver the interventions (e.g., home visits conducted by a nurse and pharmacist together). For mortality, the efficacious intervention categories varied in primary delivery personnel. MDS-HF clinic interventions (delivered by MDS teams) and STS interventions (delivered primarily by nurses or pharmacists) both reduced mortality.

Delivery Personnel Within Intervention Categories

Home-Visiting Programs

Table 16 (above) listed the included 11 home-visiting trials and delivery personnel. When more than one delivery person was involved in a major intervention component, we considered home-visiting interventions to be MDS (e.g., physician accompanies nurse on home visit or adjusts medications before discharge). We considered four interventions to be delivered primarily by MDS teams.[51,56-58] A pharmacist delivered one intervention;[59] primarily nurses delivered the interventions in the remaining trials.

63

All-Cause Readmissions

Seven trials reported all-cause readmission rates. At 30 days, variation was insufficient to determine whether delivery personnel influenced reductions in all-cause readmission. Over 3 to 6 months, our subgroup analyses found no significant difference by delivery personnel (Appendix E). However, lack of precision and disparity in when outcomes were measured limited our ability to draw definitive conclusions.

Mortality

Seven home-visiting trials reported mortality. At 30 days, variation at 30 days was insufficient to determine whether delivery personnel influenced reductions in mortality. Over 3 to 6 months, our subgroup analysis found no significant differences by delivery personnel (Appendix E).

Structured Telephone Support

Table 17 (above) listed the 10 included trials and delivery personnel. Nurses conducted the majority of STS interventions. Pharmacists conducted two interventions,[71,73] and a non-nurse case manager delivered one.[65]

All-Cause Readmissions

Among trials assessing STS interventions, our subgroup analysis found no difference in all-cause readmission by delivery personnel (Appendix E). Delivery personnel did not vary much at each time point; confidence intervals were wide and overlapped. Overall, of 10 trials, two trials found a statistically significant reduction in all-cause readmissions: one intervention was delivered by a nurse[68] and one was delivered by a pharmacist.[73]

Mortality

Mortality rates did not differ by delivery personnel (Appendix E). Delivery personnel varied little at each time point (Appendix E).

Clinic-Based Interventions

The MDS-HF interventions included a range of clinicians who had contact with patients during clinic visits. The nurse-led interventions primarily involved education and symptom monitoring from nurses. The primary-care intervention involved increased access to a primary care clinic, including contact with a primary care physician and clinic nurse.

All-Cause Readmissions

As described in KQ 1, the MDS-HF interventions did reduce all-cause readmissions at 6 months. Neither the nurse-led[83] nor the primary care intervention[91] decreased readmissions.

Mortality

As described in KQ 2, both the MDS-HF interventions and one of the nurse-led interventions reduced mortality at 6 months. The medium-intensity primary care intervention did not reduce mortality.

KQ 4c. Method of Communication

Method of Communication Across Intervention Categories

Across intervention categories, interventions were delivered primarily face-to-face or via technology (telephone, telemonitoring, video visits). Home-visiting programs and MDS-HF interventions, which are delivered primarily face-to-face, reduced all-cause readmissions; for these two categories, method of delivery did not vary within each category. STS also reduced mortality; some of the STS interventions included a face-to-face component (e.g., an educational intervention before discharge). In general, interventions primarily delivered remotely (i.e., telemonitoring, STS) were not efficacious in reducing all-cause readmission rates.

Method of Communication Within Intervention Categories

Only STS interventions varied in their method of communication. Other categories did not differ materially in their primary method of communication. STS interventions were delivered primarily via a series of structured calls to patients. Four STS interventions also had a face-to-face intervention (usually education before discharge).[65,66,71,73] Efficacy for either all-cause readmission or mortality did not differ among trials with a face-to-face component compared with those with primarily the telephone contact (Appendix E); CIs were wide and overlapped. Lack of precision (wide, overlapping CIs) and dissimilar points for measuring outcomes limited our ability to draw definitive conclusions.

One STS intervention directly compared two modes of delivery: standard telephone support and videophone (without telemonitoring technology), along with usual care. All-cause readmission did not differ in the three groups over 3 to 6 months.[69]

KQ 5. Subgroups

This KQ evaluated whether transitional care interventions differed in either benefits or harms for subgroups of patients. For this question, we searched for subgroup analyses reported by individual trials that focused on whether a particular intervention had more (or less) efficacy in reducing readmissions or mortality based on patient age, sex, race, ethnicity, socioeconomic status, disease severity (left ventricular ejection fraction or NYHA classification), or coexisting conditions.

Key Points

- Two trials, one home-visiting program and one primarily educational intervention, reported readmission rates for subgroups of patients
- No trial reported on mortality by subgroups.

Detailed Synthesis

Home-Visiting Programs

Rich and colleagues categorized patients as being at low, moderate, or high risk for readmission.[58] They used a combination of markers of disease severity and coexisting conditions: four or more prior hospitalizations within 5 years of randomization, previous history of HF, hypocholesterolemia (total cholesterol <150 mg/dL), and right bundle-branch block on the admitting electrocardiogram. Patients with none of these factors were considered low risk and excluded from the study; patients with one risk factor were considered moderate risk; those with two or more risk factors were considered to be at high risk for readmission.

Among the moderate-risk subgroup, fewer people receiving home visits were readmitted than people not receiving home visits (27.5 percent versus 47.6 percent; p=0.10). Among the high-risk subgroup, the percentage of patients readmitted over 90 days did not differ between the intervention and control groups (43.5 percent versus 42.9 percent; p-value NS).

Primarily Educational Interventions

One trial assessing a 1-hour, face-to-face inpatient educational session reported the relative risk of a composite endpoint—all-cause readmission or death at 6 months—for patient subgroups based on age, sex, race, or presence of coronary disease.[95] The p-values for relative risks were not significant for each comparison (age $\geq$ 65 versus < 65; sex; black versus white race; presence versus absence of coronary disease).[95]

Discussion

For this report, we conducted a systematic review to evaluate the evidence for transitional care interventions for adults hospitalized for heart failure (HF). Below, we summarize the main findings and strength of evidence (SOE) for the bodies of evidence pertaining to those findings. We then discuss the findings in relation to what is already known, applicability of the findings, implications for decisionmaking, limitations of the review process or evidence base, research gaps, and conclusions.

We classified interventions into six main categories based primarily on the mode and environment of delivery, as defined in the introduction: home-visiting programs; structured telephone support (STS); telemonitoring; various types of outpatient clinic interventions, including multidisciplinary (MDS) HF clinic programs, nurse-led clinic interventions and primary care clinic interventions; primarily educational programs; and "other" efforts that did not fit neatly into any of these categories. Across all these types of interventions, we had 47 trials reported in 53 articles.

Because of the health policy and clinical issues involved in recent policies intended to help reduce excessive hospital readmissions, particularly for Medicare patients, our primary outcomes were focused on 30-day readmission and mortality rates. We also included trials that reported at least one of the following outcomes at any time point before 6 months following an index hospitalization for HF: all-cause readmission, HF-readmission, composite all-cause readmission or death, and mortality. We also examined outcomes relating to health-related quality of life and caregiver or self-care burden.

Our main findings and conclusions are based on randomized controlled trials comparing transitional care interventions with usual care that we rated as low or medium risk of bias. We identified only two trials comparing one type of intervention with another (i.e., making head-to-head comparisons); we rated both as high risk of bias. Thus, direct evidence was insufficient to draw conclusions about comparative effectiveness.

When we graded evidence as insufficient, the evidence was unavailable, did not permit estimation of an effect, or did not permit us to draw a conclusion with at least a low level of confidence. An insufficient grade does not indicate that an intervention has been proven to lack efficacy.

Key Findings and Strength of Evidence

Reducing Readmissions and Mortality

Table 20 summarizes our key findings by intervention category, main outcomes (readmission rates, mortality, or the composite of all-cause readmission or death), and timing of measurement of outcomes (30 days; 3-6 months). It documents our results when data met the following three criteria: (1) sufficient evidence to grade the SOE and to draw a conclusion that evidence either supports benefit [+] or does not [-]; (2) insufficient (I) evidence to make a determination (e.g. only one trial reporting an outcome of interest); or (3) no included trials that reported an outcome (NR).

Table 21 then presents more detailed results, including relative risks (RRs) and 95% confidence intervals (CIs). We also present numbers needed to treat (NNTs, when applicable) for comparisons that included at least one trial reporting an outcome of interest.

Table 20. Summary of key findings and strength of evidence, by intervention category and outcome

Intervention Category	All-Cause Readmissions		HF-specific Readmissions		Composite Endpoint		Mortality	
	30 days	3 to 6 months	30 days	3 to 6 months	30 days	3 to 6 months	30 days	3 to 6 months
Home-visiting programs	+ low[a]	+ high	NR	+ Mod	+ low	+ mod	I	+ mod
Structured telephone support	I	- mod	I	+ High	NR	- low	NR	+ mod
Telemonitoring	I	- mod	NR	- Mod	NR	NR	NR	- low
MDS-HF clinic Interventions	NR	+ high	NR	I	NR	- mod	NR	+ mod
Nurse-led clinic interventions	NR	- low	NR	I	NR	I	NR	- low
Primary care clinic interventions	NR	I	NR	NR	NR	NR	NR	I
Primarily educational interventions	NR	I	NR	I	NR	- low	NR	- low
Other interventions	I	NR	NR	NR	NR	NR	I	NR

Note: low, mod, high and I represent strength of evidence (SOE) grades: mod = moderate, I= insufficient. + indicates that we found benefit (i.e., statistically significant reduction in readmission rate, mortality, or composite compared with usual care), - indicates that we found no benefit (i.e., no statistically significant reduction in the outcome). HR = heart failure; MDS = multidisciplinary; NR = No trials in this category reported on an eligible outcome at this time point.

[a] Two home-visiting programs reported all-cause readmission at 30 days. The intervention studied by Naylor and colleagues was of higher intensity and showed efficacy. The lower-intensity intervention studied by Jaarsma et al. did not show efficacy at 30 days (low SOE). The "+" here refers to high-intensity home-visiting programs.

Table 21. Summary of key findings and strength of evidence for transitional care interventions: Readmission, composite endpoint, and mortality

Intervention Category	Outcome	Outcome Timing	N Trials; N Subjects	Relative Risk (95% CI)[a]	Numbers Needed To Treat	Strength of Evidence
Home-visiting programs	All-cause readmission	30 days	2; 418	High intensity (1 study): 0.34 (0.19 to 0.62) Lower intensity (1 study): 0.89 (0.43 to 1.85)	6 for high intensity NA[b] for lower intensity programs	Low[c] for benefit
	All-cause readmission	3 to 6 months	9; 1,563	0.75 (0.68 to 0.86)	9	High for benefit
	HF-specific readmission	3 to 6 months	1; 282	0.51 (0.31 to 0.82)	7	Moderate[d] for benefit
	Composite endpoint[e]	30 days	1; 239	Hazard ratio (SE): 0.869 (0.033) vs. 0.737 (0.041)	NA	Low[f] for benefit
	Composite endpoint	3 to 6 months	4; 824	Hazard ratio (SE): 0.071 (0.045) vs. 0.558 (0.047) 0.78 (0.65 to 0.94)	10	Moderate[g] for benefit
	Mortality	30 days	1; 239	1.03 (0.15 to 7.16)	NA	Insufficient
	Mortality	3 to 6 months	8; 1693	0.77 (0.60 to 0.997)	33	Moderate for benefit

Table 21. Summary of key findings and strength of evidence for transitional care interventions: Readmission rates and mortality (continued)

Intervention Category	Outcome	Outcome Timing	N Trials; N Subjects	Relative Risk (95% CI)[a]	Numbers Needed To Treat	Strength of Evidence
Structured telephone support	All-cause readmission	30 days	1;134	0.80 (0.38 to 1.65)	NA	Insufficient
	All-cause readmission	3 to 6 months	8; 2166	0.92 (0.77 to 1.10)	NA	Moderate for no benefit
	HF-specific readmission	30 days	1;134	0.63 (0.24 to 1.87)	NA	Insufficient
	HF-specific readmission	3 to 6 months	7; 1790	0.74 (0.61 to 0.90)	14	High for benefit
	Composite endpoint	3 to 6 months	3; 977	0.81 (0.58 to 1.12)	NA	Low for no benefit
	Mortality	3 to 6 months	7; 2011	0.74 (0.56 to 0.97)	27	Moderate for benefit
Telemonitoring	All-cause readmission	30 days	1; 168	1.02 (0.64 to 1.63)	NA	Insufficient
	All-cause readmission	3 to 6 months	3;434	1.11 (0.87 to 1.42)	NA	Moderate[h] for no benefit
	HF-specific readmission	3 to 6 months	1; 182	1.70 (0.82 to 3.51)	NA	Moderate[h] for no benefit
	Mortality	3 to 6 months	3;564	0.93 (0.25 to 3.48)	NA	Low for no benefit
MDS-HF clinic	All-cause readmission	3 to 6 months	2; 336	0.70 (0.55 to 0.89)	8	High for benefit
	HF- specific readmission	3 to 6 months	1;106	0.70 (0.29 to 1.70)	NA	Insufficient
	Composite endpoint	3 to 6 months	2; 306	0.80 (0.43 to 1.01)	NA	Moderate for no benefit
	Mortality	3 to 6 months	3; 536	0.56 (0.34 to 0.92)	18	Moderate for benefit
Nurse-led clinic	All-cause readmission	3 to 6 months	2; 264	0.88 (0.57 to 1.37)	NA	Low for no benefit
	HF-specific readmission	3 to 6 months	1;158	0.95 (0.68 to 1.32)	NA	Insufficient
	Composite endpoint	3 to 6 months	1;106	0.66 (0.43 to 1.01)	NA	Insufficient
	Mortality	3 to 6 months	2; 264	0.59 (0.12 to 3.03)		Low for no benefit
Primary-care clinic Intervention	All-cause readmission	3 to 6 months	1; 443	1.27 (1.05 to 1.54)	NA	Insufficient
	Mortality	3 to 6 months	1; 443	1.52 (0.88 to 2.63)		Insufficient
Primarily educational interventions	All-cause readmission	3 to 6 months	1;200	1.14 (0.84 to 1.54)	NA	Insufficient
	HF-specific readmission	3 to 6 months	1; 223	0.53 (0.31 to 0.90)	NA	Insufficient
	Composite endpoint	3 to 6 months	2; 423	0.92 (0.58 to 1.47)	NA	Low
	Mortality	3 to 6 months	2; 423	1.20 (0.52 to 2.76)	NA	Low
Other (cognitive training)	All-cause readmission	30 days	1;125	1.15 (0.71 to 2.28)	NA	Insufficient
	Mortality	30 days	1;125	0.07 (0.00 to 1.12)	NA	Insufficient

[a] Entries in this column are relative risks (RRs) from our meta-analyses or RR calculations unless otherwise specified. RRs less than 1 favor interventions over controls.

[b] NA entry for numbers needed to treat (NNT) indicates that the relative risk (95% CI) was not statistically significant, so we did not calculate an NNT. NA for hazard ratios indicates that we could not calculate an NNT with the data provided by the investigators.

[c] Two home-visiting programs reported all-cause readmission at 30 days; the higher intensity showed efficacy but the lower intensity intervention did not.

[d] Although only one trial reported total number of people readmitted per group, we considered the findings consistent because one other trial reported on the number of readmissions per group and found a similar effect.[53]

[e] The composite endpoint comprises all-cause readmission or death.

[f] Although only a single trial reported the number of people alive and not readmitted at 30 days and 3 months, we considered the consistency of similar programs reducing 3-month readmissions rates when grading the SOE for this intervention at 30 days.

[g] Although evidence was limited to one trial, consistency for the 30-day outcome was unknown, and evidence was imprecise, we upgraded the SOE because this intervention category has demonstrated no effect on mortality at 3 or 6 months—thus, increasing our confidence in the results of this single trial.

[h] Although only a single trial reported on the number of people readmitted, we considered this finding consistent given that four other telemonitoring trials reported the total number of readmissions per group (rather than the number of people readmitted); all-cause readmissions did not differ between people receiving telemonitoring and those receiving usual care at 30 days, 3 months, or 6 months.

CI = confidence level; MDS-HF, multidisciplinary heart failure clinic; N = number; NA = not applicable; NNT = number needed to treat; RR = relative risk; SE = standard error; SOE = strength of evidence; STS = structured telephone support.

Outcomes at 30 Days

We found very little evidence on whether interventions reduce 30-day readmission rates. Most trials reported rates over 3 to 6 months.

The high-intensity home-visiting trial showed efficacy in reducing 30-day all-cause readmission and the composite endpoint (both low SOE).[55] Despite having only this trial, this intervention and other trials in the home-visiting category also consistently reduced readmission rates measured over 3 to 6 months. Because of those robust findings, we considered high-intensity home-visiting programs to be efficacious in reducing all-cause readmission and the composite outcome at 30 days.

Evidence was insufficient to determine whether several other intervention categories reduced 30-day all-cause readmission rates, because we found no trials or only a single trial (none of which showed efficacy).

Outcomes at 3 to 6 Months

For outcomes measured over 3 to 6 months, we found evidence of efficacy (high SOE) for improving at least one of our primary outcomes for home-visiting programs, STS, and MDS-HF clinic interventions. Specifically, home-visiting programs reduced all-cause readmission rates (high SOE), HF-specific readmission rates (moderate SOE) and the composite outcome (moderate SOE). STS interventions reduced HF-specific readmission rates (high SOE) and mortality (moderate SOE) but not all-cause readmission (moderate SOE for no benefit). MDS-HF clinic interventions reduced all-cause readmission rates (high SOE) and mortality (moderate SOE) but not HF-specific readmission (moderate SOE for no benefit).

For these outcomes, we calculated NNTs when data on a given intervention or outcome permitted (Table 21). For all-cause readmission, NNTs were 9 for home-visiting programs and 8 for MDS-HF clinic interventions. For mortality, NNTs were 33 for home-visiting programs, 27 for STS, and 18 for MDS-HF clinic interventions. An NNT of 9 means, for example, that 9 hospitalized patients with HF would need to receive a home-visiting program following discharge (rather than usual care) to prevent one additional person from being readmitted over 3 to 6 months.

Our meta-analyses did not find telemonitoring, nurse-led clinic interventions, or primarily educational interventions to be efficacious for any primary outcomes. Evidence was insufficient to determine the efficacy of the following interventions in reducing readmission rates or mortality: primary care clinic interventions, peer support interventions, and cognitive training interventions (for people with HF and coexisting mild cognitive impairment).

Some experts have cautioned that inappropriate focus on reduction of readmission rates could negatively affect patient care and perhaps mortality. However, we found no evidence of such an effect. Specifically, no interventions reduced readmission rates but increased mortality.

Utilization Outcomes

Few trials reported on emergency room (ER) visits or hospital days of subsequent readmissions. When these outcomes were reported, few trials reported measures in the same manner or at similar time points. No trial reported the number of acute outpatient (non-ER) visits.

For ER visits, evidence was generally insufficient to determine whether transitional care interventions increased or decreased such visits. The one exception was STS; these interventions had no effect on the rate of ER visits over 6 months (low SOE for no benefit).

Two intervention types significantly reduced the total number of all-cause hospital days (of subsequent readmissions) over 3 to 6 months: STS (moderate SOE) and home-visiting programs (low SOE). Otherwise, evidence was generally insufficient to determine whether other transitional care interventions increased or decreased hospital days of subsequent readmissions.

Quality of Life

Few trials measured quality of life or functional status using the same measures at similar time points. HF-specific quality of life, as measured by the Minnesota Living With Health Failure Questionnaire (MLWHFQ), showed more improvement for home-visiting programs than usual care over 3 months (low SOE). Intervention and control groups did not differ on quality of life (MLWHFQ) for patients receiving STS over 3 and 6 months (low SOE for no benefit). Evidence was insufficient to determine whether other transitional care interventions improved quality of life.

Components of Effective Interventions

No single-component intervention reduced all-cause readmissions. The two categories of interventions that reduced all-cause readmissions and the composite outcome—namely, home-visiting programs and MDS-HF clinic interventions—are multicomponent, complex interventions. As a whole, these two categories of interventions shared the following components:

- HF education emphasizing self-care, recognition of symptoms, and weight monitoring.
- HF pharmacotherapy emphasizing patient education about medications, promotion of adherence to medication regimens, and promotion of evidence-based HF pharmacotherapy before discharge or during followup (or both).
- Face-to-face contact following discharge via home-visiting personnel, MDS-HF clinic personnel (or both). In most cases, this contact occurred within 7 days of discharge.
- Streamlined mechanisms to contact care delivery personal (clinic personnel or visiting nurses or pharmacists) outside of scheduled visits (e.g., patient hotline).
- Mechanisms for postdischarge medication adjustment. In most cases, home-visiting personnel either directly recommended medication adjustment or assisted with coordination of care (e.g., with primary care provider or cardiologist) to facilitate timely medication adjustment based on a patient's needs (rather than advising patients to call for help themselves).

Three categories of interventions reduced mortality rates: home-visiting programs, STS, and MDS-HF clinic interventions. All are multicomponent interventions that include frequent patient contact following an inpatient admission for HF. As a whole, these categories shared the following components:

- HF education emphasizing self-care, recognition of symptoms, and weight monitoring.
- A series of scheduled, structured visits (via telephone or clinic followup) that focused on reinforcing education and monitoring for HF symptoms.
- A mechanism to contact providers easily outside of scheduled visits (e.g., patient hotline).

Separating out individual components from the overall categories (or "bundles") of interventions that showed efficacy was not possible.

Intensity, Delivery Personnel, and Mode of Delivery

In general, intervention categories that included higher-intensity interventions (i.e., home-visiting programs, STS, MDS-HF clinic interventions) reduced all-cause readmission or mortality. By contrast, categories with lower-intensity interventions (i.e., primarily educational interventions, nurse-led HF clinic interventions) did not.

Within most categories, evidence was generally insufficient to draw definitive conclusions about whether higher- or lower-intensity interventions are more or less efficacious in lowering all-cause readmission rates or mortality. The one exception was home-visiting programs; higher-intensity programs reduced all-cause readmission at 30 days but lower-intensity programs did not. Subgroup analyses yielded no significant difference in efficacy based on intensity for STS programs. Subgroup analyses were not possible for other categories of interventions because of either lack of variation or too few trials reporting outcomes at similar time points.

The two categories of interventions that reduced all-cause readmission and mortality (home-visiting programs and MDS-HF clinic interventions) were more likely to include teams of providers delivering the intervention (e.g., home visits that a nurse and pharmacist conducted together) than interventions that did not show efficacy (e.g., telemonitoring, primarily educational interventions). STS interventions, which were done primarily by nurses and pharmacists, did lower mortality but not all-cause readmission. Within categories, evidence was insufficient to draw definitive conclusions about whether specific delivery personnel are more or less efficacious for reducing all-cause readmission or mortality.

Across intervention categories, interventions were done mainly face-to-face or via technology (telephone, telemonitoring, video visits). The two categories of interventions delivered primarily face-to-face reduced all-cause readmission—i.e., home-visiting and MDS-HF clinic interventions. For these two categories, method of delivery did not vary within each category. STS reduced mortality; some of these interventions did include a face-to-face component (e.g., educational intervention before discharge). In general, interventions primarily delivered remotely (i.e., telemonitoring, STS) did not reduce all-cause readmission rates. Only STS interventions varied in the method of communication; our subgroup analyses for reduction in all-cause readmission and mortality found no statistically significant difference by method of communication at any time point.

Findings in Relation to What Is Already Known

The 2009 update of the American Heart Association/American College of Cardiology (AHA/ACC) guidelines addressed postdischarge HF interventions.[25 25] These guidelines focused on the importance of discharge planning, emphasizing written discharge instructions or educational material targeted to the patient or caregiver at discharge. The AHA/ACC guidelines also recommended that "postdischarge systems of care, if available, should be used to facilitate the transition to effective outpatient care for patients hospitalized with heart failure."

The 2010 Heart Failure Society of America guidelines are similar; their guidance emphasizes specific components of discharge planning. The Society does not give any specific guidance on optimal transitional care interventions aimed at preventing early readmissions for patients with HF.

As our results make clear, certain intervention categories (or combinations of components) have better efficacy than others for HF patients. For instance, categories of interventions that were delivered face-to-face (i.e., home-visiting and MDS-HF clinic interventions) reduced all-cause readmission rates, whereas other intervention categories did not. In general, intervention categories that included higher-intensity interventions, with education on self-care delivered over repeated visits through the transition from hospital to home (i.e., home-visiting programs, STS, MDS-HF clinic interventions) reduced all-cause readmission or mortality, whereas categories with lower-intensity intervention (i.e., primarily educational interventions, nurse-led HF clinic interventions) did not. Guidelines that focus on written discharge instructions and early outpatient followup may not provide sufficient guidance on optimal strategies to reduce readmission and mortality.

The interventions in the included trials were heterogeneous and could probably be categorized using a variety of approaches. We classified them in a manner that we believe is both descriptive and informative; other approaches to categorization could lead to different conclusions about the efficacy (or lack of it) for primary or other outcomes.

Other reviews have highlighted the difficulty in classifying trials into distinct categories. For example, we classified one trial by Rainville et al.[71] as STS as did a 2011 Cochrane review,[32] but a 2012 Cochrane review classified the same trial as case management, grouping it with trials that assessed home-visiting programs.[31]

The results of our current review are, in general, consistent with those in previous reviews of this literature. Unlike earlier reviews, however, we focused on shorter-term outcomes (6 months or less), with enrollment during or shortly following an admission for HF). By contrast, some other reviews included outcomes up to 12 months (or longer) following an index hospitalization or did not exclude studies in which patients had had no recent index hospitalization.[31,102,103] For these reasons, our conclusions may differ. For example, a recent meta-analysis and network meta-analysis found no statistically significant effect of remote monitoring interventions on mortality or all-cause readmission up to 1 year, but it combined STS and telemonitoring interventions.[102] At outcome timings over 3 to 6 months, we found that STS was associated with a mortality benefit while telemonitoring interventions were not.

Other reviews have used different categorization strategies (as mentioned above); a 2009 Cochrane review found that "case-management" interventions (home-visiting programs and telephone support) were associated with a reduction in all-cause mortality at 12 months (but not at 6 months) and a reduction in readmissions related to HF at 6 months and 1 year.[31] One recent review of interventions to reduce 30-day readmissions excluded interventions that were disease specific; that is, those authors did not include interventions tailored to HF patients or other chronic diseases.[33] They found that most studies tested multicomponent discharge bundles. Common components of effective interventions included postdischarge telephone calls and patient-centered discharge instructions—e.g., facilitation of patient engagement in the transition of care individually tailored for the patient's health and social circumstances.[33]

Applicability

Most trials included adults with moderate to severe HF. The mean age of subjects was generally in the 70s; very few trials enrolled patients who were, on average, either younger or older. We did not find evidence to confirm or refute whether treatments are more or less efficacious for many other subgroups, including groups defined by sex, racial or ethnic minorities, people with higher severity of HF, type of HF (e.g., diastolic vs. systolic), and patients with certain coexisting conditions. Included trials commonly excluded patients who had end-stage renal disease or severe or unstable cardiovascular disease (e.g., recent myocardial infarction [MI]). Usual-care groups of included trials experienced rates of readmission that are comparable to those found in a Medicare population: the median all-cause readmission rate at 30 days among patients receiving usual care was 19 percent (intraquartile range [IQR] 14 percent to 22 percent); over 3 to 6 months, the rate was 43 percent (IQR 35 percent to 41 percent).

Although all included studies enrolled patients with HF, some degree of population heterogeneity across intervention categories may impact our findings (e.g., variation in HF severity, etiology, or number of comorbidities). The majority of trials included patients with moderate to severe HF based on the NYHA classification; most trials did not report whether patients had a preserved versus reduced ejection fraction. The interventions included are applicable only to patients who are discharged to home. Whether interventions would benefit patients who are discharged to another institution (e.g., assisted living facility) remains unclear.

Few trials used a risk stratification scheme to determine inclusion eligibility. Two trials assessing a home-visiting program (by the same author) specified inclusion or exclusion criteria based on risk of readmission. One of these trials included only patients with one "risk factor" for early readmission[57] (prior history of HF, four or more hospitalizations for any reason in the preceding 5 years, or HF precipitated by either an acute MI or uncontrolled hypertension); the other trial excluded patients deemed "low risk."[58] Neither trial used a validated tool to assess risk.

Two other trials, one assessing a MDS-HF clinic intervention and one assessing an STS intervention, included patients deemed "high risk for readmission" but did not define how they assessed risk.[65,87] One trial testing a primarily educational intervention excluded patients who were judged to have a "noncardiac illness likely to increase 6-month mortality or hospitalization risk."[95] How such inclusion criteria based on risk affect the applicability of results remains unclear. A systematic review of validated readmission risk prediction models found that most perform poorly.[104]

Approximately one-half of the home-visiting programs were conducted in the United States; the others were conducted in Australia, the United Kingdom, and various European countries. One of three trials assessing MDS-HF clinic was conducted in the United States; the other two were conducted in Taiwan and Canada; despite the potential differences in settings and health care systems, results were similar across the three trials.

Across most included trials, the majority of patients were prescribed an angiotensin-converting enzyme inhibitor (ACEI) or angiotensin receptor blocker (ARB) (when information was reported). By contrast, the percentages of patients across trials who were prescribed beta-blockers at discharge varied widely across trials.

Whether "usual care" in trials published during the early 1990s is comparable to current practice is questionable. In general, trials did not report details of usual care; for example, they typically did not specify whether followup was scheduled soon after discharge or whether patients were receiving additional services such as home health care.

The trials we examined were conducted in a mix of inpatient settings. These settings included academic medical centers, Department of Veterans Affairs hospital settings, and community hospitals. Our findings are, therefore, generally applicable to many hospital settings in the United States.

Implications for Clinical and Policy Decisionmaking

Few trials reported readmission rates within 30 days following a HF hospitalization. Data based on Medicare claims suggest that 35.2 percent of 30-day readmissions are for HF; the remainder are for diverse indications (e.g., renal disorders, pneumonia, arrhythmias, and septicemia or shock).[5] Whether certain interventions that reduce readmissions at 3 and 6 months would also be effective in reducing earlier readmissions remains uncertain.

We found moderately strong evidence for interventions that provided relatively frequent in-person monitoring following discharge—specifically, home-visiting programs and MDS-HF clinic interventions. The one trial that showed efficacy for reducing 30-day all-cause readmission provided frequent, in-home monitoring that began within 24 hours of discharge.[55] These findings suggest, in general, the utility of such face-to-face monitoring, whether delivered at home or at an appropriate clinic.

Interventions that did not show efficacy for all-cause readmissions tended to focus more narrowly on HF self-care alone; this finding was true, for instance, for both STS and primarily educational interventions. For reducing all-cause readmissions, focusing on HF self-care training or weight monitoring alone does not appear sufficient.

Current clinical practice in the care of adults with HF after hospitalization varies greatly across the country, by hospital settings, and for other factors. A recent telephone survey of 100 U.S. hospitals found wide variation in education, discharge processes, care transition, and quality-improvement methods for patients hospitalized with HF.[17] As mentioned in the introduction to this review, readmission rates vary by both geographic location and insurance coverage.[6]

Nevertheless, our findings provide some guidance to quality-improvement efforts that try to reduce readmissions for people with HF. Specifically, systems or providers aiming to implement programs to improve transitional care for patients with HF may wish to start with the multicomponent interventions that had meaningful effects on both all-cause readmission and mortality. In this regard, we found moderately strong evidence for home-visiting programs and MDS-HF clinic interventions for reducing all-cause readmission rates; in designing quality-improvement efforts, administrators may do well to give these approaches the greatest consideration.

We did not prespecify a magnitude of effect (i.e., a specific reduction in relative risk) that clinicians or policymakers should consider a meaningful change in readmission rates. The percentage of readmissions that are preventable may differ across settings and patient populations that are not comparable with patients enrolled in the trials we examined. However, as mentioned above, the 30-day readmission rates of included trials are similar to those seen in Medicare populations.

Finally, we did not find direct evidence on whether certain types of interventions increase or decrease caregiver or self-care burden, but these issues are meaningful for patients and their families. Thus, clinicians should consider the inherent demands or expectations that some transitional care interventions may place on caregivers and patients (e.g., burden of transportation). In recommending or selecting a transitional care intervention, administrators may want to weigh the goal of minimizing additional burden that a candidate intervention might pose.

Limitations of the Comparative Effectiveness Review Process

The interventions in the included trials were quite diverse; they probably could be categorized using a variety of classification schemes or conceptual models. As explained previously, we classified them in a manner that we believe is both descriptive and informative; it accords with how numerous experts conceptualize these highly varied programs. Nonetheless, we acknowledge that other approaches to categorization could lead analysts to different conclusions.

Other reviews have highlighted the difficulty in classifying transitional care programs, particularly those aiming at specific kinds of outcomes or targeting specific types of patients, into distinct (mutually exclusive) categories. Using different categorizations for systematic reviews can place similar (or exactly the same) trials into different groupings (as noted above concerning the Rainville et al. trial). The effects of such classification decisions on findings, especially those relying on pooled data from eligible trials, are unpredictable.

We used the term "transitional care" broadly; generally, we were guided by Coleman's definition as "a set of actions designed to ensure the coordination and continuity of health care as patients transfer between different locations or different levels of care within the same location" (p. 30).[24] The included interventions are diverse in terms of whether they aimed to coordinate care at the provider level or focused more on strategies to transfer care back to the patient (e.g., through self-care training for managing HF). We did not include or exclude trials based on any specific set of components; for that reason, included trials assessed diverse interventions. We chose to cast a broad net to be able to examine a comprehensive set of strategies to reduce readmission rates, lower mortality, improve quality of life, or influence other patient-centered outcomes, on the grounds that doing so would be useful to stakeholders in different settings (hospitals, outpatient clinics, or others).

Our inclusion and exclusion criteria specified that included trials had to enroll patients during (or soon after) a hospitalization for HF and also had to measure a readmission rate over 6 months or less. We did not include readmission rates or mortality rates measured beyond 6 months; interventions that we did not find efficacious may or may not be beneficial in long-term disease management in patients with HF. Finally, publication bias and selective reporting are potential limitations. Although we searched for unpublished trials and unpublished outcomes, we did not find direct evidence of either of these biases. Many of the included trials were published before trial registries (e.g., clinicaltrials.gov) became available; had we been able to consult such registries, we would have had greater certainty about the potential for either type of bias.

Limitations of the Evidence Base

The evidence base was inadequate to draw conclusions for some of our questions or subquestions of interest. In particular, as described above, direct evidence was insufficient to permit us to draw any conclusions on comparative effectiveness of transitional care interventions.

In addition, evidence was quite limited for some outcomes (particularly readmissions within 30 days, utilization outcomes, and quality of life). Evidence was similarly insufficient to draw any definitive conclusions about whether any transitional care interventions are more or less efficacious in reducing readmissions or mortality based on patient subgroups defined by age, sex, race, ethnicity, socioeconomic status, disease severity, or coexisting conditions. We found just two eligible trials reporting information on different subgroups.

We identified little evidence on the potential harms of transitional care interventions, such as whether they increase caregiver burden or increase the rate of ER visits. None of the included trials measured caregiver burden, which is relevant given that health care interventions affect not only the health of the individual receiving the intervention but also the health of those close to the patient.

Many trials had methodological limitations introducing some risk of bias. Some trials did not clearly describe methods used for assessing utilization outcomes (e.g., readmissions, ER visits). Methods of handling missing data varied. Some trials did nothing to address missing data (i.e., analyzed only completers), but others conducted true intention-to-treat analyses and used appropriate methods of handling missing data. Some trials were limited in their ability to ascertain readmissions that were beyond a single institution.

Limitations also included inadequate sample sizes and heterogeneity of outcome measures across trials (specifically types of readmission rates). Reporting use of health services other than for the primary outcomes, such as ER visits, was variable across the included trials. This limited our ability to determine the effect of interventions on other measures of health services use (aside from readmission rates), such as an increase in ER visits or observational hospital stays.

Sometimes usual care and certain aspects of treatment interventions were not adequately described. Specifically, descriptions of whether (and how) interventions addressed medication management were often unsatisfactory. Categories of interventions that showed efficacy (e.g., the home-visiting and MDS-HF interventions) often included frequent visits with clinicians. Separating out individual components that are necessary from the overall type of interventions that showed efficacy was not possible. Moreover, some confounding components that were not described may be associated with efficacy as well, such as addressing social needs or optimizing HF pharmacotherapy.

Research Gaps

We identified important gaps in the evidence that future research could address; many are highlighted above. Of note, the gaps we highlight relate only to the key questions that we addressed in this systematic review; our suggestions to address them should not eliminate a wide range of potentially important research that falls outside the specified scope of this review. Table 22 summarizes the gaps and offers examples of potential future research that could help to close them.

Also, we identified several methodological issues that increased the risk of bias for trials, and investigators could improve them in future research. Often trials only inadequately described methods of ascertaining outcomes relating to use of health care (e.g., readmissions, ER visits). Specifically, they did not say whether measurements were based on patient report, chart review, or some combination of measurements. Masking outcome assessments raised other concerns; for example, in some trials personnel delivering the intervention also appeared to be the primary staff for measuring health care utilization. Future trials should consider methods (such as blinded outcome assessments) that guard against measurement bias.

Table 22. Evidence gaps for future research, by Key Question

KQ	Evidence Gap	Potential Future Research and Improved Methods
1	Few trials measured 30-day all-cause readmission outcomes (including those rated as high or unclear risk of bias); we found low SOE for home-visiting programs in reducing all-cause readmissions and the composite outcome (all-cause readmission or death). Evidence was insufficient to determine the efficacy of other intervention categories in reducing 30-day readmission rates.	If 30-day readmission rates remain an important metric for policy, reimbursement, and quality, then future studies should evaluate whether interventions that show efficacy in reducing 3- and 6-month readmission rates (e.g., care in an MDS-HF clinic following discharge) are also effective in reducing 30-day readmission rates. Future trials should ensure that the sample sizes and methods of ascertaining readmission outcomes are adequate to determine the effect of transitional care interventions on 30-day readmission rates. Future research could also include methods such as meta-analysis of individual patient data to ascertain whether other intervention categories reduce 30-day readmission rates.
1,2	Only one trial evaluated one intervention that was based in a primary care clinic; this intervention primarily aimed to increase access. Evidence was insufficient to determine the efficacy of this intervention in reducing readmissions or mortality.	Given that many patients do not have access to specialty care (e.g., in rural settings) or may prefer to receive care following an HF admission in primary care clinics, future studies should evaluate the efficacy of transitional care interventions based in primary care clinics. Such experimental programs could include features such as home visits or a series of clinic-based visits following discharge. In addition, future research could examine the features of patients receiving services in primary care clinics versus those of patients in cardiology-run HF clinics; these variables might include severity of HF or coexisting conditions.
1, 3-4	Key intervention components (content and process) were inconsistently described across trials. Some trials provided great detail, others very little. Researchers who aim to assess whether interventions reduce readmissions for the included time points (30 days to 6 months) do not use a common conceptual framework.	Future research of transitional care interventions could rely on guidance from the AHA statement offering a taxonomy for disease management for investigators to categorize and compare such programs.[105] Alternatively, the AHA or others might amend this taxonomy to include more specific guidance on categorizing transitional-care-type interventions; for instance, incorporating subdomains in the "environment" domain that are more specific to the transition period might be helpful.

Table 22. Evidence gaps for future research, by key question (continued)

KQ	Evidence Gap	Potential Future Research and Improved Methods
1	Evidence was insufficient to determine the comparative effectiveness of transitional care interventions. Nearly all trials examined a particular program against "usual care" of various sorts. No trial tested a single complex intervention with and without a particular component thought to be critical to the intervention.	Future RCTs should address whether certain types of interventions are more efficacious than others. Examples of head-to-head trials include: (1) home-visiting programs that are higher vs. lower intensity or that differ in specific components; and (2) MDS- HF clinic followup compared with home visits that provide similar periodicity of followup and content (e.g., education on self-care and medication reconciliation).
1	Telemonitoring interventions did not reduce readmissions over 6 months; whether this can be attributed to lack of care coordination or other factors remains unclear.	Future RCTs of telemonitoring interventions should include additional components that appear to be necessary for efficacy (based on our results for KQs 1-3). For example, conventional telemonitoring might be combined with one (or more) of three key components: (1) starts immediately after discharge, (2) is combined with initial in-person visits (in the clinic or in the home), and (3) is integrated with the patient's established outpatient care.
2	Evidence was insufficient to determine whether transitional care interventions can reduce 30-day mortality.	Future trials and observational studies should evaluate whether interventions that reduce 30-day readmission rates increase or decrease mortality rates over the same period. There remains a concern about the relationship between reductions in 30-day readmission rates and mortality, especially for vulnerable populations.
2	The literature did not adequately address the effect of interventions on burdens placed on either patients themselves or their caregivers. It also did not adequately examine the effect of interventions on health-related quality of life or physical functioning, beyond measuring changes in disease-specific outcomes (with the MLWHFQ).	Future research should include validated measures of caregiver burden, patient-reported measures of the self-care burden, or both.
2	The literature did not adequately examine the effect of interventions on health-related quality of life or physical functioning, beyond measuring changes in disease-specific outcomes (with the MLWHFQ).	Health-related quality of life (in the form of PROs) is a crucial variable for many patients, families, professional societies, and research groups. Investigators could continue to use an HF-specific--specific instrument (such as the MLWHFQ, the Kansas City Cardiomyopathy Questionnaire or the Chronic Heart Failure Assessment tool). For broader quality-of-life outcomes, researchers should also consider use of reliable and valid PRO instruments; widely administered ones include the Medical Outcomes Study Short Forms and the EURO-QOL.
5	Evidence was insufficient to determine whether certain subgroups of patients benefit from transitional care interventions.	Future research should assess whether readmission rates or other key outcomes differ by sex, racial or ethnic minority status, disease severity, literacy level, income, or socioeconomic status.

AHA = American Heart Association; HF = heart failure; KQ = Key Question; MDS-HF = multidisciplinary heart failure; MLWHFQ = Minnesota Living With Heart Failure Questionnaire; PRO = patient-reported outcome; RCT = randomized controlled trial; SOE = strength of evidence.

Conclusions

Few trials evaluating transitional care interventions for adults with HF reported 30-day readmission rates; one high-intensity home-visiting trial did reduce all-cause readmission and the composite endpoint over 30 days (low SOE). Strong evidence supported findings that three approaches improved at least one of our primary outcomes over 3 to 6 months: home-visiting programs, STS, and MDS-HF clinic interventions. Home-visiting programs reduced all-cause readmission, HF-specific readmission, the composite outcome, and mortality; STS interventions reduced HF-specific readmission and mortality; and MDS-HF clinic interventions reduced all-cause readmission and mortality. Based on current evidence, telemonitoring interventions and primarily educational interventions did not reduce readmission or mortality. Direct evidence was insufficient to conclude whether one type of intervention was better than any other type of intervention. Evidence was generally insufficient to determine whether the efficacy of interventions differed for subgroups of patients. The potential harms of transitional care interventions (e.g., higher caregiver burden) were generally not reported.

References

1. Centers for Medicare & Medicaid Service, Office of Information Services (OIS). Medicare Ranking for All Short-Stay Hospitals by Discharges. Fiscal Year 2005 Versus 2004. 2006 www.cms.hhs.gov/MedicareFeeforSvcParts AB/Downloads/SSDischarges0405.pdf. Accessed December 18, 2012.

2. Jencks SF, Williams MV, Coleman EA. Rehospitalizations among patients in the Medicare fee-for-service program. N Engl J Med. 2009 Apr 2;360(14):1418-28. Epub: 2009/04/03. PMID: 19339721.

3. Bernheim SM, Grady JN, Lin Z, et al. National patterns of risk-standardized mortality and readmission for acute myocardial infarction and heart failure. Update on publicly reported outcomes measures based on the 2010 release. Circ Cardiovasc Qual Outcomes. 2010 Sep;3(5):459-67. Epub: 2010/08/26. PMID: 20736442.

4. Bueno H, Ross JS, Wang Y, et al. Trends in length of stay and short-term outcomes among Medicare patients hospitalized for heart failure, 1993-2006. JAMA. 2010 Jun 2;303(21):2141-7. Epub: 2010/06/03. PMID: 20516414.

5. Dharmarajan K, Hsieh AF, Lin Z, et al. Diagnoses and timing of 30-day readmissions after hospitalization for heart failure, acute myocardial infarction, or pneumonia. JAMA. 2013 Jan 23;309(4):355-63. Epub: 2013/01/24. PMID: 23340637.

6. Allen LA, Tomic KE, Smith DM, et al. Rates and predictors of 30-day readmission among commercially insured and Medicaid-enrolled patients hospitalized with systolic heart failure. Circ Heart Fail. 2012 Nov 1;5(6):672-9. Epub: 2012/10/18. PMID: 23072736.

7. Naylor MD, Aiken LH, Kurtzman ET, et al. The care span: the importance of transitional care in achieving health reform. Health Aff (Millwood). 2011 Apr;30(4):746-54. Epub: 2011/04/08. PMID: 21471497.

8. Stauffer BD, Fullerton C, Fleming N, et al. Effectiveness and cost of a transitional care program for heart failure: a prospective study with concurrent controls. Arch Intern Med. 2011 Jul 25;171(14):1238-43. Epub: 2011/07/27. PMID: 21788541.

9. Centers for Medicare & Medicaid Services. Readmissions Reduction Program. August 2, 2013. www.cms.gov/Medicare/Medicare-Fee-for-Service-Payment/AcuteInpatientPPS/Readmissions-Reduction-Program.html. Accessed September 6, 2013.

10. Roger VL, Go AS, Lloyd-Jones DM, et al. Heart disease and stroke statistics--2012 update: a report from the American Heart Association. Circulation. 2012 Jan 3;125(1):e2-e220. Epub: 2011/12/20. PMID: 22179539.

11. Heidenreich PA, Trogdon JG, Khavjou OA, et al. Forecasting the future of cardiovascular disease in the United States: a policy statement from the American Heart Association. Circulation. 2011 Mar 1;123(8):933-44. Epub: 2011/01/26. PMID: 21262990.

12. Lloyd-Jones DM, Larson MG, Leip EP, et al. Lifetime risk for developing congestive heart failure: the Framingham Heart Study. Circulation. 2002 Dec 10;106(24):3068-72. Epub: 2002/12/11. PMID: 12473553.

13. Kalogeropoulos A, Georgiopoulou V, Kritchevsky SB, et al. Epidemiology of incident heart failure in a contemporary elderly cohort: the health, aging, and body composition study. Arch Intern Med. 2009 Apr 13;169(7):708-15. Epub: 2009/04/15. PMID: 19365001.

14. Roger VL, Weston SA, Redfield MM, et al. Trends in heart failure incidence and survival in a community-based population. JAMA. 2004 Jul 21;292(3):344-50. Epub: 2004/07/22. PMID: 15265849.

15. Levy D, Kenchaiah S, Larson MG, et al. Long-term trends in the incidence of and survival with heart failure. N Engl J Med. 2002 Oct 31;347(18):1397-402. Epub: 2002/11/01. PMID: 12409541.

16. Chen J, Normand SL, Wang Y, et al. National and regional trends in heart failure hospitalization and mortality rates for Medicare beneficiaries, 1998-2008. JAMA. 2011 Oct 19;306(15):1669-78. Epub: 2011/10/20. PMID: 22009099.

17. Kociol RD, Peterson ED, Hammill BG, et al. National survey of hospital strategies to reduce heart failure readmissions: findings from the Get With the Guidelines-Heart Failure registry. Circ Heart Fail. 2012 Nov 1;5(6):680-7. Epub: 2012/08/31. PMID: 22933525.

18. Goldfield NI, McCullough EC, Hughes JS, et al. Identifying potentially preventable readmissions. Health Care Financ Rev. 2008 Fall;30(1):75-91. Epub: 2008/12/02. PMID: 19040175.

19. Medicare Payment Advisory Committee (MedPAC). Report to the Congress: Promoting Greater Efficiency in Medicare. June 2007. www.medpac.gov/documents/Jun07_Entire Report.pdf.

20. Konstam MA. Home monitoring should be the central element in an effective program of heart failure disease management. Circulation. 2012 Feb 14;125(6):820-7. Epub: 2012/02/15. PMID: 22331919.

21. Krumholz HM. Post-hospital syndrome--an acquired, transient condition of generalized risk. N Engl J Med. 2013 Jan 10;368(2):100-2. Epub: 2013/01/11. PMID: 23301730.

22. Krumholz HM, Lin Z, Keenan PS, et al. Relationship between hospital readmission and mortality rates for patients hospitalized with acute myocardial infarction, heart failure, or pneumonia. JAMA. 2013;309(6):587-93. PMID: 23403683.

23. Naylor MD, Kurtzman ET, Grabowski DC, et al. Unintended consequences of steps to cut readmissions and reform payment may threaten care of vulnerable older adults. Health Aff (Millwood). 2012 July 1;31(7):1623-32. PMID: 22722702.

24. Coleman EA, Boult C. Improving the quality of transitional care for persons with complex care needs. J Am Geriatr Soc. 2003 Apr;51(4):556-7. Epub: 2003/03/27. PMID: 12657079.

25. Jessup M, Abraham WT, Casey DE, et al. 2009 focused update: ACCF/AHA Guidelines for the Diagnosis and Management of Heart Failure in Adults: a report of the American College of Cardiology Foundation/American Heart Association Task Force on Practice Guidelines: developed in collaboration with the International Society for Heart and Lung Transplantation. Circulation. 2009 Apr 14;119(14):1977-2016. Epub: 2009/03/28. PMID: 19324967.

26. Agvall B, Alehagen U, Dahlstrom U. The benefits of using a heart failure management programme in Swedish primary healthcare. Eur J Heart Fail. 2013 Feb;15(2):228-36. Epub: 2012/10/31. PMID: 23109650.

27. Lindenfeld J, Albert NM, Boehmer JP, et al. Executive Summary: HFSA 2010 Comprehensive Heart Failure Practice Guideline. J Card Fail. 2010 Jun;16(6):475-539.

28. The Joint Commission. A Comprehensive Review of Development and Testing for National Implementation of Hospital Core Measures. Oak Brook Terrace, IL; 2010 November. www.jointcommission.org/accreditation/acc reditation_main.aspx. Accessed February 14, 2014.

29. Bonow RO, Ganiats TG, Beam CT, et al. ACCF/AHA/AMA-PCPI 2011 performance measures for adults with heart failure: a report of the American College of Cardiology Foundation/American Heart Association Task Force on Performance Measures and the American Medical Association-Physician Consortium for Performance Improvement. Circulation. 2012 May 15;125(19):2382-401. Epub: 2012/04/25. PMID: 22528524.

30. Medicare Payment Advisory Commission. Report to the Congress: promoting greater efficiency in Medicare. Medicare Payment Advisory Commission Washington, DC: 2007. http://unc.summon.serialssolutions.com/link /0/eLvHCXMwTV3LCsJADFwEwYuXgu7 VH9hit_vKtdIiKCJSpdd9Hgti_x_TVcFbcgs kzDB5EEJ2jgebpBUilJ3NgymuAFnICGc81 7mf-2jq80m3jej_0LwryCKOG3Lv2v5wZN9nA Mxy2ANzCYkk1KhGJJpKxhSRnE1SwcRo BaDQcpVwMqnkIdlKei2kBh65cV5bWW3J 2s5L4-OUj8sCJcuEGY50Rl2KEVCyGoDfLgNcP2 7xc8tXvoAqnxNFkM8FwqpSvgEFdjj2.

31. Takeda A, Taylor SJ, Taylor RS, et al. Clinical service organisation for heart failure. Cochrane Database Syst Rev. 2012(9):CD002752. Epub: 2012/09/14. PMID: 22972058.

32. Inglis SC, Clark RA, Cleland JG. Telemonitoring in patients with heart failure. N Engl J Med. 2011 Mar 17;364(11):1078-9. PMID: 21410377.

33. Hansen LO, Young RS, Hinami K, et al. Interventions to reduce 30-day rehospitalization: a systematic review. Ann Intern Med. 2011 Oct 18;155(8):520-8. Epub: 2011/10/19. PMID: 22007045.

34. Lainscak M, Blue L, Clark AL, et al. Self-care management of heart failure: practical recommendations from the Patient Care Committee of the Heart Failure Association of the European Society of Cardiology. Eur J Heart Fail. 2011 Feb;13(2):115-26. Epub: 2010/12/15. PMID: 21148593.

35. Riegel B, Moser DK, Anker SD, et al. State of the science: promoting self-care in persons with heart failure: a scientific statement from the American Heart Association. Circulation. 2009 Sep 22;120(12):1141-63. Epub: 2009/09/02. PMID: 19720935.

36. Raman G, DeVine D, Lau J. Non-pharmacological interventions for post-discharge care in heart failure. Technology assessment report. Prepared by the Tufts-New England Medical Center Evidence-based Practice Center (EPC). Contract No. 290-02-0022 Rockville, MD: Agency for Healthcare Research and Quality; February 29 2008.

37. Viswanathan M, Ansari MT, Berkman ND, et al. Assessing the Risk of Bias of Individual Studies in Systematic Reviews of Health Care Interventions. Agency for Healthcare Research and Quality Methods Guide for Comparative Effectiveness Reviews AHRQ Publication No. 12-EHC047-EF. Rockville, MD: March 2012. www.effectivehealthcare.ahrq.gov.

38. West SL, Gartlehner G, Mansfield AJ, et al. Comparative effectiveness review methods: Clinical heterogeneity. Methods Research Report (Prepared by RTI International-University of North Carolina Evidence-based Practice Center under Contract No. 290-2007-10056-I) AHRQ Publication No. 11-EHC019-EF. Rockville, MD: Agency for Healthcare Research and Quality; September 2010.

39. Sutton AJ, Abrams KR, Jones DR, et al. Methods for Meta-Analysis in Medical Research (Wiley Series in Probability and Statistics - Applied Probability and Statistics Section). London: Wiley; 2000.

40. Cohen J. Statistical Power Analysis for the Behavioral Sciences. 2nd ed., Hillsdale, NJ: Erlbaum; 1988.

41. Higgins JP, Thompson SG. Quantifying heterogeneity in a meta-analysis. Stat Med. 2002 Jun 15;21(11):1539-58. Epub: 2002/07/12. PMID: 12111919.

42. Higgins JP, Thompson SG, Deeks JJ, et al. Measuring inconsistency in meta-analyses. BMJ. 2003 Sep 6;327(7414):557-60. Epub: 2003/09/06. PMID: 12958120.

43. Schünemann HJ, Oxman AD, Vist GE, et al. Chapter 12: Interpreting results and drawing conclusions. In: Higgins JPT, Green ST, eds. Cochrane Handbook for Systematic Reviews of Interventions Version 5.1.0 [updated March 2011]. The Cochrane Collaboration; 2011.

44. Owens DK, Lohr KN, Atkins D, et al. AHRQ series paper 5: grading the strength of a body of evidence when comparing medical interventions--Agency for Healthcare Research and Quality and the Effective Health Care Program. J Clin Epidemiol. 2010 May;63(5):513-23. Epub: 2009/07/15. PMID: 19595577.

45. Atkins D, Chang S, Gartlehner G, et al. Chapter 6: Assessing the Applicability of Studies When Comparing Medical Interventions. AHRQ Publication No. 11-EHC019-EF. Agency for Healthcare Research and Quality; January 11 2011. www.effectivehealthcare.ahrq.gov.

46. Moher D, Liberati A, Tetzlaff J, et al. Preferred reporting items for systematic reviews and meta-analyses: the PRISMA Statement. Open Med. 2009;3(3):21.

47. Jaarsma T, Halfens R, Huijer Abu-Saad H, et al. Effects of education and support on self-care and resource utilization in patients with heart failure. Eur Heart J. 1999 May;20(9):673-82. Epub: 1999/04/20. PMID: 10208788.

48. Sethares KA, Elliott K. The effect of a tailored message intervention on heart failure readmission rates, quality of life, and benefit and barrier beliefs in persons with heart failure. Heart Lung. 2004 Jul-Aug;33(4):249-60. Epub: 2004/07/15. PMID: 15252415.

49. Triller DM, Hamilton RA. Effect of pharmaceutical care services on outcomes for home care patients with heart failure. Am J Health Syst Pharm. 2007 Nov 1;64(21):2244-9. Epub: 2007/10/26. PMID: 17959576.

50. Stewart S, Marley JE, Horowitz JD. Effects of a multidisciplinary, home-based intervention on unplanned readmissions and survival among patients with chronic congestive heart failure: a randomised controlled study. Lancet. 1999 Sep 25;354(9184):1077-83. Epub: 1999/10/06. PMID: 10509499.

51. Stewart S, Pearson S, Horowitz JD. Effects of a home-based intervention among patients with congestive heart failure discharged from acute hospital care. Arch Intern Med. 1998 May 25;158(10):1067-72. Epub: 1998/05/30. PMID: 9605777.

52. Pugh LC, Havens DS, Xie S, et al. Case management for elderly persons with heart failure: the quality of life and cost outcomes. Medsurg Nurs. 2001;10(2):71-8.

53. Kimmelstiel C, Levine D, Perry K, et al. Randomized, controlled evaluation of short- and long-term benefits of heart failure disease management within a diverse provider network: the SPAN-CHF trial. Circulation. 2004 Sep 14;110(11):1450-5. Epub: 2004/08/18. PMID: 15313938.

54. Kwok T, Lee J, Woo J, et al. A randomized controlled trial of a community nurse-supported hospital discharge programme in older patients with chronic heart failure. J Clin Nurs. 2008 Jan;17(1):109-17. Epub: 2007/12/20. PMID: 18088263.

55. Naylor MD, Brooten DA, Campbell RL, et al. Transitional care of older adults hospitalized with heart failure: a randomized, controlled trial. J Am Geriatr Soc. 2004 May;52(5):675-84. Epub: 2004/04/17. PMID: 15086645.

56. Aldamiz-Echevarría Iraúrgui B, Muñiz J, Rodríguez-Fernández JA, et al. [Randomized controlled clinical trial of a home care unit intervention to reduce readmission and death rates in patients discharged from hospital following admission for heart failure]. Rev Esp Cardiol. 2007(9):914-22. PMID: CN-00612373.

57. Rich MW, Beckham V, Wittenberg C, et al. A multidisciplinary intervention to prevent the readmission of elderly patients with congestive heart failure. N Engl J Med. 1995 Nov 2;333(18):1190-5. Epub: 1995/11/02. PMID: 7565975.

58. Rich MW, Vinson JM, Sperry JC, et al. Prevention of readmission in elderly patients with congestive heart failure: results of a prospective, randomized pilot study. J Gen Intern Med. 1993 Nov;8(11):585-90. Epub: 1993/11/01. PMID: 8289096.

59. Holland R, Brooksby I, Lenaghan E, et al. Effectiveness of visits from community pharmacists for patients with heart failure: HeartMed randomised controlled trial. BMJ. 2007 May 26;334(7603):1098. Epub: 2007/04/25. PMID: 17452390.

60. Thompson DR, Roebuck A, Stewart S. Effects of a nurse-led, clinic and home-based intervention on recurrent hospital use in chronic heart failure. Eur J Heart Fail. 2005 Mar 16;7(3):377-84. Epub: 2005/02/19. PMID: 15718178.

61. Benatar D, Bondmass M, Ghitelman J, et al. Outcomes of chronic heart failure. Arch Intern Med. 2003 Feb 10;163(3):347-52. Epub: 2003/02/13. PMID: 12578516.

62. Barth V. A nurse-managed discharge program for congestive heart failure patients: outcomes and costs. Home Health Care Manag Pract. 2001(6):436-43. PMID: CN-00773514.

63. Riegel B, Carlson B, Kopp Z, et al. Effect of a standardized nurse case-management telephone intervention on resource use in patients with chronic heart failure. Arch Intern Med. 2002 Mar 25;162(6):705-12. Epub: 2002/03/26. PMID: 11911726.

64. Riegel B, Carlson B, Glaser D, et al. Randomized controlled trial of telephone case management in Hispanics of Mexican origin with heart failure. J Card Fail. 2006 Apr;12(3):211-9. Epub: 2006/04/21. PMID: 16624687.

65. Laramee AS, Levinsky SK, Sargent J, et al. Case management in a heterogeneous congestive heart failure population: a randomized controlled trial. Arch Intern Med. 2003 Apr 14;163(7):809-17. Epub: 2003/04/16. PMID: 12695272.

66. Angermann CE, Stork S, Gelbrich G, et al. Mode of action and effects of standardized collaborative disease management on mortality and morbidity in patients with systolic heart failure: the Interdisciplinary Network for Heart Failure (INH) study. Circ Heart Fail. 2012 Jan;5(1):25-35. Epub: 2011/10/01. PMID: 21956192.

67. Domingues FB, Clausell N, Aliti GB, et al. Education and telephone monitoring by nurses of patients with heart failure: randomized clinical trial. Arq Bras Cardiol. 2011 Mar;96(3):233-9. Epub: 2011/02/11. PMID: 21308343.

68. Dunagan WC, Littenberg B, Ewald GA, et al. Randomized trial of a nurse-administered, telephone-based disease management program for patients with heart failure. J Card Fail. 2005 Jun;11(5):358-65. Epub: 2005/06/11. PMID: 15948086.

69. Wakefield BJ, Ward MM, Holman JE, et al. Evaluation of home telehealth following hospitalization for heart failure: a randomized trial. Telemed J E Health. 2008 Oct;14(8):753-61. Epub: 2008/10/29. PMID: 18954244.

70. Jerant AF, Azari R, Nesbitt TS. Reducing the cost of frequent hospital admissions for congestive heart failure: a randomized trial of a home telecare intervention. Med Care. 2001 Nov;39(11):1234-45. Epub: 2001/10/19. PMID: 11606877.

71. Rainville EC. Impact of pharmacist interventions on hospital readmissions for heart failure. Am J Health Syst Pharm. 1999 Jul 1;56(13):1339-42. Epub: 2000/02/22. PMID: 10683133.

72. Tsuyuki RT, Fradette M, Johnson JA, et al. A multicenter disease management program for hospitalized patients with heart failure. J Card Fail. 2004 Dec;10(6):473-80. Epub: 2004/12/16. PMID: 15599837.

73. Lopez Cabezas C, Falces Salvador C, Cubi Quadrada D, et al. Randomized clinical trial of a postdischarge pharmaceutical care program vs regular follow-up in patients with heart failure. Farm Hosp. 2006 Nov-Dec;30(6):328-42. Epub: 2007/02/15. PMID: 17298190.

74. Duffy JR, Hoskins LM, Dudley-Brown S. Improving outcomes for older adults with heart failure: a randomized trial using a theory-guided nursing intervention. J Nurs Care Qual. 2010 Jan-Mar;25(1):56-64. Epub: 2009/06/11. PMID: 19512945.

75. Wakefield BJ, Holman JE, Ray A, et al. Outcomes of a home telehealth intervention for patients with heart failure. J Telemed Telecare. 2009;15(1):46-50. Epub: 2009/01/14. PMID: 19139220.

76. Jerant AF, Azari R, Martinez C, et al. A randomized trial of telenursing to reduce hospitalization for heart failure: patient-centered outcomes and nursing indicators. Home Health Care Serv Q. 2003;22(1):1-20. Epub: 2003/05/17. PMID: 12749524.

77. Dendale P, De Keulenaer G, Troisfontaines P, et al. Effect of a telemonitoring-facilitated collaboration between general practitioner and heart failure clinic on mortality and rehospitalization rates in severe heart failure: the TEMA-HF 1 (TElemonitoring in the MAnagement of Heart Failure) study. Eur J Heart Fail. 2012 Mar;14(3):333-40. Epub: 2011/11/03. PMID: 22045925.

78. Schwarz KA, Mion LC, Hudock D, et al. Telemonitoring of heart failure patients and their caregivers: a pilot randomized controlled trial. Prog Cardiovasc Nurs. 2008 Winter;23(1):18-26. Epub: 2008/03/11. PMID: 18326990.

79. Goldberg LR, Piette JD, Walsh MN, et al. Randomized trial of a daily electronic home monitoring system in patients with advanced heart failure: the Weight Monitoring in Heart Failure (WHARF) trial. Am Heart J. 2003 Oct;146(4):705-12. Epub: 2003/10/18. PMID: 14564327.

80. Dar O, Riley J, Chapman C, et al. A randomized trial of home telemonitoring in a typical elderly heart failure population in North West London: results of the Home-HF study. Eur J Heart Fail. 2009(3):319-25. PMID: CN-00681894.

81. Woodend AK, Sherrard H, Fraser M, et al. Telehome monitoring in patients with cardiac disease who are at high risk of readmission. Heart Lung. 2008 Jan-Feb;37(1):36-45. Epub: 2008/01/22. PMID: 18206525.

82. Pekmezaris R, Mitzner I, Pecinka KR, et al. The impact of remote patient monitoring (telehealth) upon Medicare beneficiaries with heart failure. Telemed J E Health. 2012 Mar;18(2):101-8. Epub: 2012/01/31. PMID: 22283360.

83. Ekman I, Andersson B, Ehnfors M, et al. Feasibility of a nurse-monitored, outpatient-care programme for elderly patients with moderate-to-severe, chronic heart failure. Eur Heart J. 1998 Aug;19(8):1254-60. Epub: 1998/09/18. PMID: 9740348.

84. McDonald K, Ledwidge M, Cahill J, et al. Elimination of early rehospitalization in a randomized, controlled trial of multidisciplinary care in a high-risk, elderly heart failure population: the potential contributions of specialist care, clinical stability and optimal angiotensin-converting enzyme inhibitor dose at discharge. Eur J Heart Fail. 2001 Mar;3(2):209-15. Epub: 2001/03/14. PMID: 11246059.

85. McDonald K, Ledwidge M, Cahill J, et al. Heart failure management: multidisciplinary care has intrinsic benefit above the optimization of medical care. J Card Fail. 2002 Jun;8(3):142-8. Epub: 2002/07/26. PMID: 12140806.

86. Ledwidge M, Barry M, Cahill J, et al. Is multidisciplinary care of heart failure cost-beneficial when combined with optimal medical care? Eur J Heart Fail. 2003(3):381-9. PMID: CN-00456908.

87. Kasper EK, Gerstenblith G, Hefter G, et al. A randomized trial of the efficacy of multidisciplinary care in heart failure outpatients at high risk of hospital readmission. J Am Coll Cardiol. 2002 Feb 6;39(3):471-80. Epub: 2002/02/02. PMID: 11823086.

88. Stromberg A, Martensson J, Fridlund B, et al. Nurse-led heart failure clinics improve survival and self-care behaviour in patients with heart failure: results from a prospective, randomised trial. Eur Heart J. 2003 Jun;24(11):1014-23. Epub: 2003/06/06. PMID: 12788301.

89. Ducharme A, Doyon O, White M, et al. Impact of care at a multidisciplinary congestive heart failure clinic: a randomized trial. CMAJ. 2005 Jul 5;173(1):40-5. Epub: 2005/07/06. PMID: 15997043.

90. Liu MH, Wang CH, Huang YY, et al. Edema index-guided disease management improves 6-month outcomes of patients with acute heart failure. Int Heart J. 2012;53(1):11-7. Epub: 2012/03/09. PMID: 22398670.

91.   Oddone EZ, Weinberger M, Giobbie-Hurder A, et al. Enhanced access to primary care for patients with congestive heart failure. Veterans Affairs Cooperative Study Group on Primary Care and Hospital Readmission. Eff Clin Pract. 1999 Sep-Oct;2(5):201-9. Epub: 2000/01/06. PMID: 10623052.

92.   Albert NM, Buchsbaum R, Li J. Randomized study of the effect of video education on heart failure healthcare utilization, symptoms, and self-care behaviors. Patient Educ Couns. 2007 Dec;69(1-3):129-39. Epub: 2007/10/05. PMID: 17913440.

93.   Nucifora G, Albanese MC, De Biaggio P, et al. Lack of improvement of clinical outcomes by a low-cost, hospital-based heart failure management programme. J Cardiovasc Med (Hagerstown). 2006 Aug;7(8):614-22. Epub: 2006/07/22. PMID: 16858241.

94.   Linne AB, Liedholm H. Effects of an interactive CD-program on 6 months readmission rate in patients with heart failure - a randomised, controlled trial [NCT00311194]. BMC Cardiovasc Disord. 2006;6:30. Epub: 2006/06/27. PMID: 16796760.

95.   Koelling TM, Johnson ML, Cody RJ, et al. Discharge education improves clinical outcomes in patients with chronic heart failure. Circulation. 2005 Jan 18;111(2):179-85. Epub: 2005/01/12. PMID: 15642765.

96.   Riegel B, Carlson B. Is individual peer support a promising intervention for persons with heart failure? J Cardiovasc Nurs. 2004 May-Jun;19(3):174-83. Epub: 2004/06/12. PMID: 15191260.

97.   Davis KK, Mintzer M, Dennison Himmelfarb CR, et al. Targeted intervention improves knowledge but not self-care or readmissions in heart failure patients with mild cognitive impairment. Eur J Heart Fail. 2012 Sep;14(9):1041-9. Epub: 2012/06/28. PMID: 22736737.

98.   Nasreddine ZS, Phillips NA, Bedirian V, et al. The Montreal Cognitive Assessment, MoCA: a brief screening tool for mild cognitive impairment. J Am Geriatr Soc. 2005 Apr;53(4):695-9. Epub: 2005/04/09. PMID: 15817019.

99.   Rodriguez-Barrientos R, López-Alcalde J, Rodríguez-Fernández C, et al. Short-course versus long-course therapy of the same antibiotic for community-acquired pneumonia in adolescent and adult outpatients. Cochrane Database of Systematic Reviews. 2011(4)PMID: CD009070.

100.   Hunt SA, Abraham WT, Chin MH, et al. 2009 focused update incorporated into the ACC/AHA 2005 Guidelines for the Diagnosis and Management of Heart Failure in Adults: a report of the American College of Cardiology Foundation/American Heart Association Task Force on Practice Guidelines: developed in collaboration with the International Society for Heart and Lung Transplantation. Circulation. 2009 Apr 14;119(14):e391-479. Epub: 2009/03/28. PMID: 19324966.

101.   Heart Failure Society of America. Executive summary: HFSA 2006 Comprehensive Heart Failure Practice Guideline. J Card Fail. 2006 Feb;12(1):10-38. Epub: 2006/02/28. PMID: 16500578.

102.   Pandor A, Gomersall T, Stevens JW, et al. Remote monitoring after recent hospital discharge in patients with heart failure: a systematic review and network meta-analysis (Provisional abstract). Database of Abstracts of Reviews of Effects. 2013(3):epub. PMID: DARE-12013029243.

103.   Inglis Sally C, Clark Robyn A, McAlister Finlay A, et al. Structured telephone support or telemonitoring programmes for patients with chronic heart failure. Cochrane Database of Systematic Reviews. 2010(8)PMID: CD007228.

104.   Kansagara D, Englander H, Salanitro A, et al. Risk prediction models for hospital readmission: a systematic review. JAMA. 2011 Oct 19;306(15):1688-98. Epub: 2011/10/20. PMID: 22009101.

105.   Krumholz HM, Currie PM, Riegel B, et al. A taxonomy for disease management: a scientific statement from the American Heart Association Disease Management Taxonomy Writing Group. Circulation. 2006 Sep 26;114(13):1432-45. Epub: 2006/09/06. PMID: 16952985.

Abbreviations and Acronyms

Abbreviation or Acronym	Definition
ACEI	Angiotensin-converting enzyme inhibitor
AF	Atrial fibrillation
AHA/ACC	American Heart Association/American College of Cardiology
AHRQ	Agency for Healthcare Research and Quality
AMA	American Medical Association
ARB	Angiotensin II receptor blocker
BB	Beta-blocker
CAD	Coronary artery disease
CD-ROM	Compact Disk Read-Only Memory
CI	Confidence interval
CINAHL	Cumulative Index to Nursing and Allied Health Literature
CMS	Centers for Medicare and Medicaid Services
COPD	Chronic obstructive pulmonary disease
DM	Diabetes mellitus
EF	Ejection fraction
EPC	Evidence-based Practice Center
ER	Emergency room
EuroQoL or EQ-5D	European Quality of Life – 5 Dimensions
HF	Heart failure
HR	Hazard ratio
HV	Home visiting
IHD	Ischemic heart disease
ITT	Intention-to-treat
KQ	Key Question
LVEF	Left ventricular ejection fraction
MCI	Mild cognitive impairment
MDS	Multidisciplinary
MDS-HF	Multidisciplinary heart failure clinic

Med	Medium
MI	Myocardial infarction
MLWHFQ	Minnesota Living With Heart Failure Questionnaire
N	Number (group or sample size)
NA	Not applicable
NNT	Number needed to treat
NR	Not reported
NS	Not significant
NYHA	New York Heart Association functional classification
PICOTS	Populations, Interventions, Comparators, Outcomes, Timing, Settings
PRISMA	Preferred Reporting Items in Systematic Reviews and Meta-Analyses
ProBNP	Probrain natriuretic peptide
QOL	Quality of life
RCT	Randomized controlled trial
RD	Risk difference
RR	Relative risk
ROB	Risk of bias
SD	Standard deviation
SE	Standard error
SF-12	Medical Outcomes Study Short Form (12 items)
SF-36	Medical Outcomes Study Short Form (36 items)
SMD	Standardized mean difference
SOE	Strength of evidence
STS	Structured telephone support
TEP	Technical Expert Panel
TM	Telemonitoring
UC	Usual care
UK	United Kingdom
Unc	Unclear
US	United States
VA	Veterans Affairs

VAMC	Veterans Affairs Medical Center
WMD	Weighted mean difference
6MWT	6 Minute Walk Test

Glossary of Terms

Term or Scale	Definition
Heart failure (HF)	A condition in which the heart muscle cannot pump sufficient blood to oxygenate the body's need for blood and oxygen. The most common hospital discharge diagnosis among the elderly in the US.[1]
Quality of life (QOL)	A multidimensional, broad-ranging concept that can be defined as an individual's perception of their position in life in the context of the culture and value systems in which they live. Factors such as physical health, mental health, and social relationships can affect a person's QOL.[2]
Minnesota Living With Heart Failure Questionnaire (MLWHFQ)	QOL measure for individuals with HF with a range of scores from 0-105, with decreasing scores indicating improvement.
6-Minute Walk Test	Measure of functional status that tests functional exercise capacity in a variety of populations. This is the distance a person can walk within 6 minutes on a flat surface, with a range of 0-400+ meters. Increasing distances indicate improvement, and an improvement of 54 meters is considered clinically significant.[3]
New York Heart Association (NYHA) Classification	Classification system for heart failure disease severity. Patients are classified in one of four categories based on the degree to which they are limited during physical activity by cardiac symptoms (e.g., fatigue, palpitation, dyspnea or anginal pain). Scores range from I-IV, with decreasing scores indicating improvement.
Medical Outcomes Study Short Form Health Survey with 36 items (SF-36)	QOL measure with a range of scores from 0-100, with increasing scores indicating improvement.
Medical Outcomes Study Short Form with 12 items (SF-12)	Shorter version of the SF-36 instrument. Also uses a range of scores from 0-100, with increasing scores indicating improvement.
European Quality of Life- 5 Dimensions (EuroQoL or EQ-5D)	QOL measure with a range of scores from 0-100, with increasing scores indicating improvement.
Risk difference (RD)	An absolute measure of how an intervention or exposure changes the risk or incidence of a dichotomous outcome, or an outcome with two potential values. Calculated as the difference in the incidence or risk of an event in an intervention or exposure group from the incidence or risk of the same event in a control or other intervention group.
Relative Risk (RR)	The ratio of the incidence of a given outcome in an intervention or exposure group compared with the incidence of that same outcome in a control or other intervention group.
Standardized mean difference (SMD)	Used in a meta-analysis when all of the analyzed studies evaluate the same continuous outcome but with different scales. Calculated as the ratio of the difference in mean outcome between groups to the standard deviation of the outcome among patients.[4]
Weighted mean difference (WMD)	Mean difference calculated for continuous data from studies in a meta-analysis in which the results of some studies make a greater contribution to the total than others.[5]

Glossary References

1. American Heart Association. About Heart Failure. http://www.heart.org/HEARTORG/Conditions/HeartFailure/AboutHeartFailure/About-Heart-Failure_UCM_002044_Article.jsp. Accessed on September 23, 2013. Last updated on September 20, 2012.

2. World Health Organization Programme on Mental Health. Measuring quality of life: The World Health Organization quality of life instruments. Geneva, Switzerland: 1997.

3. American College of Rheumatology. Six Minute Walk Test (6MWT). Accessed on September 23, 2013. Last updated on October 2011.

4. Higgins J., Green S. (editors). The standardized mean difference.Cochrane Handbook for Systematic Reviews of Interventions Version 5.1.0 [updated March 2011]: The Cochrane Collaboration; 2011. Available from http://handbook.cochrane.org/chapter_9/9_2_3_2_the_standardized_mean_difference.htm.

5. Higgins J., Green S. (editors). Principles of meta-analysis. Cochrane Handbook for Systematic Reviews of Interventions Version 5.1.0 [updated March 2011]: The Cochrane Collaboration; 2011. Available from http://handbook.cochrane.org/index.htm#front_page.htm.

Appendix A. Literature Search Strategies

Published Literature

4/26/13 PubMed: 1,295 records retrieved.

Search String	Search Terms	Number of Results
#1	Search ("congestive heart failure" OR "heart failure, congestive" OR "heart failure"[mesh])	95,131
#2	Search (Readmission OR rehospitalization OR recurrence[mesh] OR "patient readmission"[mesh])	161,929
#3	Search ("case management"[mesh] OR "rehabilitation"[mesh] OR "continuity of patient care"[mesh] OR "patient discharge"[mesh] OR "patient transfer"[mesh] OR transition* OR postdischarge OR post-discharge OR coordination OR coordinate OR transfer OR post-acute care OR postacute care OR post-hospital* OR posthospital* OR subacute care OR sub-acute care OR discharge OR referral OR continuity OR "critical pathways"[MeSH Terms] OR "critical pathways"[Text Word] OR "critical pathway"[All Fields] OR "critical path"[all fields] OR "critical paths"[all fields] OR "clinical path" [all fields] OR "clinical paths" [all fields] OR "clinical pathway" [all fields] OR "clinical pathways"[all fields] OR "telemedicine"[MeSH Terms] OR telemedicine[Text Word] OR telehealth[all fields] OR eHealth[all fields] OR "Mobile Health"[all fields] OR "Home Care Services, Hospital-Based"[MeSH] OR "Hospital Based Home Cares"[All Fields] OR "Hospital Home Care Services"[All Fields] OR "Hospital-Based Home Care"[All Fields] OR "Hospital Based Home Care"[All Fields] OR "Hospital-Based Home Cares"[All Fields] OR "home nursing"[MeSH] OR "Nonprofessional Home Care"[All Fields] OR "home nursing"[all fields] OR "Non-Professional Home Care"[All Fields] OR "Physical Therapy Modalities"[MeSH] OR "physical therapy"[All Fields] OR "physical therapies"[all fields] OR "Exercise Therapy"[MeSH] OR "exercise therapy"[All Fields])	1,132,712
#4	Search (((randomized[title/abstract] AND controlled[title/abstract] AND trial[title/abstract]) OR (controlled[title/abstract] AND trial[title/abstract]) OR "controlled clinical trial"[publication type] OR "Randomized Controlled Trial"[Publication Type] OR "Single-Blind Method"[MeSH] OR "Double-Blind Method"[MeSH] OR "Random Allocation"[MeSH]))	533,347
#5	Search ("review"[Publication Type] AND "systematic"[tiab]) OR "systematic review"[All Fields] OR ("review literature as topic"[MeSH AND "systematic"[tiab]) OR "meta-analysis"[Publication Type] OR "meta-analysis as topic"[MeSH Terms] OR "meta-analysis"[All Fields]	106,432
#6	Search ("prospective cohort" OR "prospective studies"[MeSH] OR (prospective*[All Fields] AND cohort[All Fields] AND (study[All Fields] OR studies[All Fields])) OR (controlled[title/abstract] AND trial[title/abstract]) OR "controlled clinical trial"[publication type])	520,244
#7	Search (#1 AND (#2 OR #3) AND (#5 OR #4))	1,116
#8	Search (#1 AND (#2 OR #3) AND #6)	1,123
#9	Search ((Autobiography[Publication Type] OR Bibliography[Publication Type] OR Biography[Publication Type] OR Case Reports[Publication Type] OR Classical Article[Publication Type] OR comment[Publication Type] OR Congresses[Publication Type] OR Consensus Development Conference[Publication Type] OR Dictionary[Publication Type] OR Directory[Publication Type] OR Editorial[Publication Type] OR Electronic supplementary materials[Publication Type] OR Festschrift[Publication Type] OR In Vitro[Publication Type] OR Interactive Tutorial[Publication Type] OR Interview[Publication Type] OR Lectures[Publication Type] OR Legal Cases[Publication Type] OR Legislation[Publication Type] OR Letter[Publication Type] OR News[Publication Type] OR Newspaper article[Publication Type] OR Patient Education Handout[Publication Type] OR Personal Narratives[Publication Type] OR Periodical Index[Publication Type] OR Pictorial works[Publication Type] OR Popular works[Publication Type] OR Portraits[Publication Type] OR Scientific Integrity Review[Publication Type] OR Video Audio Media[Publication Type] OR Webcasts[Publication Type]))	3,486,741
#10	Search (#7 NOT #9)	1,094

Search String	Search Terms	Number of Results
#11	Search (#7 NOT #9) Filters: Humans	1,075
#12	Search(#7 NOT #9) Filters: Humans; English	1,009
#13	Search (#7 NOT #9) Filters: Publication date from 2007/07/01; Humans; English	511
#14	Search (#8 NOT #9)	1,109
#15	Search (#8 NOT #9) Filters: Humans	1,100
#16	Search (#8 NOT #9) Filters: Humans; English	1,044
#17	Search (#8 NOT #9) Filters: Publication date from 1990/01/01; Humans; English	1,017
#18	Search (#13 OR #17)	1,295

4/26/13 Cochrane Library: 1,174 records retrieved.

Search String	Search Terms	Number of Results
#1	"congestive heart failure" or "heart failure, congestive"	3,574
#2	MeSH descriptor: [Heart Failure] explode all trees	4,968
#3	#1 or #2	7,003
#4	MeSH descriptor: [Recurrence] explode all trees	11,228
#5	MeSH descriptor: [Patient Readmission] explode all trees	651
#6	readmission or rehospitalization	2,540
#7	#4 or #5 or #6	13,619
#8	MeSH descriptor: [Case Management] explode all trees	569
#9	MeSH descriptor: [Rehabilitation] explode all trees	12,409
#10	MeSH descriptor: [Continuity of Patient Care] explode all trees	448
#11	MeSH descriptor: [Patient Discharge] explode all trees	910
#12	MeSH descriptor: [Patient Transfer] explode all trees	103
#13	MeSH descriptor: [Critical Pathways] explode all trees	223
#14	MeSH descriptor: [Telemedicine] explode all trees	961
#15	MeSH descriptor: [Home Care Services, Hospital-Based] explode all trees	227
#16	MeSH descriptor: [Home Nursing] explode all trees	297
#17	MeSH descriptor: [Physical Therapy Modalities] explode all trees	12,939
#18	MeSH descriptor: [Exercise Therapy] explode all trees	5,562
#19	transition* or postdischarge or "post-discharge" or coordination or coordinate or transfer or "post-acute care" or "postacute care" or post-hospital* or posthospital* or "subacute care" or "sub-acute care" or discharge or referral or continuity or "critical pathways" or "critical pathway" or "critical path" or "critical paths" or "clinical path" or "clinical paths" or "clinical pathway" or "clinical pathways" or telemedicine or telehealth or eHealth or "Mobile Health" or "Hospital Based Home Cares" or "Hospital Home Care Services" or "Hospital-Based Home Care" or "Hospital Based Home Care" or "Hospital-Based Home Cares" or "Nonprofessional Home Care" or "home nursing" or "Non-Professional Home Care" or "physical therapy" or "physical therapies" or "exercise therapy"	42,217
#20	#8 or #9 or #10 or #11 or #12 or #13 or #14 or #15 or #16 or #17 or #18 or #19	53,644
#21	#3 and (#7 or #20)	1,431
#22	#3 and (#7 or #20) in Trials	889
#23	#3 and (#7 or #20) from 1990, in Trials	866
#24	#3 and (#7 or #20) in Cochrane Reviews (Reviews and Protocols) and Other Reviews	375
#25	#3 and (#7 or #20) from 2007, in Cochrane Reviews (Reviews and Protocols) and Other Reviews	308
#26	#23 or #25	1,174

4/26/13 CINAHL: 283 records retrieved.

Search String	Search Terms	Number of Results
S1	(MH "Heart Failure")	16,241
S2	((MH "Recurrence") OR (MH "Readmission"))	19,303
S3	((MH "Case Management") OR (MH "Rehabilitation") OR (MH "Continuity of Patient Care") OR (MH "Patient Discharge") OR (MH "Transfer, Discharge") OR (MH "Critical Path") OR (MH "Telemedicine") OR (MH "Telehealth") OR (MH "Home Health Care") OR (MH "Home Rehabilitation") OR (MH "Home Nursing") OR (MH "Physical Therapy") OR (MH "Therapeutic Exercise"))	82,649
S4	(MH "Randomized Controlled Trials") OR (MH "Nonrandomized Trials") OR (MH "Single-Blind Studies") OR (MH "Double-Blind Studies") OR (MH "Random Assignment")	56,419
S5	((MH "Meta Analysis") OR (MH "Systematic Review"))	23,286
S6	(MH "Prospective Studies") OR (MH "Clinical Trials")	210,981
S7	S1 AND (S2 OR S3) AND (S5 OR S4)	148
S8	S1 AND (S2 OR S3) AND S6	342
S9	Search (S7) Limiters - Human	116
S10	Search(S7) Limiters - Human; Language: English	115
S11	Search (S7) Limiters - Published Date from: 20070701-20130431; Human; Language: English	70
S12	Search (S8) Limiters - Human	257
S13	Search (S8) Limiters - Human; Language: English	254
S14	Search (S8) Limiters - Published Date from: 19900101-20130431; Human; Language: English	254
S15	S11 OR S14	302
S16	(MH "Autobiographies") OR (MH "Biographies") OR (MH "Bibliography and References") OR (MH "Bibliography, Descriptive") OR (MH "Case Studies") OR (MH "Congresses and Conferences") OR (MH "Reference Books") OR (MH "Edit and Review") OR (MH "In Vitro Studies") OR (MH "Interviews") OR (MH "Lecture") OR (MH "Legal Procedure") OR (MH "Legislation") OR (MH "News") OR (MH "Newspapers") OR (MH "Historical Records") OR (MH "Narratives") OR (MH "Life Histories") OR (MH "Videorecording") OR (MH "Audiovisuals") OR (MH "Audiorecording") OR (MH "World Wide Web Applications")	191483
S17	S15 NOT S16	283

10/29/13 PubMed: 146 records retrieved.

Search String	Search Terms	Number of Results
#1	Search ("congestive heart failure" OR "heart failure, congestive" OR "heart failure"[mesh])	97,773
#2	Search (Readmission OR rehospitalization OR recurrence[mesh] OR "patient readmission"[mesh])	165,738
#3	Search ("case management"[mesh] OR "rehabilitation"[mesh] OR "continuity of patient care"[mesh] OR "patient discharge"[mesh] OR "patient transfer"[mesh] OR transition* OR postdischarge OR post-discharge OR coordination OR coordinate OR transfer OR post-acute care OR postacute care OR post-hospital* OR posthospital* OR subacute care OR sub-acute care OR discharge OR referral OR continuity OR "critical pathways"[MeSH Terms] OR "critical pathways"[Text Word] OR "critical pathway"[All Fields] OR "critical path"[all fields] OR "critical paths"[all fields] OR "clinical path" [all fields] OR "clinical paths" [all fields] OR "clinical pathway" [all fields] OR "clinical pathways"[all fields] OR "telemedicine"[MeSH Terms] OR telemedicine[Text Word] OR telehealth[all fields] OR eHealth[all fields] OR "Mobile Health"[all fields] OR "Home Care Services, Hospital-Based"[MeSH] OR "Hospital Based Home Cares"[All Fields] OR "Hospital Home Care Services"[All Fields] OR "Hospital-Based Home Care"[All Fields] OR "Hospital Based Home Care"[All Fields] OR "Hospital-Based Home Cares"[All Fields] OR "home nursing"[MeSH] OR "Nonprofessional Home Care"[All Fields] OR "home nursing"[all fields] OR "Non-Professional Home Care"[All Fields] OR "Physical Therapy Modalities"[MeSH] OR "physical therapy"[All Fields] OR "physical therapies"[all fields] OR "Exercise Therapy"[MeSH] OR "exercise therapy"[All Fields])	1,172,735
#4	Search (((randomized[title/abstract] AND controlled[title/abstract] AND trial[title/abstract]) OR	548,807

Search String	Search Terms	Number of Results
	(controlled[title/abstract] AND trial[title/abstract]) OR "controlled clinical trial"[publication type] OR "Randomized Controlled Trial"[Publication Type] OR "Single-Blind Method"[MeSH] OR "Double-Blind Method"[MeSH] OR "Random Allocation"[MeSH]))	
#5	Search ("review"[Publication Type] AND "systematic"[tiab]) OR "systematic review"[All Fields] OR ("review literature as topic"[MeSH AND "systematic"[tiab]) OR "meta-analysis"[Publication Type] OR "meta-analysis as topic"[MeSH Terms] OR "meta-analysis"[All Fields]	115,368
#6	Search ("prospective cohort" OR "prospective studies"[MeSH] OR (prospective*[All Fields] AND cohort[All Fields] AND (study[All Fields] OR studies[All Fields])) OR (controlled[title/abstract] AND trial[title/abstract]) OR "controlled clinical trial"[publication type])	538,994
#7	Search (#1 AND (#2 OR #3) AND (#5 OR #4))	1,172
#8	Search (#1 AND (#2 OR #3) AND #6)	1,171
#9	Search ((Autobiography[Publication Type] OR Bibliography[Publication Type] OR Biography[Publication Type] OR Case Reports[Publication Type] OR Classical Article[Publication Type] OR comment[Publication Type] OR Congresses[Publication Type] OR Consensus Development Conference[Publication Type] OR Dictionary[Publication Type] OR Directory[Publication Type] OR Editorial[Publication Type] OR Electronic supplementary materials[Publication Type] OR Festschrift[Publication Type] OR In Vitro[Publication Type] OR Interactive Tutorial[Publication Type] OR Interview[Publication Type] OR Lectures[Publication Type] OR Legal Cases[Publication Type] OR Legislation[Publication Type] OR Letter[Publication Type] OR News[Publication Type] OR Newspaper article[Publication Type] OR Patient Education Handout[Publication Type] OR Personal Narratives[Publication Type] OR Periodical Index[Publication Type] OR Pictorial works[Publication Type] OR Popular works[Publication Type] OR Portraits[Publication Type] OR Scientific Integrity Review[Publication Type] OR Video Audio Media[Publication Type] OR Webcasts[Publication Type]))	3,555,938
#10	Search (#7 NOT #9)	1,146
#11	Search (#7 NOT #9) Filters: Humans	1,124
#12	Search(#7 NOT #9) Filters: Humans; English	1,057
#13	Search (#7 NOT #9) Filters: Publication date from 2007/07/01; Humans; English	559
#14	Search (#8 NOT #9)	1,156
#15	Search (#8 NOT #9) Filters: Humans	1,145
#16	Search (#8 NOT #9) Filters: Humans; English	1,088
#17	Search (#8 NOT #9) Filters: Publication date from 1990/01/01; Humans; English	1,061
#18	Search (#13 OR #17)	1,370
#19	Search (#13 OR #17) AND ("2012/04/26"[Date - Entrez] : "3000"[Date - Entrez])	146

10/29/13 Cochrane: 194 records retrieved.

Search Strings	Search Terms	Results
#1	"congestive heart failure" or "heart failure, congestive"	3,664
#2	MeSH descriptor: [Heart Failure] explode all trees	5,118
#3	#1 or #2	7,233
#4	MeSH descriptor: [Recurrence] explode all trees	11,510
#5	MeSH descriptor: [Patient Readmission] explode all trees	696
#6	readmission or rehospitalization	2,638
#7	#4 or #5 or #6	13,992
#8	MeSH descriptor: [Case Management] explode all trees	591
#9	MeSH descriptor: [Rehabilitation] explode all trees	13,023
#10	MeSH descriptor: [Continuity of Patient Care] explode all trees	471
#11	MeSH descriptor: [Patient Discharge] explode all trees	953
#12	MeSH descriptor: [Patient Transfer] explode all trees	109
#13	MeSH descriptor: [Critical Pathways] explode all trees	235
#14	MeSH descriptor: [Telemedicine] explode all trees	1,046

Search Strings	Search Terms	Results
#15	MeSH descriptor: [Home Care Services, Hospital-Based] explode all trees	235
#16	MeSH descriptor: [Home Nursing] explode all trees	300
#17	MeSH descriptor: [Physical Therapy Modalities] explode all trees	13,559
#18	MeSH descriptor: [Exercise Therapy] explode all trees	5,884
#19	transition* or postdischarge or "post-discharge" or coordination or coordinate or transfer or "post-acute care" or "postacute care" or post-hospital* or posthospital* or "subacute care" or "sub-acute care" or discharge or referral or continuity or "critical pathways" or "critical pathway" or "critical path" or "critical paths" or "clinical path" or "clinical paths" or "clinical pathway" or "clinical pathways" or telemedicine or telehealth or eHealth or "Mobile Health" or "Hospital Based Home Cares" or "Hospital Home Care Services" or "Hospital-Based Home Care" or "Hospital Based Home Care" or "Hospital-Based Home Cares" or "Nonprofessional Home Care" or "home nursing" or "Non-Professional Home Care" or "physical therapy" or "physical therapies" or "exercise therapy"	43,725
#20	#8 or #9 or #10 or #11 or #12 or #13 or #14 or #15 or #16 or #17 or #18 or #19	55,669
#21	#3 and (#7 or #20)	1,506
#22	#3 and (#7 or #20) in Trials	915
#23	#3 and (#7 or #20) from 1990, in Trials	892
#24	#3 and (#7 or #20) in Cochrane Reviews (Reviews and Protocols) and Other Reviews	419
#25	#3 and (#7 or #20) from 2007, in Cochrane Reviews (Reviews and Protocols) and Other Reviews	355
#26	#23 or #25	1,247
#27	#23 or #25 from 2012	194

10/29/13 CINAHL: 51 records retrieved.

Search String	Search Terms	Number of Results
S1	(MH "Heart Failure")	16,842
S2	((MH "Recurrence") OR (MH "Readmission"))	20,137
S3	((MH "Case Management") OR (MH "Rehabilitation") OR (MH "Continuity of Patient Care") OR (MH "Patient Discharge") OR (MH "Transfer, Discharge") OR (MH "Critical Path") OR (MH "Telemedicine") OR (MH "Telehealth") OR (MH "Home Health Care") OR (MH "Home Rehabilitation") OR (MH "Home Nursing") OR (MH "Physical Therapy") OR (MH "Therapeutic Exercise"))	85,200
S4	(MH "Randomized Controlled Trials") OR (MH "Nonrandomized Trials") OR (MH "Single-Blind Studies") OR (MH "Double-Blind Studies") OR (MH "Random Assignment")	59,126
S5	((MH "Meta Analysis") OR (MH "Systematic Review"))	25,305
S6	(MH "Prospective Studies") OR (MH "Clinical Trials")	218,211
S7	S1 AND (S2 OR S3) AND (S5 OR S4)	162
S8	S1 AND (S2 OR S3) AND S6	357
S9	Search (S7) Limiters – Human	129
S10	Search(S7) Limiters - Human; Language: English	128
S11	Search (S7) Limiters - Published Date from: 20070701-; Human; Language: English	83

S12	Search (S8) Limiters – Human	271
S13	Search (S8) Limiters - Human; Language: English	268
S14	Search (S8) Limiters - Published Date from: 19900101-; Human; Language: English	268
S15	S11 OR S14	325
S16	(MH "Autobiographies") OR (MH "Biographies") OR (MH "Bibliography and References") OR (MH "Bibliography, Descriptive") OR (MH "Case Studies") OR (MH "Congresses and Conferences") OR (MH "Reference Books") OR (MH "Edit and Review") OR (MH "In Vitro Studies") OR (MH "Interviews") OR (MH "Lecture") OR (MH "Legal Procedure") OR (MH "Legislation") OR (MH "News") OR (MH "Newspapers") OR (MH "Historical Records") OR (MH "Narratives") OR (MH "Life Histories") OR (MH "Videorecording") OR (MH "Audiovisuals") OR (MH "Audiorecording") OR (MH "World Wide Web Applications")	199,321
S17	S15 NOT S16	306
S18	S15 NOT S16 Limiters – Published date from: 20120401-	51

Gray Literature

4/26/13 ClinicalTrials.gov: 455 records retrieved.

Search String	Search Terms	Number of Results
#1	Conditions: "congestive heart failure" OR "heart failure"	2,109
#2	Interventions: Readmission OR rehospitalization OR recurrence OR patient readmission	954
#3	Interventions: case management OR rehabilitation OR discharge OR transition OR post-discharge OR coordination OR transfer OR post-acute care OR post-hospital OR subacute care OR referral OR continuity OR critical path OR clinical path OR telemedicine OR telehealth	11,879
#4	Interventions: eHealth OR Mobile Health OR Hospital Based Home Care OR Nonprofessional Home Care OR home nursing OR physical therapy OR Exercise Therapy	7,650
#5	#1 AND #2	25
#6	#1 AND #3	261
#7	#1 AND #4	235
#8	#5 OR #6 OR #7	455

4/26/13 WHO ICTRP: 70 records retrieved.

Search String	Search Terms	Number of Results
#1	Condition: heart failure	2,162
#2	Intervention: Readmission OR rehospitalization OR recurrence OR "patient readmission"	306
#3	Intervention: "case management" OR "rehabilitation" OR "discharge" OR "transition" OR "post-discharge" OR "coordination" OR "transfer" OR "post-acute care" OR "post-hospital" OR "subacute care" OR "referral" OR "continuity" OR "critical path" OR "clinical path" OR "telemedicine" OR telehealth	88
#4	Interventions: eHealth OR "Mobile Health" OR "Hospital Based Home Care" OR "Nonprofessional Home Care" OR "home nursing" OR "physical therapy" OR "Exercise Therapy"	6,167
#5	#1 AND #2	6
#6	#1 AND #3	6
#7	#1 AND #4	96
#8	#5 OR #6 OR #7	102
#9	(#5 OR #6 OR #7) NOT clinicaltrials.gov	70

2/5/14 ClinicalTrials.gov: 186 records retrieved.

Search String	Search Terms	Number of Results
#1	Conditions: "congestive heart failure" OR "heart failure"	2,309
#2	Interventions: Readmission OR rehospitalization OR recurrence OR patient readmission	1,054
#3	Interventions: case management OR rehabilitation OR discharge OR transition OR post-discharge OR coordination OR transfer OR post-acute care OR post-hospital OR subacute care OR referral OR continuity OR critical path OR clinical path OR telemedicine OR telehealth	13,334
#4	Interventions: eHealth OR Mobile Health OR Hospital Based Home Care OR Nonprofessional Home Care OR home nursing OR physical therapy OR Exercise Therapy	8,667
#5	#1 AND #2	30
#6	#1 AND #3	299
#7	#1 AND #4	268
#8	#5 OR #6 OR #7	514
#9	#5 OR #6 OR #7 AND ("05/21/2013" : MAX) [LAST-RELEASE-DATE]	186

2/5/14 WHO ICTRP: 7 records retrieved.

Search String	Search Terms	Number of Results
#1	Condition: heart failure	2,408
#2	Intervention: Readmission OR rehospitalization OR recurrence OR "patient readmission"	265
#3	Intervention: "case management" OR "rehabilitation" OR "discharge" OR "transition" OR "post-discharge" OR "coordination" OR "transfer" OR "post-acute care" OR "post-hospital" OR "subacute care" OR "referral" OR "continuity" OR "critical path" OR "clinical path" OR "telemedicine" OR telehealth	2,627
#4	Intervention: eHealth OR "Mobile Health" OR "Hospital Based Home Care" OR "Nonprofessional Home Care" OR "home nursing" OR "physical therapy" OR "Exercise Therapy"	360
#5	#1 AND #2	3
#6	#1 AND #3	60
#7	#1 AND #4	3
#8	#5 OR #6 OR #7	64
#9	#5 OR #6 OR #7 AND Date of Registration from 21/05/2013	14
#10	(#9) NOT clinicaltrials.gov	7

Appendix B. Studies Excluded After Full-Text Level Review

Reasons for exclusion signify only the usefulness of the articles for this study and are not intended as criticisms of the articles.

Exclusion codes:
X1   Ineligible publication type
X2   Ineligible population
X3   Ineligible or no intervention
X4   Ineligible comparator
X5   Ineligible outcomes
X6   Ineligible timing
X8   Ineligible study design

1. . CHF education saved this hospital $173,000. RN. 1998 Nov;61(11):24C-F, H. PMID: 10205572. Exclusion Code: X1.

2. . Solid outcomes show e-health and chronically ill senior populations are compatible. Dis Manag Advis. 2001 Jul;7(7):103-6, 97. PMID: 11496438. Exclusion Code: X1.

3. . Telehealth helps hospital cut readmissions by 75%. Healthcare Benchmarks Qual Improv. 2007 Aug;14(8):92-4. PMID: 17715882. Exclusion Code: X1.

4. . Development and implementation of a standard congestive heart failure education guide and evaluation of the impact on medical therapy, hospital readmission rates and patient outcomes. J Cardiovasc Nurs. 2012;27(5):376-7. PMID: 2011720618. Language: English. Entry Date: 20121102. Publication Type: journal article. Exclusion Code: X8.

5. Agren S, Evangelista LS, Hjelm C, et al. Dyads affected by chronic heart failure: a randomized study evaluating effects of education and psychosocial support to patients with heart failure and their partners. J Card Fail. 2012 May;18(5):359-66. PMID: 22555264. Exclusion Code: X2.

6. Aguado O, Morcillo C, Delas J, et al. Long-term implications of a single home-based educational intervention in patients with heart failure. Heart Lung. 2010 Nov-Dec;39(6 Suppl):S14-22. PMID: 20598745. Exclusion Code: X6.

7. Agvall B, Alehagen U, Dahlstrom U. The benefits of using a heart failure management programme in Swedish primary healthcare. Eur J Heart Fail. 2013 Feb;15(2):228-36. PMID: 23109650. Exclusion Code: X2.

8. Aimonino N, Tibaldi V, Barale S, et al. Depressive symptoms and quality of life in elderly patients with exacerbation of chronic obstructive pulmonary disease or cardiac heart failure: preliminary data of a randomized controlled trial. Arch Gerontol Geriatr. 2007;44 Suppl 1:7-12. PMID: 17317428. Exclusion Code: X3.

9. Albanese MC, Bulfoni A, Rossi P, et al. [The SCOOP II trial in heart failure]. Italian heart journal. Supplement : official journal of the Italian Federation of Cardiology. 2001(4):390-5. PMID: CN-00699305. Exclusion Code: X1.

10. Albert NM, Nutter B, Forney J, et al. A randomized controlled pilot study of outcomes of strict allowance of fluid therapy in hyponatremic heart failure (SALT-HF). J Card Fail. 2013 Jan;19(1):1-9. PMID: 23273588. Exclusion Code: X3.

11. Aliti GB, Rabelo ER, Clausell N, et al. Aggressive fluid and sodium restriction in acute decompensated heart failure: a randomized clinical trial. JAMA Intern Med. 2013 Jun 24;173(12):1058-64. PMID: 23689381. Exclusion Code: X3.

12. Anderson C, Deepak BV, Amoateng-Adjepong Y, et al. Benefits of comprehensive inpatient education and discharge planning combined with outpatient support in elderly patients with congestive heart failure. Congest Heart Fail. 2005;11(6):315-21. Exclusion Code: X8.

13. Andryukhin A, Frolova E, Vaes B, et al. The impact of a nurse-led care programme on events and physical and psychosocial parameters in patients with heart failure with preserved ejection fraction: a randomized clinical trial in primary care in Russia. Eur J Gen Pract. 2010 Dec;16(4):205-14. PMID: 21073267. Exclusion Code: X2.

14. Anguita M, Esteban F, Castillo JC, et al. [Usefulness of brain natriuretic peptide levels, as compared with usual clinical control, for the treatment monitoring of patients with heart failure]. Med Clin (Barc). 2010(10):435-40. PMID: CN-00770147. Exclusion Code: X1.

15. Antonicelli R, Mazzanti I, Abbatecola AM, et al. Impact of home patient telemonitoring on use of beta-blockers in congestive heart failure. Drugs Aging. 2010 Oct 1;27(10):801-5. PMID: 20883060. Exclusion Code: X6.

16. Antonicelli R, Testarmata P, Spazzafumo L, et al. Impact of telemonitoring at home on the management of elderly patients with congestive heart failure. J Telemed Telecare. 2008;14(6):300-5. PMID: 18776075. Exclusion Code: X6.

17. Artinian NT, Harden JK, Kronenberg MW, et al. Pilot study of a Web-based compliance monitoring device for patients with congestive heart failure. Heart Lung. 2003 Jul-Aug;32(4):226-33. PMID: 12891162. Exclusion Code: X2.

18. Atienza F, Anguita M, Martinez-Alzamora N, et al. Multicenter randomized trial of a comprehensive hospital discharge and outpatient heart failure management program. Eur J Heart Fail. 2004 Aug;6(5):643-52. PMID: 15302014. Exclusion Code: X6.

19. Austin J, Williams R, Ross L, et al. Randomised controlled trial of cardiac rehabilitation in elderly patients with heart failure. Eur J Heart Fail. 2005 Mar 16;7(3):411-7. PMID: 15718182. Exclusion Code: X2.

20. Azad N, Molnar F, Byszewski A. Lessons learned from a multidisciplinary heart failure clinic for older women: a randomised controlled trial. Age Ageing. 2008 May;37(3):282-7. PMID: 18285347. Exclusion Code: X2.

21. Azad NA, Molnar FJ, Byszewski AM. Multidisciplinary congestive heart failure clinic for older women: a randomized, controlled trial. J Am Geriatr Soc. 2006(5):874-5. PMID: CN-00556312. Exclusion Code: X2.

22. Azevedo A, Pimenta J, Dias P, et al. Effect of a heart failure clinic on survival and hospital readmission in patients discharged from acute hospital care. Eur J Heart Fail. 2002 Jun;4(3):353-9. PMID: 12034162. Exclusion Code: X8.

23. Bakan G, Akyol AD. Theory-guided interventions for adaptation to heart failure. J Adv Nurs. 2008 Mar;61(6):596-608. PMID: 18302601. Exclusion Code: X2.

24. Baker DW, Dewalt DA, Schillinger D, et al. The effect of progressive, reinforcing telephone education and counseling versus brief educational intervention on knowledge, self-care behaviors and heart failure symptoms. J Card Fail. 2011 Oct;17(10):789-96. PMID: 21962415. Exclusion Code: X2.

25. Balk AH, Davidse W, Dommelen P, et al. Tele-guidance of chronic heart failure patients enhances knowledge about the disease. A multi-centre, randomised controlled study. Eur J Heart Fail. 2008 Nov;10(11):1136-42. PMID: 18790668. Exclusion Code: X2.

26. Barnason S, Zimmerman L, Nieveen J, et al. Impact of a home communication intervention for coronary artery bypass graft patients with ischemic heart failure on self-efficacy, coronary disease risk factor modification, and functioning. Heart Lung. 2003 May-Jun;32(3):147-58. PMID: 12827099. Exclusion Code: X5.

27. Barnason S, Zimmerman L, Young L. An integrative review of interventions promoting self-care of patients with heart failure (Structured abstract). J Clin Nurs. 2012(3/4):448-75. PMID: DARE-12012005438. Exclusion Code: X5.

28. Basford JR, Oh JK, Allison TG, et al. Safety, acceptance, and physiologic effects of sauna bathing in people with chronic heart failure: a pilot report. Arch Phys Med Rehabil. 2009 Jan;90(1):173-7. PMID: 19154844. Exclusion Code: X2.

29. Belardinelli R, Capestro F, Misiani A, et al. Moderate exercise training improves functional capacity, quality of life, and endothelium-dependent vasodilation in chronic heart failure patients with implantable cardioverter defibrillators and cardiac resynchronization therapy. Eur J Cardiovasc Prev Rehabil. 2006 Oct;13(5):818-25. PMID: 17001224. Exclusion Code: X2.

30. Berger R, Moertl D, Peter S, et al. N-terminal pro-B-type natriuretic peptide-guided, intensive patient management in addition to multidisciplinary care in chronic heart failure a 3-arm, prospective, randomized pilot study. J Am Coll Cardiol. 2010 Feb 16;55(7):645-53. PMID: 20170790. Exclusion Code: X6.

31. Bernardi L. Modifying breathing patterns in chronic heart failure. Eur Heart J. 1999(2):83-4. PMID: CN-00161282. Exclusion Code: X1.

32. Blue L, Lang E, McMurray JJ, et al. Randomised controlled trial of specialist nurse intervention in heart failure. BMJ. 2001 Sep 29;323(7315):715-8. PMID: 11576977. Exclusion Code: X6.

33. Blue L, Lang E, McMurray JJV, et al. Randomized controlled trial of specialist nurse intervention in heart failure. BMJ: British Medical Journal (International Edition). 2001;323(7315):715-8. PMID: 2002021276. Language: English. Entry Date: 20020201. Revision Date: 20121228. Publication Type: journal article. Exclusion Code: X6.

34. Bocalini DS, dos Santos L, Serra AJ. Physical exercise improves the functional capacity and quality of life in patients with heart failure. Clinics (Sao Paulo). 2008 Aug;63(4):437-42. PMID: 18719752. Exclusion Code: X3.

35. Bocchi EA, Cruz F, Guimaraes G, et al. Long-term prospective, randomized, controlled study using repetitive education at six-month intervals and monitoring for adherence in heart failure outpatients: the REMADHE trial. Circ Heart Fail. 2008 Jul;1(2):115-24. PMID: 19808281. Exclusion Code: X2.

36. Bondmass M, Bolger N, Castro G, et al. The effect of physiological home monitoring and telemanagement on chronic heart failure outcomes. Int J Asthm, Allerg, Immunolog [online]. 1999;3(2). Exclusion Code: X8.

37. Boren SA, Wakefield BJ, Gunlock TL, et al. Heart failure self-management education: a systematic review of the evidence (Structured abstract). International Journal of Evidence-Based Healthcare. 2009(3):159-68. PMID: DARE-12009108816. Exclusion Code: X8 (SR).

38. Bouvy ML, Heerdink ER, Urquhart J, et al. Effect of a pharmacist-led intervention on diuretic compliance in heart failure patients: a randomized controlled study. J Card Fail. 2003(5):404-11. PMID: CN-00471819. Exclusion Code: X2.

39. Bowles KH, Holland DE, Horowitz DA. A comparison of in-person home care, home care with telephone contact and home care with telemonitoring for disease management. J Telemed Telecare. 2009;15(7):344-50. PMID: 19815903. Exclusion Code: X2.

40. Boyde M, Turner C, Thompson DR, et al. Educational interventions for patients with heart failure: a systematic review of randomized controlled trials. J Cardiovasc Nurs. 2011 Jul-Aug;26(4):E27-35. PMID: 21076308. Exclusion Code: X8 (SR).

41. Boyne JJ, Vrijhoef HJ, Crijns HJ, et al. Tailored telemonitoring in patients with heart failure: results of a multicentre randomized controlled trial. Eur J Heart Fail. 2012 Jul;14(7):791-801. PMID: 22588319. Exclusion Code: X2.

42. Brodie DA, Inoue A, Shaw DG. Motivational interviewing to change quality of life for people with chronic heart failure: a randomised controlled trial. Int J Nurs Stud. 2008 Apr;45(4):489-500. PMID: 17258218. Exclusion Code: X5.

43. Brotons C, Falces C, Alegre J, et al. Randomized clinical trial of the effectiveness of a home-based intervention in patients with heart failure: the IC-DOM study. Rev Esp Cardiol. 2009 Apr;62(4):400-8. PMID: 19401125. Exclusion Code: X6.

44. Brumley R, Enguidanos S. Findings from a multisite in-home palliative care study. J Palliat Care. 2006;22(3):199-. PMID: 2009325546. Language: English. Entry Date: 20070119. Revision Date: 20101231. Publication Type: journal article. Exclusion Code: X3.

45. Byszewski A, Azad N, Molnar FJ, et al. Clinical pathways: adherence issues in complex older female patients with heart failure (HF). Arch Gerontol Geriatr. 2010 Mar-Apr;50(2):165-70. PMID: 19406488. Exclusion Code: X5.

46. Caldwell MA, Peters KJ, Dracup KA. A simplified education program improves knowledge, self-care behavior, and disease severity in heart failure patients in rural settings. Am Heart J. 2005 Nov;150(5):983. PMID: 16290977. Exclusion Code: X2.

47. Capomolla S, Febo O, Ceresa M, et al. Cost/utility ratio in chronic heart failure: comparison between heart failure management program delivered by day-hospital and usual care. J Am Coll Cardiol. 2002 Oct 2;40(7):1259-66. PMID: 12383573. Exclusion Code: X6.

48. Capomolla S, Pinna G, La Rovere MT, et al. Heart failure case disease management program: a pilot study of home telemonitoring versus usual care. European Heart Journal Supplements. 2004 November 1, 2004;6(suppl F):F91-F8. Exclusion Code: X6.

49. Cartwright M, Hirani SP, Rixon L, et al. Effect of telehealth on quality of life and psychological outcomes over 12 months (Whole Systems Demonstrator telehealth questionnaire study): nested study of patient reported outcomes in a pragmatic, cluster randomised controlled trial. BMJ. 2013;346:f653. PMID: 23444424. Exclusion Code: X2.

50. Chan C, Tang D, Jones A. Clinical outcomes of a cardiac rehabilitation and maintenance program for Chinese patients with congestive heart failure. Disabil Rehabil. 2008;30(17):1245-53. PMID: 2010057566. Language: English. Entry Date: 20090116. Revision Date: 20101231. Publication Type: journal article. Exclusion Code: X8.

51. Chang BH, Hendricks AM, Slawsky MT, et al. Patient recruitment to a randomized clinical trial of behavioral therapy for chronic heart failure. BMC Med Res Methodol. 2004 Apr 17;4:8. PMID: 15090073. Exclusion Code: X2.

52. Chang BH, Jones D, Hendricks A, et al. Relaxation response for Veterans Affairs patients with congestive heart failure: results from a qualitative study within a clinical trial. Preventive cardiology. 2004(2):64-70. PMID: CN-00468815. Exclusion Code: X8.

53. Chaudhry SI, Barton B, Mattera J, et al. Randomized trial of Telemonitoring to Improve Heart Failure Outcomes (Tele-HF): study design. J Card Fail. 2007 Nov;13(9):709-14. PMID: 17996818. Exclusion Code: X2.

54. Chaudhry SI, Mattera JA, Curtis JP, et al. Telemonitoring in patients with heart failure. N Engl J Med. 2010 Dec 9;363(24):2301-9. PMID: 21080835. Exclusion Code: X2.

55. Chaudhry SI, Phillips CO, Stewart SS, et al. Telemonitoring for patients with chronic heart failure: a systematic review (Provisional abstract). J Card Fail. 2007(1):56-62. PMID: DARE-12007001099. Exclusion Code: X8 (SR).

56. Chen YH, Ho YL, Huang HC, et al. Assessment of the clinical outcomes and cost-effectiveness of the management of systolic heart failure in Chinese patients using a home-based intervention. J Int Med Res. 2010 Jan-Feb;38(1):242-52. PMID: 20233536. Exclusion Code: X8.

57. Chetney R. The Cardiac Connection program: home care that doesn't miss a beat. Home Healthc Nurse. 2003;21(10):680-6. Exclusion Code: X2.

58. Chien CL, Lee CM, Wu YW, et al. Home-based exercise increases exercise capacity but not quality of life in people with chronic heart failure: a systematic review. Aust J Physiother. 2008;54(2):87-93. PMID: 18491999. Exclusion Code: X2.

59. Clark RA, Inglis SC, McAlister FA, et al. Telemonitoring or structured telephone support programmes for patients with chronic heart failure: systematic review and meta-analysis. BMJ. 2007 May 5;334(7600):942. PMID: 17426062. Exclusion Code: X8 (SR).

60. Cleland JG, Louis AA, Rigby AS, et al. Noninvasive home telemonitoring for patients with heart failure at high risk of recurrent admission and death: the Trans-European Network-Home-Care Management System (TEN-HMS) study. J Am Coll Cardiol. 2005 May 17;45(10):1654-64. PMID: 15893183. Exclusion Code: X2.

61. Coleman EA, Boult C. Improving the quality of transitional care for persons with complex care needs. J Am Geriatr Soc. 2003 Apr;51(4):556-7. PMID: 12657079. Exclusion Code: X1.

62. Copeland LA, Berg GD, Johnson DM, et al. An intervention for VA patients with congestive heart failure. Am J Manag Care. 2010 Mar;16(3):158-65. PMID: 20225911. Exclusion Code: X2.

63. Cordisco ME, Benjaminovitz A, Hammond K, et al. Use of telemonitoring to decrease the rate of hospitalization in patients with severe congestive heart failure. Am J Cardiol. 1999 Oct 1;84(7):860-2, A8. PMID: 10513789. Exclusion Code: X2.

64. Cutrona SL, Choudhry NK, Fischer MA, et al. Modes of delivery for interventions to improve cardiovascular medication adherence (Structured abstract). Am J Manag Care. 2010(12):929-42. PMID: DARE-12011000969. Exclusion Code: X2.

65. Dall'Ago P, Chiappa GR, Guths H, et al. Inspiratory muscle training in patients with heart failure and inspiratory muscle weakness: a randomized trial. J Am Coll Cardiol. 2006(4):757-63. PMID: CN-00555241. Exclusion Code: X2.

66. Dansky K, Vasey J. Managing heart failure patients after formal homecare. Telemed J E Health. 2009 Dec;15(10):983-91. PMID: 19929234. Exclusion Code: X2.

67. Dansky KH, Vasey J, Bowles K. Use of telehealth by older adults to manage heart failure. Res Gerontol Nurs. 2008 Jan;1(1):25-32. PMID: 20078015. Exclusion Code: X2.

68. Dansky KH, Vasey J, Bowles K. Impact of telehealth on clinical outcomes in patients with heart failure. Clin Nurs Res. 2008 Aug;17(3):182-99. PMID: 18617707. Exclusion Code: X2.

69. Davidson PM, Cockburn J, Newton PJ, et al. Can a heart failure-specific cardiac rehabilitation program decrease hospitalizations and improve outcomes in high-risk patients? Eur J Cardiovasc Prev Rehabil. 2010 Aug;17(4):393-402. PMID: 20498608. Exclusion Code: X5.

70. Davies P, Taylor F, Beswick A, et al. Promoting patient uptake and adherence in cardiac rehabilitation. Cochrane Database of Systematic Reviews. 2010(7)PMID: CD007131. Exclusion Code: X3.

71. de la Porte PW, Lok DJ, van Veldhuisen DJ, et al. Added value of a physician-and-nurse-directed heart failure clinic: results from the Deventer-Alkmaar heart failure study. Heart. 2007 Jul;93(7):819-25. PMID: 17065182. Exclusion Code: X2.

72. de Lusignan S, Wells S, Johnson P, et al. Compliance and effectiveness of 1 year's home telemonitoring. The report of a pilot study of patients with chronic heart failure. Eur J Heart Fail. 2001 Dec;3(6):723-30. PMID: 11738225. Exclusion Code: X2.

73. DeBusk RF, Miller NH, Parker KM, et al. Care management for low-risk patients with heart failure: a randomized, controlled trial. Ann Intern Med. 2004 Oct 19;141(8):606-13. PMID: 15492340. Exclusion Code: X6.

74. Del Sindaco D, Pulignano G, Minardi G, et al. Two-year outcome of a prospective, controlled study of a disease management programme for elderly patients with heart failure. J Cardiovasc Med (Hagerstown). 2007 May;8(5):324-9. PMID: 17443097. Exclusion Code: X6.

75. Delagardelle C, Feiereisen P, Vaillant M, et al. Reverse remodelling through exercise training is more pronounced in non-ischemic heart failure. Clin Res Cardiol. 2008 Dec;97(12):865-71. PMID: 18696023. Exclusion Code: X2.

76. Delaney C, Apostolidis B. Pilot testing of a multicomponent home care intervention for older adults with heart failure: an academic clinical partnership. J Cardiovasc Nurs. 2010 Sep-Oct;25(5):E27-40. PMID: 20671564. Exclusion Code: X8.

77. Delaney C, Apostolidis B, Bartos S, et al. A Randomized Trial of Telemonitoring and Self-Care Education in Heart Failure Patients Following Home Care Discharge. Home Health Care Management & Practice. 2013;25(5):187-95. PMID: 2012309911. Language: English. Entry Date: 20131004. Revision Date: 20131025. Publication Type: journal article. Exclusion Code: X6.

78. DeWalt DA, Malone RM, Bryant ME, et al. A heart failure self-management program for patients of all literacy levels: a randomized, controlled trial [ISRCTN11535170]. BMC Health Serv Res. 2006;6:30. PMID: 16533388. Exclusion Code: X2.

79. DeWalt DA, Schillinger D, Ruo B, et al. Multisite randomized trial of a single-session versus multisession literacy-sensitive self-care intervention for patients with heart failure. Circulation. 2012 Jun 12;125(23):2854-62. PMID: 22572916. Exclusion Code: X2.

80. Ditewig JB, Blok H, Havers J, et al. Effectiveness of self-management interventions on mortality, hospital readmissions, chronic heart failure hospitalization rate and quality of life in patients with chronic heart failure: a systematic review (Structured abstract). Patient Educ Couns. 2010(3):297-315. PMID: DARE-12010002763. Exclusion Code: X8 (SR).

81. Domingo M, Lupón J, González B, et al. [Noninvasive remote telemonitoring for ambulatory patients with heart failure: effect on number of hospitalizations, days in hospital, and quality of life. CARME (CAtalan Remote Management Evaluation) study]. Rev Esp Cardiol. 2011(4):277-85. PMID: CN-00786543. Exclusion Code: X2.

82. Doughty RN, Wright SP, Pearl A, et al. Randomized, controlled trial of integrated heart failure management: The Auckland Heart Failure Management Study. Eur Heart J. 2002 Jan;23(2):139-46. PMID: 11785996. Exclusion Code: X6.

83. Dracup K, Evangelista LS, Hamilton MA, et al. Effects of a home-based exercise program on clinical outcomes in heart failure. Am Heart J. 2007 Nov;154(5):877-83. PMID: 17967593. Exclusion Code: X2.

84. Duffy JR, Hoskins LM, Chen MC. Nonpharmacological strategies for improving heart failure outcomes in the community: a systematic review. J Nurs Care Qual. 2004 Oct-Dec;19(4):349-60. PMID: 15535541. Exclusion Code: X8 (SR).

85. Duffy JR, Hoskins LM, Dudley-Brown S. Development and testing of a caring-based intervention for older adults with heart failure. The Journal of cardiovascular nursing. 2005(5):325-33. PMID: CN-00529955. Exclusion Code: X1.

86. Duncan K, Pozehl B. Effects of an exercise adherence intervention on outcomes in patients with heart failure. Rehabil Nurs. 2003 Jul-Aug;28(4):117-22. PMID: 12875144. Exclusion Code: X2.

87. Engel Mark E, Matchaba Patrice T, Volmink J. Corticosteroids for tuberculous pleurisy: John Wiley & Sons, Ltd; 2007. Exclusion Code: Corticosteroids for tuberculous pleurisy.

88. Evengelista L, Doering L, Dracup K. Exercise training and weight control in patients with chronic heart failure. Commun Nurs Res. 2005;38:245-. PMID: 2009901972. Language: English. Entry Date: 20080613. Revision Date: 20101231. Publication Type: journal article. Exclusion Code: X3.

89. Fabbri G, Gorini M, Maggioni AP, et al. [Heart failure: the importance of a disease management program]. Giornale italiano di cardiologia (2006). 2007(6):353-8. PMID: CN-00704189. Exclusion Code: X1.

90. Falces C, López-Cabezas C, Andrea R, et al. [An educative intervention to improve treatment compliance and to prevent readmissions of elderly patients with heart failure]. Med Clin (Barc). 2008(12):452-6. PMID: CN-00687356. Exclusion Code: X1.

91. Feaster SJ. Tips, tools, and techniques. Nursing, technology, and patient care: a home-based model. Nurs Case Manag. 1998 1998 Jan-Feb;3(1):7-10. PMID: 1998042640. Language: English. Entry Date: 19980701. Revision Date: 20101231. Publication Type: journal article. Exclusion Code: X1.

92. Feldman PH, Murtaugh CM, Pezzin LE, et al. Just-in-time evidence-based e-mail "reminders" in home health care: impact on patient outcomes. Health Serv Res. 2005 Jun;40(3):865-85. PMID: 15960695. Exclusion Code: X2.

93. Finkelstein SM, Speedie SM, Potthoff S. Home telehealth improves clinical outcomes at lower cost for home healthcare. Telemed J E Health. 2006 Apr;12(2):128-36. PMID: 16620167. Exclusion Code: X2.

94. Flynn KE, Pina IL, Whellan DJ, et al. Effects of exercise training on health status in patients with chronic heart failure: HF-ACTION randomized controlled trial. JAMA. 2009 Apr 8;301(14):1451-9. PMID: 19351942. Exclusion Code: X2.

95. Fredericks S, Beanlands H, Spalding K, et al. Effects of the characteristics of teaching on the outcomes of heart failure patient education interventions: a systematic review. Eur J Cardiovasc Nurs. 2010 Mar;9(1):30-7. PMID: 19734100. Exclusion Code: X8 (SR).

96. Fursse J, Clarke M, Jones R, et al. Early experience in using telemonitoring for the management of chronic disease in primary care. J Telemed Telecare. 2008;14(3):122-4. Exclusion Code: X8.

97. Gardner-Bonneau D. Remote patient monitoring: a human factors assessment. Biomed Instrum Technol. 2010:71-7. PMID: 2010918553. Language: English. Entry Date: 20110311. Revision Date: 20120622. Publication Type: journal article. Exclusion Code: X5.

98. Gary R. Exercise self-efficacy in older women with diastolic heart failure: results of a walking program and education intervention. J Gerontol Nurs. 2006 Jul;32(7):31-9; quiz 40-1. PMID: 16863044. Exclusion Code: X2.

99. Gary RA, Sueta CA, Dougherty M, et al. Home-based exercise improves functional performance and quality of life in women with diastolic heart failure. Heart Lung. 2004 Jul-Aug;33(4):210-8. PMID: 15252410. Exclusion Code: X2.

100. Gattis WA, Hasselblad V, Whellan DJ, et al. Reduction in heart failure events by the addition of a clinical pharmacist to the heart failure management team: results of the Pharmacist in Heart Failure Assessment Recommendation and Monitoring (PHARM) Study. Arch Intern Med. 1999 Sep 13;159(16):1939-45. PMID: 10493325. Exclusion Code: X2.

101. Gellis ZD, Kenaley B, McGinty J, et al. Outcomes of a telehealth intervention for homebound older adults with heart or chronic respiratory failure: a randomized controlled trial. Gerontologist. 2012 Aug;52(4):541-52. PMID: 22241810. Exclusion Code: X2.

102. GESICA Investigators. Randomised trial of telephone intervention in chronic heart failure: DIAL trial. BMJ. 2005 Aug 20;331(7514):425. PMID: 16061499. Exclusion Code: X2.

103. Giannuzzi P, Temporelli PL, Corra U, et al. Antiremodeling effect of long-term exercise training in patients with stable chronic heart failure: results of the Exercise in Left Ventricular Dysfunction and Chronic Heart Failure (ELVD-CHF) Trial. Circulation. 2003 Aug 5;108(5):554-9. PMID: 12860904. Exclusion Code: X2.

104. Giliarevski SR, Orlov VA, Khamaganova LK, et al. [Effect of therapeutic education of patients with chronic heart failure on quality of life and requirement of rehospitalizations. Results of 12-months randomized study]. Kardiologiia. 2002(5):56-61. PMID: CN-00434818. Exclusion Code: X1.

105. Giordano A, Scalvini S, Zanelli E, et al. Multicenter randomised trial on home-based telemanagement to prevent hospital readmission of patients with chronic heart failure. Int J Cardiol. 2009 Jan 9;131(2):192-9. PMID: 18222552. Exclusion Code: X6.

106. Godfrey CM, Harrison MB, Friedberg E, et al. The symptom of pain in individuals recently hospitalized for heart failure. J Cardiovasc Nurs. 2007 Sep-Oct;22(5):368-74; discussion 6-7. PMID: 17724418. Exclusion Code: X4.

107. Gohler A, Januzzi JL, Worrell SS, et al. A systematic meta-analysis of the efficacy and heterogeneity of disease management programs in congestive heart failure. J Card Fail. 2006 Sep;12(7):554-67. PMID: 16952790. Exclusion Code: X8 (SR).

108. Gomez-Soto FM, Puerto JL, Andrey JL, et al. Consultation between specialists in Internal Medicine and Family Medicine improves management and prognosis of heart failure. Eur J Intern Med. 2008 Nov;19(7):548-54. PMID: 19013386. Exclusion Code: X8.

109. Gonseth J, Guallar-Castillon P, Banegas JR, et al. The effectiveness of disease management programmes in reducing hospital re-admission in older patients with heart failure: a systematic review and meta-analysis of published reports. Eur Heart J. 2004 Sep;25(18):1570-95. PMID: 15351157. Exclusion Code: X8 (SR).

110. Grady KL. Self-care and quality of life outcomes in heart failure patients (Structured abstract). J Cardiovasc Nurs. 2008(3):285-92. PMID: DARE-12008103868. Exclusion Code: X8 (SR).

111. Grancelli HO. [Disease management programs in heart failure. Findings of the DIAL study]. Rev Esp Cardiol. 2007:15-22. PMID: CN-00628926. Exclusion Code: X1.

112. Gregory D, Kimmelstiel C, Perry K, et al. Hospital cost effect of a heart failure disease management program: the Specialized Primary and Networked Care in Heart Failure (SPAN-CHF) trial. Am Heart J. 2006 May;151(5):1013-8. PMID: 16644325. Exclusion Code: X8.

113. Guadagnoli E, Normand SL, DiSalvo TG, et al. Effects of treatment recommendations and specialist intervention on care provided by primary care physicians to patients with myocardial infarction or heart failure. Am J Med. 2004 Sep 15;117(6):371-9. PMID: 15380493. Exclusion Code: X5.

114. Guimaraes GV, Carvalho VO, Bocchi EA, et al. Pilates in heart failure patients: a randomized controlled pilot trial. Cardiovasc Ther. 2012 Dec;30(6):351-6. PMID: 21884019. Exclusion Code: X2.

115. Gwadry-Sridhar F, Guyatt G, O'Brien B, et al. TEACH: Trial of Education And Compliance in Heart dysfunction chronic disease and heart failure (HF) as an increasing problem. Contemp Clin Trials. 2008 Nov;29(6):905-18. PMID: 18703166. Exclusion Code: X5.

116. Gwadry-Sridhar FH, Arnold JM, Zhang Y, et al. Pilot study to determine the impact of a multidisciplinary educational intervention in patients hospitalized with heart failure. Am Heart J. 2005 Nov;150(5):982. PMID: 16290975. Exclusion Code: X6.

117. Gwadry-Sridhar FH, Flintoft V, Lee DS, et al. A systematic review and meta-analysis of studies comparing readmission rates and mortality rates in patients with heart failure. Arch Intern Med. 2004 Nov 22;164(21):2315-20. PMID: 15557409. Exclusion Code: X8 (SR).

118. Hailey D, Ohinmaa A, Roine R. Published evidence on the success of telecardiology: a mixed record. J Telemed Telecare. 2004;10 Suppl 1:36-8. PMID: 15603604. Exclusion Code: X2.

119. Hamner JB. State of the science: posthospitalization nursing interventions in congestive heart failure. ANS Adv Nurs Sci. 2005 Apr-Jun;28(2):175-90. PMID: 15920363. Exclusion Code: X8.

120. Harrison MB. Providing supportive care during hospital to home transfer: implementing and evaluating clinical practice guidelines on supportive care for individuals with heart failure [abstract]. Annual Meeting of International Society of Technology Assessment in Health Care. 1998:52. PMID: CN-00598189. Exclusion Code: X1.

121. Harrison MB, Browne GB, Roberts J, et al. Quality of life of individuals with heart failure: a randomized trial of the effectiveness of two models of hospital-to-home transition. Med Care. 2002 Apr;40(4):271-82. PMID: 12021683. Exclusion Code: X5.

122. Heisler M, Halasyamani L, Cowen ME, et al. Randomized controlled effectiveness trial of reciprocal peer support in heart failure. Circ Heart Fail. 2013 Mar;6(2):246-53. PMID: 23388114. Exclusion Code: X2.

123. Hershberger RE, Ni H, Nauman DJ, et al. Prospective evaluation of an outpatient heart failure management program. J Card Fail. 2001 Mar;7(1):64-74. PMID: 11264552. Exclusion Code: X2.

124. Holst DP, Kaye D, Richardson M, et al. Improved outcomes from a comprehensive management system for heart failure. Eur J Heart Fail. 2001 Oct;3(5):619-25. PMID: 11595611. Exclusion Code: X2.

125. Hopp F, Woodbridge P, Subramanian U, et al. Outcomes associated with a home care telehealth intervention. Telemed J E Health. 2006 Jun;12(3):297-307. PMID: 16796497. Exclusion Code: X2.

126. Hughes S, Weaver F, Manheim L, et al. Cost-effectiveness of team-managed home care in the VA: an update from a multi-site randomized trial [abstract]. Abstract Book/Association for Health Services Research. 1997:110-1. PMID: CN-00270902. Exclusion Code: X2.

127. Hughes SL, Weaver FM, Giobbie-Hurder A, et al. Effectiveness of team-managed home-based primary care: a randomized multicenter trial. JAMA. 2000 Dec 13;284(22):2877-85. PMID: 11147984. Exclusion Code: X2.

128. Hwang R, Marwick T. Efficacy of home-based exercise programmes for people with chronic heart failure: a meta-analysis. Eur J Cardiovasc Prev Rehabil. 2009 Oct;16(5):527-35. PMID: 20054288. Exclusion Code: X5.

129. Inglis Sally C, Clark Robyn A, McAlister Finlay A, et al. Structured telephone support or telemonitoring programmes for patients with chronic heart failure. Cochrane Database of Systematic Reviews. 2010(8)PMID: CD007228. Exclusion Code: X8 (SR).

130. Inglis SC, Clark RA, Cleland JG. Telemonitoring in patients with heart failure. N Engl J Med. 2011 March 17;364(11):1078-9. PMID: 21410377. Exclusion Code: X1.

131. Inglis SC, Clark RA, McAlister FA, et al. Which components of heart failure programmes are effective? A systematic review and meta-analysis of the outcomes of structured telephone support or telemonitoring as the primary component of chronic heart failure management in 8323 patients: Abridged Cochrane Review. Eur J Heart Fail. 2011 Sep;13(9):1028-40. PMID: 21733889. Exclusion Code: X8 (SR).

132. Jaarsma T, Brons M, Kraai I, et al. Components of heart failure management in home care; a literature review. European Journal of Cardiovascular Nursing. 2013;12(3):230-41. PMID: 2012114095. Language: English. Entry Date: 20130531. Revision Date: 20130531. Publication Type: journal article. Exclusion Code: X8.

133. Jaarsma T, Halfens R, Tan F, et al. Self-care and quality of life in patients with advanced heart failure: the effect of a supportive educational intervention. Heart Lung. 2000 Sep-Oct;29(5):319-30. PMID: 10986526. Exclusion Code: X5.

134. Jaarsma T, Lvan-Der-Wal M, Lesman LI. [Value of basic or intensive management of patients with heart failure confirmed in a randomised controlled clinical trial]. Ned Tijdschr Geneeskd. 2008;152:2016-21. Exclusion Code: X1.

135. Jaarsma T, Van Der Wal MH, Hogenhuis J, et al. Design and methodology of the COACH study: a multicenter randomised Coordinating study evaluating Outcomes of Advising and Counselling in Heart failure. Eur J Heart Fail. 2004 Mar 1;6(2):227-33. PMID: 14984731. Exclusion Code: X1.

136. Jaarsma T, van der Wal MH, Lesman-Leegte I, et al. Effect of moderate or intensive disease management program on outcome in patients with heart failure: Coordinating Study Evaluating Outcomes of Advising and Counseling in Heart Failure (COACH). Arch Intern Med. 2008 Feb 11;168(3):316-24. PMID: 18268174. Exclusion Code: X6.

137. Jaarsma T, van Veldhuisen DJ. When, how and where should we "coach" patients with heart failure: the COACH results in perspective. Eur J Heart Fail. 2008;10(4):331-3. PMID: 18353718. Exclusion Code: X1.

138. Jaarsma T, van Veldhuisen DJ, van der Wal MH. NHF-COACH multicenter trial in The Netherlands: searching for underlying potentially beneficial mechanisms in nurse led heart failure management. Prog Cardiovasc Nurs. 2002 Spring;17(2):96-8. PMID: 11986543. Exclusion Code: X1.

139. Jaarsma T, Veldhuisen DJ. [Research set-up concerning the effectiveness of heart failure clinics in the Netherlands]. Ned Tijdschr Geneeskd. 2003(11):513-4. PMID: CN-00558540. Exclusion Code: X1.

140. Jackson RA. Internet and telephone-based congestive heart failure program as effective as and cheaper than traditional one, study says. Rep Med Guidel Outcomes Res. 2001 Feb 22;12(4):9-10, 2. PMID: 11767797. Exclusion Code: X1.

141. Jayadevappa R, Johnson JC, Bloom BS, et al. Effectiveness of transcendental meditation on functional capacity and quality of life of African Americans with congestive heart failure: a randomized control study. Ethn Dis. 2007(1):72-7. PMID: CN-00575174. Exclusion Code: X3.

142. Jerant AF, Nesbitt TS. Heart failure disease management incorporating telemedicine: a critical review. Journal of Clinical Outcomes Management. 2005;12(4):207-17. PMID: 2005098853. Language: English. Entry Date: 20050624. Revision Date: 20101231. Publication Type: journal article. Exclusion Code: X8 (SR).

143. Johnson MJ, Oxberry SG, Cleland JG, et al. Measurement of breathlessness in clinical trials in patients with chronic heart failure: the need for a standardized approach: a systematic review. Eur J Heart Fail. 2010 Feb;12(2):137-47. PMID: 20083623. Exclusion Code: X3.

144. Jolly K, Taylor RS, Lip GY, et al. A randomized trial of the addition of home-based exercise to specialist heart failure nurse care: the Birmingham Rehabilitation Uptake Maximisation study for patients with Congestive Heart Failure (BRUM-CHF) study. Eur J Heart Fail. 2009 Feb;11(2):205-13. PMID: 19168520. Exclusion Code: X2.

145. Jonsdottir S, Andersen KK, Sigurosson AF, et al. The effect of physical training in chronic heart failure. Eur J Heart Fail. 2006 Jan;8(1):97-101. PMID: 16194620. Exclusion Code: X2.

146. Jovicic A, Chignell M, Wu R, et al. Is Web-only self-care education sufficient for heart failure patients? AMIA Annu Symp Proc. 2009;2009:296-300. PMID: 20351868. Exclusion Code: X5.

147. Jovicic A, Holroyd-Leduc JM, Straus SE. Effects of self-management intervention on health outcomes of patients with heart failure: a systematic review of randomized controlled trials. BMC Cardiovasc Disord. 2006;6:43. PMID: 17081306. Exclusion Code: X8 (SR).

148. Karapolat H, Demir E, Bozkaya YT, et al. Comparison of hospital-based versus home-based exercise training in patients with heart failure: effects on functional capacity, quality of life, psychological symptoms, and hemodynamic parameters. Clin Res Cardiol. 2009 Oct;98(10):635-42. PMID: 19641843. Exclusion Code: X2.

149. Karlsson MR, Edner M, Henriksson P, et al. A nurse-based management program in heart failure patients affects females and persons with cognitive dysfunction most. Patient Educ Couns. 2005 Aug;58(2):146-53. PMID: 16009290. Exclusion Code: X5.

150. Kashem A, Droogan MT, Santamore WP, et al. Managing heart failure care using an internet-based telemedicine system. J Card Fail. 2008 Mar;14(2):121-6. PMID: 18325458. Exclusion Code: X2.

151. Kashem A, Droogan MT, Santamore WP, et al. Web-based Internet telemedicine management of patients with heart failure. Telemedicine journal and e-health : the official journal of the American Telemedicine Association. 2006(4):439-47. PMID: CN-00571916. Exclusion Code: X2.

152. Kayanakis JG, Page E, Aros F, et al. [Rehabilitation of patients with chronic cardiac insufficiency. Immediate and midterm effects]. Presse médicale (Paris, France : 1983). 1994(3):121-6. PMID: CN-00101144. Exclusion Code: X1.

153. Kessing D, Denollet J, Widdershoven J, et al. Investigating a TELEmedicine solution to improve MEDication adherence in chronic Heart Failure (TELEMED-HF): study protocol for a randomized controlled trial. Trials. 2011;12:227. PMID: 21999637. Exclusion Code: X2.

154. Keteyian SJ, Isaac D, Thadani U, et al. Safety of symptom-limited cardiopulmonary exercise testing in patients with chronic heart failure due to severe left ventricular systolic dysfunction. Am Heart J. 2009(4 Suppl):S72-7. PMID: CN-00722507. Exclusion Code: X2.

155. Khunti K, Stone M, Paul S, et al. Disease management programme for secondary prevention of coronary heart disease and heart failure in primary care: a cluster randomised controlled trial. Heart. 2007 Nov;93(11):1398-405. PMID: 17309907. Exclusion Code: X2.

156. Kim YJ, Soeken KL. A meta-analysis of the effect of hospital-based case management on hospital length-of-stay and readmission. Nurs Res. 2005 Jul-Aug;54(4):255-64. PMID: 16027568. Exclusion Code: X8 (SR).

157. Klersy C, De Silvestri A, Gabutti G, et al. Economic impact of remote patient monitoring: an integrated economic model derived from a meta-analysis of randomized controlled trials in heart failure. Eur J Heart Fail. 2011 Apr;13(4):450-9. PMID: 21193439. Exclusion Code: X8.

158. Klersy C, De Silvestri A, Gabutti G, et al. A meta-analysis of remote monitoring of heart failure patients. J Am Coll Cardiol. 2009 Oct 27;54(18):1683-94. PMID: 19850208. Exclusion Code: X8 (SR).

159. Kline KS, Scott LD, Britton AS. The use of supportive-educative and mutual goal-setting strategies to improve self-management for patients with heart failure. Home Healthc Nurse. 2007 Sep;25(8):502-10. PMID: 17828004. Exclusion Code: X2.

160. Köhler F, Nettlau H, Schweizer T, et al. The research project of the German Federal Ministry of Economics and Technology: 'Partnership for the Heart' -- a new approach in telemedicine. Disease Management & Health Outcomes. 2006;14:37-41. PMID: 2009326473. Language: English. Entry Date: 20080208. Revision Date: 20101231. Publication Type: journal article. Exclusion Code: X1.

161. Kommuri NV, Johnson ML, Koelling TM. Relationship between improvements in heart failure patient disease specific knowledge and clinical events as part of a randomized controlled trial. Patient Educ Couns. 2012 Feb;86(2):233-8. PMID: 21705170. Exclusion Code: X5.

162. Konstam MA. Home monitoring should be the central element in an effective program of heart failure disease management. Circulation. 2012 Feb 14;125(6):820-7. PMID: 22331919. Exclusion Code: X1.

163. Konstam V, Gregory D, Chen J, et al. Health-related quality of life in a multicenter randomized controlled comparison of telephonic disease management and automated home monitoring in patients recently hospitalized with heart failure: SPAN-CHF II trial. J Card Fail. 2011 Feb;17(2):151-7. PMID: 21300305. Exclusion Code: X5.

164. Kothe K, Ullmann K, Daiss W. Risk score modifications in congestive heart failure-focus on exercise therapy and women. Int J Sports Med. 1996(Suppl 1):S13. PMID: CN-00506784. Exclusion Code: X3.

165. Koukouvou G, Kouidi E, Iacovides A, et al. Quality of life, psychological and physiological changes following exercise training in patients with chronic heart failure. J Rehabil Med. 2004 Jan;36(1):36-41. PMID: 15074436. Exclusion Code: X2.

166. Kozak AT, Rucker-Whitaker C, Basu S, et al. Elements of nonpharmacologic interventions that prevent progression of heart failure: a meta-analysis. Congest Heart Fail. 2007 Sep-Oct;13(5):280-7. PMID: 17917495. Exclusion Code: X8 (SR).

167. Kraai IH, Luttik ML, de Jong RM, et al. Heart failure patients monitored with telemedicine: patient satisfaction, a review of the literature. J Card Fail. 2011;17(8):684-90. PMID: 2011233563. Language: English. Entry Date: 20120615. Revision Date: 20120615. Publication Type: journal article. Exclusion Code: X5.

168. Krantz MJ, Havranek EP, Haynes DK, et al. Inpatient initiation of beta-blockade plus nurse management in vulnerable heart failure patients: a randomized study. J Card Fail. 2008 May;14(4):303-9. PMID: 18474343. Exclusion Code: X3.

169. Krumholz HM, Amatruda J, Smith GL, et al. Randomized trial of an education and support intervention to prevent readmission of patients with heart failure. J Am Coll Cardiol. 2002 Jan 2;39(1):83-9. PMID: 11755291. Exclusion Code: X6.

170. Kulcu DG, Kurtais Y, Tur BS, et al. The effect of cardiac rehabilitation on quality of life, anxiety and depression in patients with congestive heart failure. A randomized controlled trial, short-term results. Europa Medicophysica. 2007;43(4):489-97. PMID: 2009776771. Language: English. Entry Date: 20080418. Revision Date: 20101231. Publication Type: journal article. Exclusion Code: X2.

171. Kutzleb J, Reiner D. The impact of nurse-directed patient education on quality of life and functional capacity in people with heart failure. J Am Acad Nurse Pract. 2006 Mar;18(3):116-23. PMID: 16499744. Exclusion Code: X2.

172. LaFramboise LM, Todero CM, Zimmerman L, et al. Comparison of Health Buddy with traditional approaches to heart failure management. Fam Community Health. 2003 Oct-Dec;26(4):275-88. PMID: 14528134. Exclusion Code: X2.

173. Lainchbury JG, Troughton RW, Strangman KM, et al. N-terminal pro-B-type natriuretic peptide-guided treatment for chronic heart failure: results from the BATTLESCARRED (NT-proBNP-Assisted Treatment To Lessen Serial Cardiac Readmissions and Death) trial. J Am Coll Cardiol. 2009 Dec 29;55(1):53-60. PMID: 20117364. Exclusion Code: X4.

174. Lambrinou E, Kalogirou F, Lamnisos D, et al. Effectiveness of heart failure management programmes with nurse-led discharge planning in reducing re-admissions: a systematic review and meta-analysis. Int J Nurs Stud. 2012 May;49(5):610-24. PMID: 22196054. Exclusion Code: X8 (SR).

175. Landolina M, Perego GB, Lunati M, et al. Remote monitoring reduces healthcare use and improves quality of care in heart failure patients with implantable defibrillators: the evolution of management strategies of heart failure patients with implantable defibrillators (EVOLVO) study. Circulation. 2012 Jun 19;125(24):2985-92. PMID: 22626743. Exclusion Code: X2.

176. Laoutaris I, Dritsas A, Brown MD, et al. Inspiratory muscle training using an incremental endurance test alleviates dyspnea and improves functional status in patients with chronic heart failure. Eur J Cardiovasc Prev Rehabil. 2004 Dec;11(6):489-96. PMID: 15580060. Exclusion Code: X2.

177. LaPointe NM, DeLong ER, Chen A, et al. Multifaceted intervention to promote beta-blocker use in heart failure. Am Heart J. 2006 May;151(5):992-8. PMID: 16644320. Exclusion Code: X2.

178. Ledwidge M, Ryan E, O'Loughlin C, et al. Heart failure care in a hospital unit: a comparison of standard 3-month and extended 6-month programs. Eur J Heart Fail. 2005 Mar 16;7(3):385-91. PMID: 15718179. Exclusion Code: X2.

179. Ledwidge MT, O'Hanlon R, Lalor L, et al. Can individualized weight monitoring using the HeartPhone algorithm improve sensitivity for clinical deterioration of heart failure? Eur J Heart Fail. 2013 Apr;15(4):447-55. PMID: 23204211. Exclusion Code: X2.

180. Leff B, Burton L, Mader S, et al. Satisfaction with hospital at home care. J Am Geriatr Soc. 2006 Sep;54(9):1355-63. PMID: 16970642. Exclusion Code: X2.

181. Leff B, Burton L, Mader SL, et al. Comparison of functional outcomes associated with hospital at home care and traditional acute hospital care. J Am Geriatr Soc. 2009 Feb;57(2):273-8. PMID: 19170781. Exclusion Code: X3.

182. Leff B, Burton L, Mader SL, et al. Comparison of stress experienced by family members of patients treated in hospital at home with that of those receiving traditional acute hospital care. J Am Geriatr Soc. 2008 Jan;56(1):117-23. PMID: 17979955. Exclusion Code: X3.

183. Leventhal ME, Denhaerynck K, Brunner-La Rocca HP, et al. Swiss Interdisciplinary Management Programme for Heart Failure (SWIM-HF): a randomised controlled trial study of an outpatient inter-professional management programme for heart failure patients in Switzerland. Swiss Med Wkly. 2011;141:w13171. PMID: 21384285. Exclusion Code: X6.

184. Lin SJ, McElfresh J, Hall B, et al. Inspiratory muscle training in patients with heart failure: a systematic review (Provisional abstract). Database of Abstracts of Reviews of Effects. 2012(3):29-36. PMID: DARE-12012057718. Exclusion.

185. Lloyd-Williams F, Mair FS, Leitner M. Exercise training and heart failure: a systematic review of current evidence. Br J Gen Pract. 2002 Jan;52(474):47-55. PMID: 11791816. Exclusion Code: X3.

186. Louis AA, Turner T, Gretton M, et al. A systematic review of telemonitoring for the management of heart failure. Eur J Heart Fail. 2003 Oct;5(5):583-90. PMID: 14607195. Exclusion Code: X8 (SR).

187. Lusignan S, Meredith K, Wells S, et al. A controlled pilot study in the use of telemedicine in the community on the management of heart failure--a report of the first three months. Stud Health Technol Inform. 1999:126-37. PMID: CN-00371805. Exclusion Code: X2.

188. Lynga P, Persson H, Hagg-Martinell A, et al. Weight monitoring in patients with severe heart failure (WISH). A randomized controlled trial. Eur J Heart Fail. 2012 Apr;14(4):438-44. PMID: 22371525. Exclusion Code: X2.

189. Madigan EA, Schott D, Matthews CR. Rehospitalization among home healthcare patients: results of a prospective study. Home Healthc Nurse. 2001 May;19(5):298-305. PMID: 11985040. Exclusion Code: X8.

190. Mainardi L, Iazzolino E, Asteggiano R, et al. [Comparison between telephone and outpatient nursing management in patients with chronic heart failure in a large territorial area in Piedmont, Italy]. Giornale italiano di cardiologia (2006). 2010(1):35-42. PMID: CN-00743369. Exclusion Code: X1.

191. Maric B, Kaan A, Ignaszewski A, et al. A systematic review of telemonitoring technologies in heart failure. Eur J Heart Fail. 2009 May;11(5):506-17. PMID: 19332417. Exclusion Code: X3.

192. Martinez A, Everss E, Rojo-Alvarez JL, et al. A systematic review of the literature on home monitoring for patients with heart failure. J Telemed Telecare. 2006;12(5):234-41. PMID: 16848935. Exclusion Code: X8 (SR).

193. Mau J, Kolk M, Pelon J, et al. Nurse-directed home-based heart failure management program decreases death/readmission rates and increases dietary and medication compliance. Prog Cardiovasc Nurs. 2006(2):112. PMID: CN-00614843. Exclusion Code: X8.

194. McAlister FA, Lawson FM, Teo KK, et al. A systematic review of randomized trials of disease management programs in heart failure. Am J Med. 2001 Apr 1;110(5):378-84. PMID: 11286953. Exclusion Code: X8 (SR).

195. McBride MG, Binder TJ, Paridon SM. Safety and feasibility of inpatient exercise training in pediatric heart failure: a preliminary report. Journal of Cardiopulmonary Rehabilitation & Prevention. 2007;27(4):219-22. PMID: 2009653090. Language: English. Entry Date: 20080215. Revision Date: 20101231. Publication Type: journal article. Exclusion Code: X2.

196. McCauley KM, Bixby MB, Naylor MD. Advanced practice nurse strategies to improve outcomes and reduce cost in elders with heart failure. Dis Manag. 2006;9(5):302-10. Exclusion Code: X5.

197. McKelvie RS, Teo KK, Roberts R, et al. Effects of exercise training in patients with heart failure: the Exercise Rehabilitation Trial (EXERT). Am Heart J. 2002 Jul;144(1):23-30. PMID: 12094184. Exclusion Code: X2.

198. McManus SG. A Telehealth Program to Reduce Readmission Rates Among Heart Failure Patients: One Agency's Experience. Home Health Care Management & Practice. 2004 June 1, 2004;16(4):250-4. Exclusion Code: X2.

199. Mehra MR, Uber PA, Chomsky DB, et al. Emergence of electronic home monitoring in chronic heart failure: rationale, feasibility, and early results with the HomMed Sentry-Observer system. Congest Heart Fail. 2000;6(3):137-9. Exclusion Code: X2.

200. Mejhert M, Kahan T, Persson H, et al. Limited long term effects of a management programme for heart failure. Heart. 2004 Sep;90(9):1010-5. PMID: 15310688. Exclusion Code: X5.

201. Mello PR, Guerra GM, Borile S, et al. Inspiratory muscle training reduces sympathetic nervous activity and improves inspiratory muscle weakness and quality of life in patients with chronic heart failure: a clinical trial. J Cardiopulm Rehabil Prev. 2012 Sep-Oct;32(5):255-61. PMID: 22785143. Exclusion Code: X2.

202. Mendoza H, Martin MJ, Garcia A, et al. 'Hospital at home' care model as an effective alternative in the management of decompensated chronic heart failure. Eur J Heart Fail. 2009 Dec;11(12):1208-13. PMID: 19875400. Exclusion Code: X3.

203. Metten L, Zueca F, Haver Y, et al. 22 Effects of intensified care for heart failure patients by telemonitoring. European Journal of Cardiovascular Nursing. 2011;10(s):S26-S. PMID: 2012031743. Language: English. Entry Date: 20130322. Revision Date: 20130419. Publication Type: journal article. Exclusion Code: X2.

204. Moertl D, Berger R, Hammer A, et al. B-type natriuretic peptide predicts benefit from a home-based nurse care in chronic heart failure. J Card Fail. 2009 Apr;15(3):233-40. PMID: 19327625. Exclusion Code: X2.

205. Molloy GJ, Johnston DW, Gao C, et al. Effects of an exercise intervention for older heart failure patients on caregiver burden and emotional distress. Eur J Cardiovasc Prev Rehabil. 2006 Jun;13(3):381-7. PMID: 16926668. Exclusion Code: X2.

206. Morcillo C, Valderas JM, Aguado O, et al. [Evaluation of a home-based intervention in heart failure patients. Results of a randomized study]. Rev Esp Cardiol. 2005(6):618-25. PMID: CN-00528602. Exclusion Code: X1 (May be excluded).

207. Morguet AJ, Kuhnelt P, Kallel A, et al. Impact of telemedical care and monitoring on morbidity in mild to moderate chronic heart failure. Cardiology. 2008;111(2):134-9. PMID: 18376125. Exclusion Code: X2.

208. Mortara A, Pinna GD, Johnson P, et al. Home telemonitoring in heart failure patients: the HHH study (Home or Hospital in Heart Failure). Eur J Heart Fail. 2009;11(3):312-8. Exclusion Code: X2.

209. Mudge A, Denaro C, Scott I, et al. The paradox of readmission: effect of a quality improvement program in hospitalized patients with heart failure. J Hosp Med. 2010 Mar;5(3):148-53. PMID: 20235283. Exclusion Code: X6.

210. Mueller TM, Vuckovic KM, Knox DA, et al. Telemanagement of heart failure: a diuretic treatment algorithm for advanced practice nurses. Heart Lung. 2002 Sep-Oct;31(5):340-7. PMID: 12487012. Exclusion Code: X1.

211. Murphy SA. Initiation Management Predischarge: Process for Assessment of Carvedilol Therapy in Heart Failure (IMPACT-HF). ACC Current Journal Review. 2004;13(7):41-2. PMID: 2005114409. Language: English. Entry Date: 20050729. Revision Date: 20101231. Publication Type: journal article. Exclusion Code: X3.

212. Murray MD, Young J, Hoke S, et al. Pharmacist intervention to improve medication adherence in heart failure: a randomized trial. Ann Intern Med. 2007 May 15;146(10):714-25. PMID: 17502632. Exclusion Code: X2.

213. Murray MD, Young JM, Morrow DG, et al. Methodology of an ongoing, randomized, controlled trial to improve drug use for elderly patients with chronic heart failure. The American journal of geriatric pharmacotherapy. 2004(1):53-65. PMID: CN-00492778. Exclusion Code: X2.

214. Nanevicz T, Piette J, Zipkin D, et al. The feasibility of a telecommunications service in support of outpatient congestive heart failure care in a diverse patient population. Congest Heart Fail. 2000;6(3):140-5. Exclusion Code: X2.

215. Naylor M, Brooten D, Jones R, et al. Comprehensive discharge planning for the hospitalized elderly. A randomized clinical trial. Ann Intern Med. 1994 Jun 15;120(12):999-1006. PMID: 8185149. Exclusion Code: X2.

216. Naylor MD, Aiken LH, Kurtzman ET, et al. The care span: the importance of transitional care in achieving health reform. Health Aff (Millwood). 2011 Apr;30(4):746-54. PMID: 21471497. Exclusion Code: X2.

217. Nechwatal RM, Duck C, Gruber G. [Physical training as interval or continuous training in chronic heart failure for improving functional capacity, hemodynamics and quality of life--a controlled study]. Z Kardiol. 2002(4):328-37. PMID: CN-00389580. Exclusion Code: X3.

218. Nguyen V, Ducharme A, White M, et al. Lack of long-term benefits of a 6-month heart failure disease management program. J Card Fail. 2007(4):287-93. PMID: CN-00589076. Exclusion Code: X6.

219. Nieboer AP, Schulz R, Matthews KA, et al. Spousal caregivers' activity restriction and depression: a model for changes over time. Soc Sci Med. 1998 Nov;47(9):1361-71. PMID: 9783879. Exclusion Code: X2.

220. Nobel JJ, Norman GK. Emerging information management technologies and the future of disease management. Dis Manag. 2003 Winter;6(4):219-31. PMID: 14736346. Exclusion Code: X2.

221. Nundy S, Razi RR, Dick JJ, et al. A text messaging intervention to improve heart failure self-management after hospital discharge in a largely African-American population: before-after study. J Med Internet Res. 2013;15(3):e53. PMID: 23478028. Exclusion Code: X5.

222. O'Connor CM, Whellan DJ, Lee KL, et al. Efficacy and safety of exercise training in patients with chronic heart failure: HF-ACTION randomized controlled trial. JAMA. 2009 Apr 8;301(14):1439-50. PMID: 19351941. Exclusion Code: X2.

223. Ojeda S, Anguita M, Delgado M, et al. Short- and long-term results of a programme for the prevention of readmissions and mortality in patients with heart failure: are effects maintained after stopping the programme? Eur J Heart Fail. 2005 Aug;7(5):921-6. PMID: 16051519. Exclusion Code: X6.

224. Pandor A, Gomersall T, Stevens JW, et al. Remote monitoring after recent hospital discharge in patients with heart failure: a systematic review and network meta-analysis (Provisional abstract). Database of Abstracts of Reviews of Effects. 2013(3):epub. PMID: DARE-12013029243. Exclusion.

225. Panella M, Marchisio S, Demarchi ML, et al. Reduced in-hospital mortality for heart failure with clinical pathways: the results of a cluster randomised controlled trial. Qual Saf Health Care. 2009 Oct;18(5):369-73. PMID: 19812099. Exclusion Code: X3.

226. Panella M, Marchisio S, Di Mario G, et al. The effectiveness of an integrated care pathway for inpatient heart failure treatment: results of a trial in a community hospital. Journal of Integrated Care Pathways. 2005;9(1):21-8. PMID: 2009061993. Language: English. Entry Date: 20051202. Revision Date: 20101231. Publication Type: journal article. Exclusion Code: X3.

227. Panella M, Marchisio S, Gardini A, et al. A cluster randomized controlled trial of a clinical pathway for hospital treatment of heart failure: study design and population. BMC Health Serv Res. 2007;7:179. PMID: 17986361. Exclusion Code: X3.

228. Pantilat SZ, O'Riordan DL, Dibble SL, et al. Hospital-based palliative medicine consultation: a randomized controlled trial. Arch Intern Med. 2010(22):2038-40. PMID: CN-00770681. Exclusion Code: X2.

229. Paradis V, Cossette S, Frasure-Smith N, et al. The efficacy of a motivational nursing intervention based on the stages of change on self-care in heart failure patients. J Cardiovasc Nurs. 2010 Mar-Apr;25(2):130-41. PMID: 20168193. Exclusion Code: X2.

230. Pare G, Moqadem K, Pineau G, et al. Clinical effects of home telemonitoring in the context of diabetes, asthma, heart failure and hypertension: a systematic review. J Med Internet Res. 2010;12(2):e21. PMID: 20554500. Exclusion Code: X2.

231. Parry C, Min SJ, Chugh A, et al. Further application of the care transitions intervention: results of a randomized controlled trial conducted in a fee-for-service setting. Home Health Care Serv Q. 2009;28(2-3):84-99. PMID: 20182958. Exclusion Code: X2.

232. Pascual CR, Galán EP, Guerrero JL, et al. Rationale and methods of the multicenter randomised trial of a heart failure management programme among geriatric patients (HF-Geriatrics). BMC Public Health. 2011:627. PMID: CN-00806731. Exclusion Code: X1.

233. Patel H, Shafazand M, Ekman I, et al. Home care as an option in worsening chronic heart failure -- a pilot study to evaluate feasibility, quality adjusted life years and cost-effectiveness. Eur J Heart Fail. 2008 Jul;10(7):675-81. PMID: 18573692. Exclusion Code: X3.

234. Paterna S, Gaspare P, Fasullo S, et al. Normal-sodium diet compared with low-sodium diet in compensated congestive heart failure: is sodium an old enemy or a new friend? Clin Sci (Lond). 2008 Feb;114(3):221-30. PMID: 17688420. Exclusion Code: X6.

235. Patja K, Absetz P, Auvinen A, et al. Health coaching by telephony to support self-care in chronic diseases: clinical outcomes from The TERVA randomized controlled trial. BMC Health Serv Res. 2012;12:147. PMID: 22682298. Exclusion Code: X5.

236. Peacock WFt, Remer EE, Aponte J, et al. Effective observation unit treatment of decompensated heart failure. Congest Heart Fail. 2002 Mar-Apr;8(2):68-73. PMID: 11927779. Exclusion Code: X8.

237. Pearl A, Wright SP, Gamble GD, et al. The effect of an integrated care approach for heart failure on general practice. Fam Pract. 2003 Dec;20(6):642-5. PMID: 14701886. Exclusion Code: X6.

238. Pearson S, Inglis SC, McLennan SN, et al. Prolonged effects of a home-based intervention in patients with chronic illness. Arch Intern Med. 2006 Mar 27;166(6):645-50. PMID: 16567604. Exclusion Code: X6.

239. Pecchia L, Schiraldi F, Verde S, et al. Evaluation of short-term effectiveness of the disease management program "Di.Pro.Di." on continuity of care of patients with congestive heart failure. J Am Geriatr Soc. 2010(8):1603-4. PMID: CN-00760374. Exclusion Code: X8.

240. Peters-Klimm F, Campbell S, Hermann K, et al. Case management for patients with chronic systolic heart failure in primary care: the HICMan exploratory randomised controlled trial. Trials. 2010;11:56. PMID: 20478035. Exclusion Code: X2.

241. Peters-Klimm F, Muller-Tasch T, Schellberg D, et al. Rationale, design and conduct of a randomised controlled trial evaluating a primary care-based complex intervention to improve the quality of life of heart failure patients: HICMan (Heidelberg Integrated Case Management). BMC Cardiovasc Disord. 2007;7:25. PMID: 17716364. Exclusion Code: X2.

242. Philbin EF, Rocco TA, Lindenmuth NW, et al. The results of a randomized trial of a quality improvement intervention in the care of patients with heart failure. The MISCHF Study Investigators. Am J Med. 2000 Oct 15;109(6):443-9. PMID: 11042232. Exclusion Code: X3.

243. Philbin EF, Weil HF, Erb TA, et al. Cardiology or primary care for heart failure in the community setting: process of care and clinical outcomes. Chest. 1999 Aug;116(2):346-54. PMID: 10453861. Exclusion Code: X8.

244. Phillips CO, Singa RM, Rubin HR, et al. Complexity of program and clinical outcomes of heart failure disease management incorporating specialist nurse-led heart failure clinics. A meta-regression analysis. Eur J Heart Fail. 2005 Mar 16;7(3):333-41. PMID: 15718173. Exclusion Code: X8 (SR).

245. Phillips CO, Wright SM, Kern DE, et al. Comprehensive discharge planning with postdischarge support for older patients with congestive heart failure: a meta-analysis. JAMA. 2004 Mar 17;291(11):1358-67. PMID: 15026403. Exclusion Code: X8 (SR).

246. Pihl E, Cider Å, Strömberg A, et al. Exercise in elderly patients with chronic heart failure in primary care: Effects on physical capacity and health-related quality of life. European Journal of Cardiovascular Nursing. 2011;10(3):150-8. PMID: 2011213329. Language: English. Entry Date: 20110916. Revision Date: 20120727. Publication Type: journal article. Exclusion Code: X2.

247. Pinna GD, Maestri R, Andrews D, et al. Home telemonitoring of vital signs and cardiorespiratory signals in heart failure patients: system architecture and feasibility of the HHH model. Int J Cardiol. 2007 Sep 3;120(3):371-9. PMID: 17189654. Exclusion Code: X2.

248. Piotrowicz E, Baranowski R, Bilinska M, et al. A new model of home-based telemonitored cardiac rehabilitation in patients with heart failure: effectiveness, quality of life, and adherence. Eur J Heart Fail. 2010 Feb;12(2):164-71. PMID: 20042423. Exclusion Code: X2.

249. Polisena J, Tran K, Cimon K, et al. Home telemonitoring for congestive heart failure: a systematic review and meta-analysis. J Telemed Telecare. 2010;16(2):68-76. PMID: 20008054. Exclusion Code: X8 (SR).

250. Powell LH, Calvin JE, Jr., Richardson D, et al. Self-management counseling in patients with heart failure: the heart failure adherence and retention randomized behavioral trial. JAMA. 2010 Sep 22;304(12):1331-8. PMID: 20858878. Exclusion Code: X6.

251. Prescott E, Hjardem-Hansen R, Dela F, et al. Effects of a 14-month low-cost maintenance training program in patients with chronic systolic heart failure: a randomized study. Eur J Cardiovasc Prev Rehabil. 2009 Aug;16(4):430-7. PMID: 19491687. Exclusion Code: X5.

252. Proctor EK, Morrow-Howell N, Kaplan SJ. Implementation of discharge plans for chronically ill elders discharged home. Health Soc Work. 1996 Feb;21(1):30-40. PMID: 8626156. Exclusion Code: X5.

253. Proctor EK, Morrow-Howell N, Li H, et al. Adequacy of home care and hospital readmission for elderly congestive heart failure patients. Health Soc Work. 2000 May;25(2):87-96. PMID: 10845143. Exclusion Code: X3.

254. Pugh LC, Tringali RA, Boehmer J, et al. Partners in care: a model of collaboration. Holist Nurs Pract. 1999;13(2):61-5. PMID: 1999048053. Language: English. Entry Date: 19990701. Revision Date: 20101231. Publication Type: journal article. Exclusion Code: X1.

255. Quinn C. Low-technology heart failure care in home health: improving patient outcomes. Home Healthc Nurse. 2006 Sep;24(8):533-40. PMID: 17012959. Exclusion Code: X2.

256. Radhakrishnan K, Jacelon C. Impact of Telehealth on Patient Self-management of Heart Failure: A Review of Literature. J Cardiovasc Nurs. 2012 2012 Jan-Feb;27(1):33-43. PMID: 2011419631. Language: English. Entry Date: 20120217. Revision Date: 20120217. Publication Type: journal article. Exclusion Code: X5.

257. Ramaekers BL, Janssen-Boyne JJ, Gorgels AP, et al. Adherence among telemonitored patients with heart failure to pharmacological and nonpharmacological recommendations. Telemed J E Health. 2009 Jul-Aug;15(6):517-24. PMID: 19566401. Exclusion Code: X5.

258. Ritchie C, Richman J, Sobko H, et al. The E-coach transition support computer telephony implementation study: protocol of a randomized trial. Contemp Clin Trials. 2012 Nov;33(6):1172-9. PMID: 22922245. Exclusion Code: X5.

259. Rosenman MB, Holmes AM, Ackermann RT, et al. The Indiana Chronic Disease Management Program. Milbank Q. 2006;84(1):135-63. PMID: 16529571. Exclusion Code: X1.

260. Roth A, Kajiloti I, Elkayam I, et al. Telecardiology for patients with chronic heart failure: the 'SHL' experience in Israel. Int J Cardiol. 2004 Oct;97(1):49-55. PMID: 15336806. Exclusion Code: X2.

261. Roth A, Korb H, Gadot R, et al. Telecardiology for patients with acute or chronic cardiac complaints: the 'SHL' experience in Israel and Germany. Int J Med Inform. 2006 Sep;75(9):643-5. PMID: 16765634. Exclusion Code: X8.

262. Savard LA, Thompson DR, Clark AM. A meta-review of evidence on heart failure disease management programs: the challenges of describing and synthesizing evidence on complex interventions. Trials. 2011;12:194. PMID: 21846340. Exclusion Code: X8 (SR).

263. Scalvini S, Capomolla S, Zanelli E, et al. Effect of home-based telecardiology on chronic heart failure: costs and outcomes. J Telemed Telecare. 2005;1:16-8. Exclusion Code: X2.

264. Scalvini S, Zanelli E, Paletta L, et al. Chronic heart failure home-based management with a telecardiology system: a comparison between patients followed by general practitioners and by a cardiology department. J Telemed Telecare. 2006;1:46-8. Exclusion Code: X8.

265. Scalvini S, Zanelli E, Volterrani M, et al. A pilot study of nurse-led, home-based telecardiology for patients with chronic heart failure. J Telemed Telecare. 2004;10(2):113-7. Exclusion Code: X2.

266. Scherr D, Kastner P, Kollmann A, et al. Effect of home-based telemonitoring using mobile phone technology on the outcome of heart failure patients after an episode of acute decompensation: randomized controlled trial. J Med Internet Res. 2009;11(3):e34. PMID: 19687005. Exclusion Code: X2.

267. Schmidt S, Schuchert A, Krieg T, et al. Home telemonitoring in patients with chronic heart failure: a chance to improve patient care? Dtsch Arztebl Int. 2010 Feb;107(8):131-8. PMID: 20300221. Exclusion Code: X8 (SR).

268. Schneider JK, Hornberger S, Booker J, et al. A medication discharge planning program: measuring the effect on readmissions. Clin Nurs Res. 1993 Feb;2(1):41-53. PMID: 8453387. Exclusion Code: X8.

269. Schou M, Gustafsson F, Videbaek L, et al. Extended heart failure clinic follow-up in low-risk patients: a randomized clinical trial (NorthStar). Eur Heart J. 2013 Feb;34(6):432-42. PMID: 22875412. Exclusion Code: X2.

270. Scott LD, Setter-Kline K, Britton AS. The effects of nursing interventions to enhance mental health and quality of life among individuals with heart failure. Appl Nurs Res. 2004 Nov;17(4):248-56. PMID: 15573333. Exclusion Code: X2.

271. Seibert PS, Whitmore TA, Patterson C, et al. Telemedicine facilitates CHF home health care for those with systolic dysfunction. Int J Telemed Appl. 2008;235031(10):235031. Exclusion Code: X2.

272. Senden PJ, Sabelis LW, Zonderland ML, et al. The effect of physical training on workload, upper leg muscle function and muscle areas in patients with chronic heart failure. Int J Cardiol. 2005 Apr 20;100(2):293-300. PMID: 15823638. Exclusion Code: X2.

273. Seto E. Cost comparison between telemonitoring and usual care of heart failure: a systematic review. Telemed J E Health. 2008 Sep;14(7):679-86. PMID: 18817497. Exclusion Code: X1.

274. Seto E, Leonard KJ, Cafazzo JA, et al. Mobile phone-based telemonitoring for heart failure management: a randomized controlled trial. J Med Internet Res. 2012;14(1):e31. PMID: 22356799. Exclusion Code: X2.

275. Seto E, Leonard KJ, Cafazzo JA, et al. Developing healthcare rule-based expert systems: case study of a heart failure telemonitoring system. Int J Med Inform. 2012 Aug;81(8):556-65. PMID: 22465288. Exclusion Code: X2.

276. Shah MR, Flavell CM, Weintraub JR, et al. Intensity and focus of heart failure disease management after hospital discharge. Am Heart J. 2005 Apr;149(4):715-21. PMID: 15990758. Exclusion Code: X5.

277. Shah MR, Whellan DJ, Peterson ED, et al. Delivering heart failure disease management in 3 tertiary care centers: key clinical components and venues of care. Am Heart J. 2008 Apr;155(4):764 e1-5. PMID: 18371490. Exclusion Code: X5.

278. Shah NB, Der E, Ruggerio C, et al. Prevention of hospitalizations for heart failure with an interactive home monitoring program. Am Heart J. 1998;135(3):373-8. Exclusion Code: X2.

279. Shearer NB, Cisar N, Greenberg EA. A telephone-delivered empowerment intervention with patients diagnosed with heart failure. Heart Lung. 2007 May-Jun;36(3):159-69. PMID: 17509423. Exclusion Code: X5.

280. Sisk JE, Hebert PL, Horowitz CR, et al. Effects of nurse management on the quality of heart failure care in minority communities: a randomized trial. Ann Intern Med. 2006 Aug 15;145(4):273-83. PMID: 16908918. Exclusion Code: X2.

281. Smart NA, Steele M. A comparison of 16 weeks of continuous vs intermittent exercise training in chronic heart failure patients. Congest Heart Fail. 2012 Jul-Aug;18(4):205-11. PMID: 22809258. Exclusion Code: X2.

282. Smeulders ES, van Haastregt JC, Ambergen T, et al. The impact of a self-management group programme on health behaviour and healthcare utilization among congestive heart failure patients. Eur J Heart Fail. 2009 Jun;11(6):609-16. PMID: 19359326. Exclusion Code: X2.

283. Smeulders ES, van Haastregt JC, Ambergen T, et al. Nurse-led self-management group programme for patients with congestive heart failure: randomized controlled trial. J Adv Nurs. 2010 Jul;66(7):1487-99. PMID: 20492026. Exclusion Code: X2.

284. Smeulders ES, van Haastregt JC, Janssen-Boyne JJ, et al. Feasibility of a group-based self-management program among congestive heart failure patients. Heart Lung. 2009 Nov-Dec;38(6):499-512. PMID: 19944874. Exclusion Code: X5.

285. Sochalski J, Jaarsma T, Krumholz HM, et al. What works in chronic care management: the case of heart failure. Health Aff (Millwood). 2009 2009 Jan-Feb;28(1):179-89. PMID: 2010153617. Language: English. Entry Date: 20090306. Revision Date: 20110513. Publication Type: journal article. Exclusion Code: X8.

286. Sofer D. APNs: improved outcomes at lower costs: older adults with heart failure fare better with transitional care after hospitalization. Am J Nurs. 2004 Sep;104(9):19. PMID: 15365321. Exclusion Code: X1.

287. Soran OZ, Feldman AM, Pina IL, et al. Cost of medical services in older patients with heart failure: those receiving enhanced monitoring using a computer-based telephonic monitoring system compared with those in usual care: the Heart Failure Home Care trial. J Card Fail. 2010 Nov;16(11):859-66. PMID: 21055649. Exclusion Code: X2.

288. Soran OZ, Pina IL, Lamas GA, et al. A randomized clinical trial of the clinical effects of enhanced heart failure monitoring using a computer-based telephonic monitoring system in older minorities and women. J Card Fail. 2008 Nov;14(9):711-7. PMID: 18995174. Exclusion Code: X2.

289. Spruit MA, Eterman RM, Hellwig VA, et al. Effects of moderate-to-high intensity resistance training in patients with chronic heart failure. Heart. 2009 Sep;95(17):1399-408. PMID: 19342376. Exclusion Code: X5.

290. Stauffer BD, Fullerton C, Fleming N, et al. Effectiveness and cost of a transitional care program for heart failure: a prospective study with concurrent controls. Arch Intern Med. 2011 Jul 25;171(14):1238-43. PMID: 21788541. Exclusion Code: X8.

291. Stewart, Vandenbroek, Pearson. Prolonged beneficial effects of a home-based intervention on unplanned readmissions and mortality among congestive heart failure patients. [abstract]. Aust N Z J Med. 1999:112. PMID: CN-00319319. Exclusion Code: X6.

292. Stewart S, Carrington MJ, Marwick TH, et al. Impact of home versus clinic-based management of chronic heart failure: the WHICH? (Which Heart Failure Intervention Is Most Cost-Effective & Consumer Friendly in Reducing Hospital Care) multicenter, randomized trial. J Am Coll Cardiol. 2012 Oct 2;60(14):1239-48. PMID: 23017533. Exclusion Code: X2.

293. Stewart S, Horowitz JD. Home-based intervention in congestive heart failure: long-term implications on readmission and survival. Circulation. 2002 Jun 18;105(24):2861-6. PMID: 12070114. Exclusion Code: X6.

294. Stewart S, Horowitz JD. Detecting early clinical deterioration in chronic heart failure patients post-acute hospitalisation-a critical component of multidisciplinary, home-based intervention? Eur J Heart Fail. 2002 Jun;4(3):345-51. PMID: 12034161. Exclusion Code: X8.

295. Stewart S, Vandenbroek AJ, Pearson S, et al. Prolonged beneficial effects of a home-based intervention on unplanned readmissions and mortality among patients with congestive heart failure. Arch Intern Med. 1999 Feb 8;159(3):257-61. PMID: 9989537. Exclusion Code: X6.

296. Stewart S, Vandenbroek AJ, Pearson S, et al. A home-based intervention reduced out-of-hospital deaths and hospitalizations in CHF... including commentary by Farmer A. Evidence Based Medicine. 1999;4(4):115-. PMID: 1999066451. Language: English. Entry Date: 19991001. Revision Date: 20101231. Publication Type: journal article. Exclusion Code: X1.

297. Stromberg A, Dahlstrom U, Fridlund B. Computer-based education for patients with chronic heart failure. A randomised, controlled, multicentre trial of the effects on knowledge, compliance and quality of life. Patient Educ Couns. 2006 Dec;64(1-3):128-35. PMID: 16469469. Exclusion Code: X2.

298. Subramanian U, Hopp F, Lowery J, et al. Research in home-care telemedicine: challenges in patient recruitment. Telemed J E Health. 2004 Summer;10(2):155-61. PMID: 15319045. Exclusion Code: X1.

299. Sullivan MJ, Wood L, Terry J, et al. The Support, Education, and Research in Chronic Heart Failure Study (SEARCH): a mindfulness-based psychoeducational intervention improves depression and clinical symptoms in patients with chronic heart failure. Am Heart J. 2009 Jan;157(1):84-90. PMID: 19081401. Exclusion Code: X3.

300. Supervia A, Aranda D, Marquez MA, et al. Predicting length of hospitalisation of elderly patients, using the Barthel Index. Age Ageing. 2008 May;37(3):339-42. PMID: 18339617. Exclusion Code: X3.

301. Swanson KS, Gevirtz RN, Brown M, et al. The effect of biofeedback on function in patients with heart failure. Appl Psychophysiol Biofeedback. 2009 Jun;34(2):71-91. PMID: 19205870. Exclusion Code: X2.

302. Tabidze GA, Kobaladze NI, Tsibadze TA. [Assessment of efficiency of patients' therapeutic education in chronic heart failure treatment]. Georgian medical news. 2009(175):35-8. PMID: CN-00743741. Exclusion Code: X1.

303. Tai M, Meininger JC, Frazier LQ. A systematic review of exercise interventions in patients with heart failure. Biological Research for Nursing. 2008;10(2):156-82. PMID: 2010064952. Language: English. Entry Date: 20090116. Revision Date: 20101231. Publication Type: journal article. Exclusion Code: X3.

304. Takeda A, Taylor SJ, Taylor RS, et al. Clinical service organisation for heart failure. Cochrane Database Syst Rev. 2012;9:CD002752. PMID: 22972058. Exclusion Code: X8 (SR).

305. Taylor Rod S, Dalal H, Jolly K, et al. Home-based versus centre-based cardiac rehabilitation. Cochrane Database of Systematic Reviews. 2010(1)PMID: CD007130. Exclusion Code: X2.

306. Thomas R, Huntley A, Mann M, et al. Specialist clinics for reducing emergency admissions in patients with heart failure: a systematic review and meta-analysis of randomised controlled trials. Heart. 2013 Feb;99(4):233-9. PMID: 23355639. Exclusion Code: X8 (SR).

307. Tomita MR, Tsai BM, Fisher NM, et al. Improving adherence to exercise in patients with heart failure through internet-based self-management. J Am Geriatr Soc. 2008(10):1981-3. PMID: CN-00667339. Exclusion Code: X5.

308. Tompkins C, Orwat J. A Randomized Trial of Telemonitoring Heart Failure Patients. J Healthc Manag. 2010;55(5):312-22. PMID: 2010862502. Language: English. Entry Date: 20110107. Revision Date: 20110805. Publication Type: journal article. Exclusion Code: X2.

309. Topp R, Tucker D, Weber C. Effect of a clinical case manager/clinical nurse specialist on patients hospitalized with congestive heart failure. Nurs Case Manag. 1998(4):140-7. PMID: CN-00497710. Exclusion Code: X8.

310. Tran K, Polisena J, Coyle D, et al. Home telehealth for chronic disease management (Structured abstract). Database of Abstracts of Reviews of Effects. 2008(1):1. PMID: DARE-12010008017. Exclusion Code: X2.

311. Tribouilloy C, Rusinaru D, Mahjoub H, et al. Impact of echocardiography in patients hospitalized for heart failure: a prospective observational study. Arch Cardiovasc Dis. 2008 Jul-Aug;101(7-8):465-73. PMID: 18848689. Exclusion Code: X3.

312. Tsuchihashi-Makaya M, Matsuo H, Kakinoki S, et al. Home-based disease management program to improve psychological status in patients with heart failure in Japan. Circ J. 2013;77(4):926-33. PMID: 23502992. Exclusion Code: X6.

313. Turner DA, Paul S, Stone MA, et al. Cost-effectiveness of a disease management programme for secondary prevention of coronary heart disease and heart failure in primary care. Heart. 2008;94(12):1601-6. PMID: 2010121302. Language: English. Entry Date: 20090213. Revision Date: 20101231. Publication Type: journal article. Exclusion Code: X2.

314. Tyni-Lenné R, Gordon A, Sylvén C. Improved quality of life in chronic heart failure patients following local endurance training with leg muscles. J Card Fail. 1996(2):111-7. PMID: CN-00129813. Exclusion Code: X2.

315. Valle R, Canali C, Giovinazzo P, et al. [Is early discharge possible in patients with uncomplicated heart failure? Cost-efficacy analysis]. Italian heart journal. Supplement : official journal of the Italian Federation of Cardiology. 2003(12):965-72. PMID: CN-00489029. Exclusion Code: X1.

316. Valle R, Carbonieri E, Tenderini P, et al. [Proposed protocol for the ambulatory management of patients discharged with heart failure diagnosis: collaborative project Venice-HF]. Italian heart journal. Supplement : official journal of the Italian Federation of Cardiology. 2004(4):282-91. PMID: CN-00489742. Exclusion Code: X1.

317. Vallina H, Effken J. Telemonitoring and heart failure outcomes. Commun Nurs Res. 2010;43:433-. PMID: 2010750401. Language: English. Entry Date: 20101210. Revision Date: 20101231. Publication Type: journal article. Exclusion Code: X8.

318. van der Meer S, Zwerink M, van Brussel M, et al. Effect of outpatient exercise training programmes in patients with chronic heart failure: a systematic review. Eur J Prev Cardiol. 2012 Aug;19(4):795-803. PMID: 22988592. Exclusion Code: X3.

319. Varma S, McElnay JC, Hughes CM, et al. Pharmaceutical care of patients with congestive heart failure: interventions and outcomes. Pharmacotherapy. 1999 Jul;19(7):860-9. PMID: 10417035. Exclusion Code: X2.

320. Vavouranakis I, Lambrogiannakis E, Markakis G, et al. Effect of home-based intervention on hospital readmission and quality of life in middle-aged patients with severe congestive heart failure: a 12-month follow up study. European Journal of Cardiovascular Nursing. 2003;2(2):105-11. PMID: 2003138521. Language: English. Entry Date: 20031017. Revision Date: 20101231. Publication Type: journal article. Exclusion Code: X6.

321. Veroff DR, Sullivan LA, Shoptaw EJ, et al. Improving self-care for heart failure for seniors: the impact of video and written education and decision aids. Popul Health Manag. 2012 Feb;15(1):37-45. PMID: 22004181. Exclusion Code: X2.

322. Villani A, Malfatto G, Della Rosa F, et al. [Disease management for heart failure patients: role of wireless technologies for telemedicine. The ICAROS project]. Giornale italiano di cardiologia (2006). 2007(2):107-14. PMID: CN-00579624. Exclusion Code: X1.

323. Vinson JM, Rich MW, Sperry JC, et al. Early readmission of elderly patients with congestive heart failure. J Am Geriatr Soc. 1990 Dec;38(12):1290-5. PMID: 2254567. Exclusion Code: X3.

324. Wade MJ, Desai AS, Spettell CM, et al. Telemonitoring with case management for seniors with heart failure. Am J Manag Care. 2011 Mar;17(3):e71-9. PMID: 21504262. Exclusion Code: X2.

325. Wakefield BJ, Boren SA, Groves PS, et al. Heart Failure Care Management Programs: A Review of Study Interventions and Meta-Analysis of Outcomes. J Cardiovasc Nurs. 2013 2013 Jan-Feb;28(1):8-19. PMID: 2011883998. Language: English. Entry Date: 20130215. Revision Date: 20130215. Publication Type: journal article. Exclusion Code: X8 (SR).

326. Wall HK, Ballard J, Troped P, et al. Impact of home-based, supervised exercise on congestive heart failure. Int J Cardiol. 2010(2):267-70. PMID: CN-00813626. Exclusion Code: X2.

327. Wang SP, Lin LC, Lee CM, et al. Effectiveness of a self-care program in improving symptom distress and quality of life in congestive heart failure patients: a preliminary study. J Nurs Res. 2011 Dec;19(4):257-66. PMID: 22089651. Exclusion Code: X8.

328. Weinberger M, Oddone EZ, Henderson WG. Does increased access to primary care reduce hospital readmissions? Veterans Affairs Cooperative Study Group on Primary Care and Hospital Readmission. N Engl J Med. 1996 May 30;334(22):1441-7. PMID: 8618584. Exclusion Code: X2.

329. Weintraub A, Gregory D, Patel AR, et al. A multicenter randomized controlled evaluation of automated home monitoring and telephonic disease management in patients recently hospitalized for congestive heart failure: the SPAN-CHF II trial. J Card Fail. 2010 Apr;16(4):285-92. PMID: 20350694. Exclusion Code: X2.

330. Wheeler EC, Waterhouse JK. Telephone interventions by nursing students: improving outcomes for heart failure patients in the community. J Community Health Nurs. 2006 Fall;23(3):137-46. PMID: 16863399. Exclusion Code: X2.

331. Whellan DJ, Hasselblad V, Peterson E, et al. Metaanalysis and review of heart failure disease management randomized controlled clinical trials. Am Heart J. 2005 Apr;149(4):722-9. PMID: 15990759. Exclusion Code: X8 (SR).

332. White M, Garbez R, Carroll M, et al. Is "teach-back" associated with knowledge retention and hospital readmission in hospitalized heart failure patients? J Cardiovasc Nurs. 2013 Mar-Apr;28(2):137-46. PMID: 22580624. Exclusion Code: X4.

333. Whitten P, Bergman A, Meese MA, et al. St. Vincent's Home telehealth for congestive heart failure patients. Telemed J E Health. 2009;15(2):148-53. Exclusion Code: X2.

334. Whitten P, Mickus M. Home telecare for COPD/CHF patients: outcomes and perceptions. J Telemed Telecare. 2007(2):69-73. PMID: CN-00609354. Exclusion Code: X2.

335. Wielenga RP, Huisveld IA, Bol E, et al. Exercise training in elderly patients with chronic heart failure [corrected] [published erratum appears in CORONARY ARTERY DIS 1999; 10(1): 57]. Coron Artery Dis. 1998;9(11):765-70. PMID: 1999072500. Language: English. Entry Date: 19991101. Revision Date: 20101231. Publication Type: journal article. Exclusion Code: X2.

336. Wierzchowiecki M, Poprawski K, Nowicka A, et al. [New multidisciplinary heart failure care program (six-month preliminary observation)]. Polski merkuriusz lekarski : organ Polskiego Towarzystwa Lekarskiego. 2006(126):511-5. PMID: CN-00587715. Exclusion Code: X1.

337. Wierzchowiecki M, Poprawski K, Nowicka A, et al. A new programme of multidisciplinary care for patients with heart failure in Poznan: one-year follow-up. Kardiol Pol. 2006 Oct;64(10):1063-70; discussion 71-2. PMID: 17089238. Exclusion Code: X6.

338. Winkelmann ER, Chiappa GR, Lima CO, et al. Addition of inspiratory muscle training to aerobic training improves cardiorespiratory responses to exercise in patients with heart failure and inspiratory muscle weakness. Am Heart J. 2009 Nov;158(5):768 e1-7. PMID: 19853695. Exclusion Code: X2.

339. Witham MD, Fulton RL, Greig CA, et al. Efficacy and cost of an exercise program for functionally impaired older patients with heart failure: a randomized controlled trial. Circ Heart Fail. 2012 Mar 1;5(2):209-16. PMID: 22271753. Exclusion Code: X2.

340. Wongpiriyayothar A, Pothiban L, Liehr P, et al. Effects of home-based care program on symptom alleviation and well-being among persons with chronic heart failure. Thai Journal of Nursing Research. 2008 2008 Jan-Mar;12(1):25-39. PMID: 2009811975. Language: English. Entry Date: 20080606. Revision Date: 20101231. Publication Type: journal article. Exclusion Code: X5.

341. Wootton R, Gramotnev H, Hailey D. A randomized controlled trial of telephone-supported care coordination in patients with congestive heart failure. J Telemed Telecare. 2009;15(4):182-6. PMID: 19471029. Exclusion Code: X2.

342. Wright SP, Walsh H, Ingley KM, et al. Uptake of self-management strategies in a heart failure management programme. Eur J Heart Fail. 2003 Jun;5(3):371-80. PMID: 12798837. Exclusion Code: X6.

343. Yamada S, Shimizu Y, Suzuki M, et al. Functional limitations predict the risk of rehospitalization among patients with chronic heart failure. Circ J. 2012;76(7):1654-61. PMID: 22484978. Exclusion Code: X2.

344. Yancy CW, Abraham WT, Albert NM, et al. Quality of care of and outcomes for African Americans hospitalized with heart failure: findings from the OPTIMIZE-HF (Organized Program to Initiate Lifesaving Treatment in Hospitalized Patients With Heart Failure) registry. J Am Coll Cardiol. 2008 Apr 29;51(17):1675-84. PMID: 18436120. Exclusion Code: X4.

345. Yehle KS, Plake KS. Self-efficacy and educational interventions in heart failure: a review of the literature. J Cardiovasc Nurs. 2010 May-Jun;25(3):175-88. PMID: 20386241. Exclusion Code: X5.

346. Yu DS, Thompson DR, Lee DT. Disease management programmes for older people with heart failure: crucial characteristics which improve post-discharge outcomes. Eur Heart J. 2006 Mar;27(5):596-612. PMID: 16299021. Exclusion Code: X6.

347. Zugck C, Nelles M, Frankenstein L, et al. [Telemonitoring in chronic heart failure patients. Which diagnostic finding prevents hospital readmission?]. Herzschrittmachertherapie & Elektrophysiologie. 2005(3):176-82. PMID: CN-00530465. Exclusion Code: X1.

348. Zwisler AD, Schou L, Soja AM, et al. A randomized clinical trial of hospital-based, comprehensive cardiac rehabilitation versus usual care for patients with congestive heart failure, ischemic heart disease, or high risk of ischemic heart disease (the DANREHAB trial)--design, intervention, and population. Am Heart J. 2005(5):899. PMID: CN-00531971. Exclusion Code: X1.

349. Zwisler AD, Soja AM, Rasmussen S, et al. Hospital-based comprehensive cardiac rehabilitation versus usual care among patients with congestive heart failure, ischemic heart disease, or high risk of ischemic heart disease: 12-month results of a randomized clinical trial. Am Heart J. 2008 Jun;155(6):1106-13. PMID: 18513526. Exclusion Code: X2.

Appendix C. Characteristics of Interventions

Table C1. Intervention components for primarily educational interventions

Author, Year	Risk of Bias	Intensity	Primary Mode of Delivery	Delivery Personnel	Self-Care Management Education/Promotion	Weight Monitoring Education or Promotion	Diet/Sodium Restriction Education or Promotion	Promotion of Medication Adherence	Exercise Education or Promotion	Other or Unspecified HF Education	Medication Reconciliation	Setting/Timing of Education[a]	Planned Telephone Follow-up Post d/c	Timing of First Phone or TM Follow-up (Days)	Phone Follow-up Conducted by Same Personnel Delivering Inpatient Intervention Component	Patient Phone HF Hotline	Timing of First Clinic Visit Post d/c
Albert et al., 2007[1]	High	Low	Video	NA	x	x	x	x	x	-	-	Post-d/c	-	-	-	-	-
Koelling et al., 2005[2]	Low	Low	Face-to-Face	Nurse	x	x	x	x	-	x	-	Pre-d/c	-	-	-	-	-
Linne et al., 2006[3]	Unclear	Low	Interactive CD-ROM	NA	x	x	-	x	x	-	-	Both	-	-	-	-	-
Nucifora et al., 2006[4]	Med	Med.	Face-to-Face	Nurse	x	x	x	x	-	-	-	Both	x	> 7 days	x	x	> 14 days

Note: x = this component was part of the study intervention and "-" = this component was not included in the intervention

[a] Both = both pre- and post-d/c.

Abbreviations: CD-ROM = compact disk read-only memory; d/c = discharge; HF = heart failure; MDS = multidisciplinary; Med = Medium; NA = not applicable.

Table C2. Intervention components for home visiting interventions (Part 1)

Author, Year	Risk of Bias	Intensity	Primary Mode of Delivery	Delivery Personnel	Self-Care Management Education/Promotion	Weight-Monitoring Education or Promotion	Diet/Sodium Restriction Education or Promotion	Promotion of Medication Adherence	Exercise Education or Promotion	Other or Unspecified HF Education	Medication Reconciliation	Setting/Timing of Education[a]
Aldamiz-Echevarria Iraúrgui et al., 2007[5]	Med	High	Face-to-Face	MDS	x	x	x	x	-	x	x	Post-d/c
Holland et al., 2007[6]	Med	Med	Face-to-Face	Pharm.	x	x	x	x	x	x	x	Post-d/c
Jaarsma et al., 1999[7]	Med	Med	Face-to-Face	Nurse	x	-	x	x	-	x	-	Both
Kimmelstiel et al., 2004[8]	Med	Med	Face-to-Face	Nurse	x	x	x	x	-	x	-	Post-d/c
Kwok et al., 2007[9]	Med	High	Face-to-Face	Nurse	x	-	x	x	x	-	x	Both
Naylor et al., 2004[10]	Low	High	Face-to-Face	Nurse	x	x	x	x	-	-	x	Both
Pugh et al., 2001[11]	High	Med	Face-to-Face	Nurse	x	-	-	-	-	x	-	Other
Rich et al., 1993[12]	Med	High	Face-to-Face	MDS	x	x	x	x	-	x	x	Both
Rich et al., 1995[13]	Med	High	Face-to-Face	MDS	x	x	x	x	-	x	x	Both
Sethares et al., 2004[14]	High	Med	Face-to-Face	Nurse	x	x	x	x	-	-	-	Both
Stewart et al., 1998[15]	Med	Med	Face-to-Face	Nurse	x	-	-	x	-	-	-	Both
Stewart et al., 1999[16]	Med	Med	Face-to-Face	Nurse	x	x	-	x	x	-	-	Post-d/c (based on assessment)
Thompson et al., 2005[17]	High	High	Face-to-Face	Nurse	x	x	x	x	x	x	x	Both
Triller et al., 2008[18]	Unclear	Med	Face-to-Face	Pharm.	x	x	x	x	-	-	x	Post-d/c

Note: x = this component was part of the study intervention and "-" = this component was not included in the intervention.

[a] Both = both pre- and post-d/c.

Abbreviations: d/c= discharge; HF = heart failure; MDS = multidisciplinary; Med = Medium; Pharm. = Pharmacist

Table C3. Intervention components for home visiting interventions (Part 2)

Author, Year	Risk of Bias	Transition Coach or Coordination Between Inpatient/ Outpatient Providers	Individua-lized D/C Plan	Provider Continuity	Planned Tele-phone Follow-up Post D/C	Timing of First Phone or TM Follow-up (Days)	Phone Follow-up Conducted by Same Personnel Delivering Inpatient Intervention Component	Series of Structured Calls	Patient Phone Hotline	Timing of First Home Visit (Days)
Aldamiz-Echevarría Iraúrgui et al., 2007[5]	Med	-	-	-	-	-	-	-	x	1-2
Holland et al., 2007[6]	Med	-	-	-	-	-	-	-	-	<14
Jaarsma et al., 1999[7]	Med	-	x	-	x	≤7	x	-	x	<7
Kimmelstiel et al., 2004[8]	Med	-	-	-	-	-	-	x (as needed)	x	<7
Kwok et al., 2007[9]	Med	x	-	x	-	-	-	-	x	<7
Naylor et al., 2004[10]	Low	x	x	-	-	-	-	-	x	<1
Pugh et al., 2001[11]	High	-	x	-	x	-	-	x	-	unclear
Rich et al., 1993[12]	Med	x	x	-	x (as needed)	-	x	-	x	1-2
Rich et al., 1995[13]	Med	x	x	-	x (as needed)	-	x	-	x	1-2
Sethares et al., 2004[14]	High	x	-	-	-	-	-	-	-	>7
Stewart et al., 1998[15]	Med	x	-	-	-	-	-	-	-	<7
Stewart et al., 1999[16]	Med	-	-	-	-	-	-	-	-	>7
Thompson et al., 2005[17]	High	x	-	-	-	-	-	-	x	>7
Triller et al., 2008[18]	Unclear	-	-	-	-	-	-	-	-	<7

Note: x = this component was part of the study intervention and "-" = this component was not included in the intervention.

Abbreviations: d/c = discharge; HF = heart failure; hrs = hours; Med = Medium; TM = telemonitoring.

Table C4. Intervention components for home visiting interventions (Part 3)

Author, Year	Risk of Bias	Number of Scheduled Home Visits	Medication Reconciliation During Home Visit	Unspecified HF Education/ Promotion During Home Visit	Symptom Checklist or Clinical Assessment During Home Visit (e.g. History, Symptoms)	Physical Exam During Home Visit	Home Visiting Personnel Coordinates Care or Collaborates With Outpatient Provider	Clinic Personnel On-Call/ Available for Acute Symptom Management (Outside of Scheduled Appt)	Medication Optimization; Pre-D/C or During Intervention
Aldamiz-Echevarría Iraúrgui et al., 2007[5]	Med	2 to 3	x	x	x	x	-	-	x
Holland et al., 2007[6]	Med	2	x	x	x	-	x	-	x
Jaarsma et al., 1999[7]	Med	1	-	x	-	-	-	-	-
Kimmelstiel et al., 2004[8]	Med	1	x	x	x	-	x	-	-
Kwok et al., 2007[9]	Med	6[a]	x	-	x	x	x	-	x
Naylor et al., 2004[10]	Low	8	x	x	x	-	x	-	-
Pugh et al., 2001[11]	High	1[b]	x	x	-	-	-	-	-
Rich et al., 1993[12]	Med	>3	x	x	-	x	-	-	x
Rich et al., 1995[13]	Med	>3	x	x	-	x	-	-	x
Sethares et al., 2004[14]	High	2 to 3	x	-	-	-	-	-	-
Stewart et al., 1998[15]	Med	1	x	x	-	-	x	-	-
Stewart et al., 1999[16]	Med	1	-	x	x	x	x	-	-
Thompson et al., 2005[17]	High	1	-	x	x	x	-	x	x
Triller et al., 2008[18]	Unclear	other	x	x	-	x	x	-	x

Note: x = this component was part of the study intervention and "-" = this component was not included in the intervention.

[a] In Kwok et al., an average of 6 visits took place, including the initial inpatient visit, but more visits were scheduled for individual patients if needed.[9]

[b] Additional visits were scheduled at home or in a clinic based on individual need.[19]

Abbreviations: appt = appointment; d/c = discharge; HF = heart failure; Med = Medium.

C-4

Table C5. Intervention components for clinic-based interventions (Part 1)

Author, Year	Risk of Bias	Intensity	Primary Mode of Delivery	Delivery Personnel	Self-Care Management Education/Promotion	Weight-Monitoring Education or Promotion	Diet/Sodium Restriction Education or Promotion	Promotion of Medication Adherence	Other or Unspecified HF Education	Medication Reconciliation	Setting/Timing of Education[a]	Transition Coach or Coordination Between Inpatient/Outpatient Providers
Ekman et al., 1998[20]	Med	Med	Face-to-Face	Nurse	-	x	-	x	-	-	Post-d/c	-
Stromberg et al., 2003[21]	Low	Med	Face-to-Face	Nurse	x	x	x	x	-	-	Post-d/c	-
Ducharme et al., 2005[22]	Low	High	Face-to-Face	MDS	x	x	x	x	x	x	Post-d/c	-
Kasper et al., 2002[23]	Low	High	Face-to-Face	MDS	x	-	-	-	x	-	Post-d/c	-
Liu et al., 2012[24]	Low	High	Face-to-Face	MDS	x	-	-	x	-	x	Both	x
McDonald et al., 2001[25]; McDonald et al., 2002[26]; Ledwidge et al., 2003[27]	Unclear	High	Face-to-Face	MDS	-	x	x	x	-	-	Both	-
Oddone et al., 1999[28]	Med	Med	Face-to-Face	PCP	-	-	-	-	-	-	Pre-d/c	-

Note: x = this component was part of the study intervention and "-" = this component was not included in the intervention.

[a] Both = both pre- and post-d/c.

Abbreviations: *d/c* = discharge; HF = heart failure; MDS = multidisciplinary; Med = Medium; PCP = primary care (physician, nurse in clinic).

C-5

Table C6. Intervention components for clinic-based interventions (Part 2)

Author, Year	Risk of Bias	Individualized D/C Plan	Provider Continuity	Medications Adjusted During Inpatient Stay	Planned Telephone Follow-Up Post D/C	Timing of First Phone or TM Follow-Up (Days)	Phone Follow-up Conducted by Same Personnel Delivering Inpatient Intervention Component	Series of Structured Calls	Patient Phone Hotline	Timing of First Clinic Visit Post D/C (Days)	Consultation With a Dietician	Clinic Personnel On-Call/ Available for Acute Symptom Management (Outside of Scheduled Appt)	Cardiac Rehab Component	Clinical Pharmacist Visit/ Consultation	Medication Optimization; Pre-D/C or During Intervention
Ekman et al., 1998[20]	Med	-	-	-	x	<7	-	-	x	NR	-	x	-	-	-
Stromberg et al., 2003[21]	Low	-	-	-	-	-	-	-	-	>14	x	x	x	x	-
Ducharme et al., 2005[22]	Low	-	-	-	x	≤3	-	x	-	≤14	x	x	-	x	x
Kasper et al., 2002[23]	Low	-	-	-	x	≤7	-	x	x	Unclear	-	-	-	-	x
Liu et al., 2012[24]	Low	x	-	-	x	≤7	unclear	x	x	≤7	x	x	-	-	x
McDonald et al., 2001[25]; McDonald et al., 2002[26]; Ledwidge et al., 2003[27]	Unclear	-	-	-	x	<7	x	x	x	<14	x	x	-	-	-
Oddone et al., 1999[28]	Med	x	-	-	x	1-2	-	-	-	<7	-	-	-	-	-

Note: x = this component was part of the study intervention and "-" = this component was not included in the intervention.

Abbreviations: d/c= discharge; hrs = hours; Med = Medium; NR = not reported; TM= telemonitoring.

C-6

Table C7. Intervention components for other interventions

Author, Year	Specific Type of Intervention	Risk of Bias	Intensity	Primary Mode of Delivery	Delivery Personnel	Self-Care Management Education/ Promotion	Weight Monitoring Education or Promotion	Diet/sodium Restriction Education or Promotion	Promotion of Medication Adherence	Exercise Education or Promotion	Other or Unspecified HF Education	Medication Reconciliation	Setting/ Timing of Education[a]	Planned Telephone Follow-up Post D/C	Timing of First Phone or TM Follow-up (Days)	Phone Follow-up Conducted by Same Personnel Delivering Inpatient Intervention Component
Davis et al., 2012[29]	Other (Cognitive Training)	Med	Med	Face-to-Face	Nurse	x	x	x	x	-	-	-	Both	x	≤7	x
Riegel et al., 2004[30]	Other (Peer Support)	High	Med	Face-to-Face; Telephone	Peer Support	x	x	x	x	-	-	-	Post-d/c	x	<7	-

Note: x = this component was part of the study intervention and "-" = this component was not included in the intervention.

[a] Both = both pre- and post-d/c.

Abbreviations: d/c= discharge; HF = heart failure; hrs = hours; Med = Medium.

Table C8. Intervention components for STS interventions (Part 1)

Author, Year	Risk of Bias	Intensity	Primary Mode of Delivery	Delivery Personnel	Self-care Management Education/Promotion	Weight-Monitoring Education or Promotion	Diet/Sodium Restriction Education or Promotion	Promotion of Medication Adherence	Exercise Education or promotion	Other or Unspecified HF Education	Medication Reconciliation	Setting/Timing of Education[a]	Transition Coach or Coordination Between Inpatient/Outpatient Providers
Angermann et al., 2011[31]	Med	High	Telephone; Face-to-Face	Nurse	x	x	x	X	x	x	-	Both	x
Barth et al., 2001[32]	High	Low	Telephone	Nurse	x	x	x	X	x	-	x	Post-d/c	-
Cabezas et al., 2006[33]	Med	Med	Telephone; Face-to-Face	Pharmacist	-	-	x	X	x	x	-	Both	-
Domingues et al., 2010[34]	Med	Low	Telephone	Nurse	x	x	-	X	x	x	-	Post-d/c	-
Duffy et al., 2010[35]	High	Med	Face-to-Face; Telephone	Nurse	x	x	-	X	-	x	-	Post-d/c	-
Dunagan et al., 2005[36]	Med	High	Telephone	Nurse	x	x	x	X	x	-	x	Post-d/c	-
Jerant et al., 2001[37], Jerant et al., 2003[38]	High	Med	Videophone; Telephone	Nurse	x	x	x	X	-	-	-	Both	-
Laramee et al., 2003[39]	Med	High	Telephone; Face-to-Face	Nurse-Case Manager	x	x	x	X	-	-	x	Both	x
Rainville et al., 1999[40]	Med	Med	Telephone; Face-to-Face	Pharmacist	-	x	-	X	-	x	-	Both	x
Riegel et al., 2002[41]	Med	Med	Telephone	Nurse	x	-	x	X	x	x	x	Post-d/c	-
Riegel et al., 2006[42]	Med	Med	Telephone	Nurse	x	-	x	X	-	x	-	Post-d/c	-
Tsuyuki et al., 2004[43]	Med	High	Telephone	Nurse	x	x	x	X	x	x	x	Both	-
Wakefield et al., 2008[44], Wakefield et al.,	Med	Med	Telephone	Nurse	x	x	x	x	-	-	-	Both	-

Table C8. Intervention components for STS interventions (Part 1) (continued)

Author, Year	Risk of Bias	Intensity	Primary Mode of Delivery	Delivery Personnel	Self-care Management Education/Promotion	Weight-Monitoring Education or Promotion	Diet/Sodium Restriction Education or Promotion	Promotion of Medication Adherence	Exercise Education or promotion	Other or Unspecified HF Education	Medication Reconciliation	Setting/Timing of Education[a]	Transition Coach or Coordination Between Inpatient/Outpatient Providers
Wakefield et al., 2008[44], Wakefield et al., 2009[45]	Med	Med	Videophone	Nurse	x	x	x	X	-	-	-	Both	-

Note: x = this component was part of the study intervention and "-" = this component was not included in the intervention.

[a] Both = both pre- and post-d/c.

Abbreviations: d/c= discharge; HF = heart failure; Med = Medium; STS = Structured Telephone Support.

Table C9. Intervention components for STS interventions (Part 2)

Author, Year	Risk of Bias	Individualized D/C Plan	Medications Adjusted During Inpatient Stay	Planned Telephone Follow-up Post D/C	Timing of First Phone or TM Follow-up (Days)	Phone Follow-up Conducted by Same Personnel Delivering Inpatient Intervention Component	Series of Structured Calls	Patient Phone Hotline	Unspecified HF Education/Promotion During Home Visit	Symptom Checklist or Clinical Assessment During Home Visit (e.g. History, symptoms)	Timing of First Clinic Visit Post D/C (Days)	Clinical Pharmacist Visit/Consultation
Angermann et al., 2011[31]	Med	-	-	x	≤7	x	x	x	-	-	-	-
Barth et al., 2001[32]	High	-	-	x	≤7	-	x	x	-	-	-	-
Cabezas et al., 2006[33]	Med	-	-	x	≤7	unclear	x	-	-	-	≥14	x
Domingues et al., 2010[34]	Med	-	-	x	≤7	-	x	-	-	-	-	-
Duffy et al., 2010[35]	High	-	-	x	NR	-	x	x	x	x	-	-
Dunagan et al., 2005[36]	Med	-	-	x	≤7	-	x	x	-	-	-	-
Jerant et al., 2001[37], Jerant et al., 2003[38]	High	-	-	x	>7	x	x	x	-	-	-	-
Laramee et al., 2003[39]	Med	x	-	x	≤7	x	x	x	-	-	-	-
Rainville et al., 1999[40]	Med	-	x	x	≤2	x	x	x	-	-	-	-
Riegel et al., 2002[41]	Med	-	-	x	≤7	-	x	-	-	-	-	-
Riegel et al., 2006[42]	Med	-	-	x	≤7	-	x	-	-	-	-	-
Tsuyuki et al., 2004[43]	Med	-	x	x	≤14	x	x	x	-	-	-	-
Wakefield et al., 2008[44], Wakefield et al., 2009[45]	Med	-	-	x	≤7	-	x	x	-	-	-	-
Wakefield et al., 2008[44],	Med	-	-	x	≤7	-	x	-	-	-	-	-

Wakefield et al.,
2009[45]

Note: x = this component was part of the study intervention and "-" = this component was not included in the intervention.

Abbreviations: CND = cannot determine; d/c= discharge; HF = heart failure; hrs = hours; Med = Medium; NR = not reported; STS = Structured Telephone Support; TM= telemonitoring.

Table C10. Intervention components for STS interventions (Part 3)

Author, Year	Risk of Bias	Medication Optimization; Pre-d/c or During Intervention	Timing of First Telehealth Contact After d/c	Intervention Involves Reinforcement of D/C Plan	Prescribed Protocol Used to Guide Assessment And/or Plan	Telehealth Service Coordinates Care With Outpatient Provider	TM Device has Automated Adherence Reminder	Device Can Transmit Vital Signs	Device Can Transmit Symptoms	Device Utilizes Technology That Allows Physical Exam
Angermann et al., 2011[31]	Med	-	-	-	x	x	-	-	-	-
Barth et al., 2001[32]	High	x	≤7	x	x	x	-	-	-	-
Cabezas et al., 2006[33]	Med	-	-	x	-	-	-	-	-	-
Domingues et al., 2010[34]	Med	-	-	-	-	-	-	-	-	-
Duffy et al., 2010[35]	High	-	-	-	x	-	-	-	-	-
Dunagan et al., 2005[36]	Med	-	-	-	-	x	-	-	x	x
Jerant et al., 2001[37]; Jerant et al., 2003[38]	High	-	>7	-	x	-	-	x	x	x
Laramee et al., 2003[39]	Med	-	≤7	x	x	x	-	x	-	-
Rainville et al., 1999[40]	Med	-	-	-	-	-	-	-	-	-
Riegel et al., 2002[41]	Med	-	≤7	x	x	x	-	-	-	-
Riegel et al., 2006[42]	Med	-	≤7	x	x	x (as needed)	-	-	-	-
Tsuyuki et al., 2004[43]	Med	-	-	-	-	-	-	-	-	-
Wakefield et al., 2008[44]; Wakefield et al., 2009[45]	Med	-	-	-	-	-	-	-	-	-
Wakefield et al., 2008[44]; Wakefield et al., 2009[45]	Med	-	≤7	x	x	x	-	-	x	x

Note: x = this component was part of the study intervention and "-" = this component was not included in the intervention.

Abbreviations: d/c= discharge; Med = Medium; STS = Structured Telephone Support; TM= telemonitoring.

Table C11. Intervention components for telemonitoring interventions (Part 1)

Author, Year	Risk of Bias	Intensity	Primary Mode of Delivery	Delivery Personnel	Self-Management Education/Promotion	Weight-Monitoring Education or Promotion	Diet/Sodium Restriction Education or Promotion	Promotion of Medication Adherence	Exercise Education or Promotion	Other or Unspecified HF Education	Medication Reconciliation	Setting/Timing of Education
Benatar et al., 2003[46]	Unclear	Med	Telephone	Nurse	-	-	X	x	-	-	-	Post-d/c
Dar et al., 2008[47]	Med	High	Remote monitoring	Nurse	x	-	-	-	-	-	-	Post-d/c
Dendale et al., 2012[48]	Unclear	Med	Remote monitoring	Nurse	x	x	X	x	x	-	-	Pre-d/c
Goldberg et al., 2003[49]	Med	High	Remote monitoring	Nurse	x	x	X	-	-	-	-	Pre-d/c
Jerant et al., 2001[37]; Jerant et al., 2003[38]	High	Med	Videophone, telephone	Nurse	x	x	X	x	-	-	-	Post-d/c
Pekmezaris et al., 2012[50]	Med	Med	Videophone	Nurse	x	-	X	x	-	-	-	Post-d/c
Schwarz et al., 2008[51]	Med	Med	Remote monitoring	Nurse	-	x	-	-	-	-	-	Post-d/c
Woodend et al., 2008[52]	High	High	Remote monitoring and videophone	Nurse	x	-	-	-	-	-	-	Post-d/c

Note: x = this component was part of the study intervention and "-" = this component was not included in the intervention.

Abbreviations: d/c= discharge; HF = heart failure; Med = Medium.

Table C12. Intervention components for telemonitoring interventions (Part 2)

Author, Year	Risk of Bias	Transition Coach or Coordination Between Inpatient/Outpatient Providers	Planned Telephone Follow-up Post d/c	Timing of First Phone or TM Follow-up (Days)	Phone Follow-up Conducted by Same Personnel Delivering Inpatient Intervention Component	Series of Structured Calls	Patient Phone Hotline	Timing of First Home Visit (Days)	Number of Scheduled Home Visits	Symptom Checklist or Clinical Assessment During Home Visit (e.g. History, Symptoms)	Physical Exam During Home Visit	Timing of First Clinic Visit Post D/C (Days)
Benatar et al., 2003[46]	Unclear	x	-	-	-	-	-	-	-	-	-	-
Dar et al., 2008[47]	Med	-	-	-	-	-	-	-	-	-	-	-
Dendale et al., 2012[48]	Unclear	x	x	≤7	x	-	-	-	-	-	-	> 14
Goldberg et al., 2003[49]	Med	-	-	-	-	-	-	-	-	-	-	-
Jerant et al., 2001[37], Jerant et al., 2003[38]	High	-	x	>7	-	x	x	>7	other	x	-	-
Pekmezaris et al., 2012[50]	Med	-	-	-	-	-	-	-	-	-	-	-
Schwarz et al., 2008[51]	Med	-	-	-	-	-	-	>7	2 to 3	-	x	-
Woodend et al., 2008[52]	High	-	-	-	-	-	-	-	-	-	-	-

Note: x = this component was part of the study intervention and "-" = this component was not included in the intervention.

Abbreviations: d/c= discharge; Med = Medium; TM = telemonitoring.

C-15

Table C13. Intervention components for telemonitoring interventions (Part 3)

Author, Year	Risk of Bias	Clinic Personnel on-Call/ Available for Acute Symptom Management (Outside of Scheduled Appt)	Timing of First Telehealth Contact After D/C (Days)	Intervention Involves Reinforcement of D/C Plan	Prescribed Protocol Used to Guide Assessment and/or Plan	Telehealth Service Coordinates Care With Outpatient Provider	TM Device has Automated Adherence Reminder	Device Can Transmit Vital Signs	Device Can Transmit Symptoms	Device Utilizes Technology that Allows Physical Exam
Benatar et al., 2003[46]	Unclear	-	> 7	-	x	-	-	x	-	-
Dar et al., 2008[47]	Med	-	-	-	x	-	-	x	x	-
Dendale et al., 2012[48]	Unclear	x	≤1	-	-	-	-	x	-	-
Goldberg et al., 2003[49]	Med	-	> 7	x	x	x	x	x	x	-
Jerant et al., 2001[37]; Jerant et al., 2003[38]	High	-	> 7	-	x	-	-	x	x	x
Pekmezaris et al., 2012[50]	Med	-	> 7	-	-	-	-	x	-	x
Schwarz et al., 2008[51]	Med	-	-	-	x	x	-	x	x	-
Woodend et al., 2008[52]	High	-	1-2	-	x	-	-	x	-	x

Note: x = this component was part of the study intervention and "-" = this component was not included in the intervention.

Abbreviations: appt = appointment; d/c= discharge; hrs = hours; Med = Medium; TM = telemonitoring.

Appendix C. References

1. Albert NM, Buchsbaum R, Li J. Randomized study of the effect of video education on heart failure healthcare utilization, symptoms, and self-care behaviors. Patient Educ Couns. 2007 Dec;69(1-3):129-39. PMID: 17913440.

2. Koelling TM, Johnson ML, Cody RJ, et al. Discharge education improves clinical outcomes in patients with chronic heart failure. Circulation. 2005 Jan 18;111(2):179-85. PMID: 15642765.

3. Linne AB, Liedholm H. Effects of an interactive CD-program on 6 months readmission rate in patients with heart failure - a randomised, controlled trial [NCT00311194]. BMC Cardiovasc Disord. 2006;6:30. PMID: 16796760.

4. Nucifora G, Albanese MC, De Biaggio P, et al. Lack of improvement of clinical outcomes by a low-cost, hospital-based heart failure management programme. J Cardiovasc Med (Hagerstown). 2006 Aug;7(8):614-22. PMID: 16858241.

5. Aldamiz-Echevarría Iraúrgui B, Muñiz J, Rodríguez-Fernández JA, et al. [Randomized controlled clinical trial of a home care unit intervention to reduce readmission and death rates in patients discharged from hospital following admission for heart failure]. Rev Esp Cardiol. 2007(9):914-22. PMID: CN-00612373.

6. Holland R, Brooksby I, Lenaghan E, et al. Effectiveness of visits from community pharmacists for patients with heart failure: HeartMed randomised controlled trial. BMJ. 2007 May 26;334(7603):1098. PMID: 17452390.

7. Jaarsma T, Halfens R, Huijer Abu-Saad H, et al. Effects of education and support on self-care and resource utilization in patients with heart failure. Eur Heart J. 1999 May;20(9):673-82. PMID: 10208788.

8. Phillips CO, Wright SM, Kern DE, et al. Comprehensive discharge planning with postdischarge support for older patients with congestive heart failure: a meta-analysis. JAMA. 2004 Mar 17;291(11):1358-67. PMID: 15026403.

9. Kwok T, Lee J, Woo J, et al. A randomized controlled trial of a community nurse-supported hospital discharge programme in older patients with chronic heart failure. J Clin Nurs. 2008 Jan;17(1):109-17. PMID: 18088263.

10. Naylor MD, Brooten DA, Campbell RL, et al. Transitional care of older adults hospitalized with heart failure: a randomized, controlled trial. J Am Geriatr Soc. 2004 May;52(5):675-84. PMID: 15086645.

11. Pugh LC, Havens DS, Xie S, et al. Case management for elderly persons with heart failure: the quality of life and cost outcomes. Medsurg Nurs. 2001;10(2):71-8.

12. Rich MW, Vinson JM, Sperry JC, et al. Prevention of readmission in elderly patients with congestive heart failure: results of a prospective, randomized pilot study. J Gen Intern Med. 1993 Nov;8(11):585-90. PMID: 8289096.

13. Rich MW, Beckham V, Wittenberg C, et al. A multidisciplinary intervention to prevent the readmission of elderly patients with congestive heart failure. N Engl J Med. 1995 Nov 2;333(18):1190-5. PMID: 7565975.

14. Sethares KA, Elliott K. The effect of a tailored message intervention on heart failure readmission rates, quality of life, and benefit and barrier beliefs in persons with heart failure. Heart Lung. 2004 Jul-Aug;33(4):249-60. PMID: 15252415.

15. Stewart S, Pearson S, Horowitz JD. Effects of a home-based intervention among patients with congestive heart failure discharged from acute hospital care. Arch Intern Med. 1998 May 25;158(10):1067-72. PMID: 9605777.

16. Stewart S, Marley JE, Horowitz JD. Effects of a multidisciplinary, home-based intervention on unplanned readmissions and survival among patients with chronic congestive heart failure: a randomised controlled study. Lancet. 1999 Sep 25;354(9184):1077-83. PMID: 10509499.

17. Thompson DR, Roebuck A, Stewart S. Effects of a nurse-led, clinic and home-based intervention on recurrent hospital use in chronic heart failure. Eur J Heart Fail. 2005 Mar 16;7(3):377-84. PMID: 15718178.

18. Triller DM, Hamilton RA. Effect of pharmaceutical care services on outcomes for home care patients with heart failure. Am J Health Syst Pharm. 2007 Nov 1;64(21):2244-9. PMID: 17959576.

19. Blaha C, Robinson JM, Pugh LC, et al. Longitudinal nursing case management for elderly heart failure patients: notes from the field. Nurs Case Manag. 2000 Jan-Feb;5(1):32-6. PMID: 10855156.

20. Kasper EK, Gerstenblith G, Hefter G, et al. A randomized trial of the efficacy of multidisciplinary care in heart failure outpatients at high risk of hospital readmission. J Am Coll Cardiol. 2002 Feb 6;39(3):471-80. PMID: 11823086.

21. Stromberg A, Martensson J, Fridlund B, et al. Nurse-led heart failure clinics improve survival and self-care behaviour in patients with heart failure: results from a prospective, randomised trial. Eur Heart J. 2003 Jun;24(11):1014-23. PMID: 12788301.

22. Ducharme A, Doyon O, White M, et al. Impact of care at a multidisciplinary congestive heart failure clinic: a randomized trial. CMAJ. 2005 Jul 5;173(1):40-5. PMID: 15997043.

23. Ekman I, Andersson B, Ehnfors M, et al. Feasibility of a nurse-monitored, outpatient-care programme for elderly patients with moderate-to-severe, chronic heart failure. Eur Heart J. 1998 Aug;19(8):1254-60. PMID: 9740348.

24. Liu MH, Wang CH, Huang YY, et al. Edema index-guided disease management improves 6-month outcomes of patients with acute heart failure. Int Heart J. 2012;53(1):11-7. PMID: 22398670.

25. McDonald K, Ledwidge M, Cahill J, et al. Elimination of early rehospitalization in a randomized, controlled trial of multidisciplinary care in a high-risk, elderly heart failure population: the potential contributions of specialist care, clinical stability and optimal angiotensin-converting enzyme inhibitor dose at discharge. Eur J Heart Fail. 2001 Mar;3(2):209-15. PMID: 11246059.

26. McDonald K, Ledwidge M, Cahill J, et al. Heart failure management: multidisciplinary care has intrinsic benefit above the optimization of medical care. J Card Fail. 2002 Jun;8(3):142-8. PMID: 12140806.

27. Ledwidge M, Barry M, Cahill J, et al. Is multidisciplinary care of heart failure cost-beneficial when combined with optimal medical care? Eur J Heart Fail. 2003(3):381-9. PMID: CN-00456908.

28. Oddone EZ, Weinberger M, Giobbie-Hurder A, et al. Enhanced access to primary care for patients with congestive heart failure. Veterans Affairs Cooperative Study Group on Primary Care and Hospital Readmission. Eff Clin Pract. 1999 Sep-Oct;2(5):201-9. PMID: 10623052.

29. Davis KK, Mintzer M, Dennison Himmelfarb CR, et al. Targeted intervention improves knowledge but not self-care or readmissions in heart failure patients with mild cognitive impairment. Eur J Heart Fail. 2012 Sep;14(9):1041-9. PMID: 22736737.

30. Riegel B, Carlson B. Is individual peer support a promising intervention for persons with heart failure? J Cardiovasc Nurs. 2004 May-Jun;19(3):174-83. PMID: 15191260.

31. Angermann CE, Stork S, Gelbrich G, et al. Mode of action and effects of standardized collaborative disease management on mortality and morbidity in patients with systolic heart failure: the Interdisciplinary Network for Heart Failure (INH) study. Circ Heart Fail. 2012 Jan;5(1):25-35. PMID: 21956192.

32. Barth V. A nurse-managed discharge program for congestive heart failure patients: outcomes and costs. Home Health Care Manag Pract. 2001(6):436-43. PMID: CN-00773514.

33. Lopez Cabezas C, Falces Salvador C, Cubi Quadrada D, et al. Randomized clinical trial of a postdischarge pharmaceutical care program vs regular follow-up in patients with heart failure. Farm Hosp. 2006 Nov-Dec;30(6):328-42. PMID: 17298190.

34. Domingues FB, Clausell N, Aliti GB, et al. Education and telephone monitoring by nurses of patients with heart failure: randomized clinical trial. Arq Bras Cardiol. 2011 Mar;96(3):233-9. PMID: 21308343.

35. Duffy JR, Hoskins LM, Dudley-Brown S. Improving outcomes for older adults with heart failure: a randomized trial using a theory-guided nursing intervention. J Nurs Care Qual. 2010 Jan-Mar;25(1):56-64. PMID: 19512945.

36. Dunagan WC, Littenberg B, Ewald GA, et al. Randomized trial of a nurse-administered, telephone-based disease management program for patients with heart failure. J Card Fail. 2005 Jun;11(5):358-65. PMID: 15948086.

37. Jerant AF, Azari R, Nesbitt TS. Reducing the cost of frequent hospital admissions for congestive heart failure: a randomized trial of a home telecare intervention. Med Care. 2001 Nov;39(11):1234-45. PMID: 11606877.

38. Jerant AF, Azari R, Martinez C, et al. A randomized trial of telenursing to reduce hospitalization for heart failure: patient-centered outcomes and nursing indicators. Home Health Care Serv Q. 2003;22(1):1-20. PMID: 12749524.

39. Laramee AS, Levinsky SK, Sargent J, et al. Case management in a heterogeneous congestive heart failure population: a randomized controlled trial. Arch Intern Med. 2003 Apr 14;163(7):809-17. PMID: 12695272.

40. Rainville EC. Impact of pharmacist interventions on hospital readmissions for heart failure. Am J Health Syst Pharm. 1999 Jul 1;56(13):1339-42. PMID: 10683133.

41. Riegel B, Carlson B, Kopp Z, et al. Effect of a standardized nurse case-management telephone intervention on resource use in patients with chronic heart failure. Arch Intern Med. 2002 Mar 25;162(6):705-12. PMID: 11911726.

42. Riegel B, Carlson B, Glaser D, et al. Randomized controlled trial of telephone case management in Hispanics of Mexican origin with heart failure. J Card Fail. 2006 Apr;12(3):211-9. PMID: 16624687.

43. Tsuyuki RT, Fradette M, Johnson JA, et al. A multicenter disease management program for hospitalized patients with heart failure. J Card Fail. 2004 Dec;10(6):473-80. PMID: 15599837.

44. Wakefield BJ, Ward MM, Holman JE, et al. Evaluation of home telehealth following hospitalization for heart failure: a randomized trial. Telemed J E Health. 2008 Oct;14(8):753-61. PMID: 18954244.

45. Wakefield BJ, Holman JE, Ray A, et al. Outcomes of a home telehealth intervention for patients with heart failure. J Telemed Telecare. 2009;15(1):46-50. PMID: 19139220.

46. Benatar D, Bondmass M, Ghitelman J, et al. Outcomes of chronic heart failure. Arch Intern Med. 2003 Feb 10;163(3):347-52. PMID: 12578516.

47. Dar O, Riley J, Chapman C, et al. A randomized trial of home telemonitoring in a typical elderly heart failure population in North West London: results of the Home-HF study. Eur J Heart Fail. 2009(3):319-25. PMID: CN-00681894.

48. Dendale P, De Keulenaer G, Troisfontaines P, et al. Effect of a telemonitoring-facilitated collaboration between general practitioner and heart failure clinic on mortality and rehospitalization rates in severe heart failure: the TEMA-HF 1 (TElemonitoring in the MAnagement of Heart Failure) study. Eur J Heart Fail. 2012 Mar;14(3):333-40. PMID: 22045925.

49. Goldberg LR, Piette JD, Walsh MN, et al. Randomized trial of a daily electronic home monitoring system in patients with advanced heart failure: the Weight Monitoring in Heart Failure (WHARF) trial. Am Heart J. 2003 Oct;146(4):705-12. PMID: 14564327.

50. Pekmezaris R, Mitzner I, Pecinka KR, et al. The impact of remote patient monitoring (telehealth) upon Medicare beneficiaries with heart failure. Telemed J E Health. 2012 Mar;18(2):101-8. PMID: 22283360.

51.   Schwarz KA, Mion LC, Hudock D, et al. Telemonitoring of heart failure patients and their caregivers: a pilot randomized controlled trial. Prog Cardiovasc Nurs. 2008 Winter;23(1):18-26. PMID: 18326990.

52.   Woodend AK, Sherrard H, Fraser M, et al. Telehome monitoring in patients with cardiac disease who are at high risk of readmission. Heart Lung. 2008 Jan-Feb;37(1):36-45. PMID: 18206525.

Appendix D. Risk of Bias Assessments for Included Studies

Table D1. Risk of bias evaluations and rationale

Author, Year Trial Name[a]	Randomization Method Adequate?	Allocation Concealment Adequate?	Are Groups Similar at Baseline?	Outcome Assessors Blinded?	Overall Attrition / Differential Attrition	Does High Attrition Rate Raise Concern for Bias?	Intervention Fidelity Adequate?	ITT Analysis? / Appropriate Method for Handling Missing Data?	Utilization Outcomes: Valid, Reliable, Consistent?	Health and Social Outcomes: Valid, Reliable, Consistent?	Risk of Bias	Rationale for Any High or Unclear Risk of Bias Ratings
Albert et al., 2007[1]	Yes	Yes	No	NR/CND	19% lost to follow-up; 29% died or were lost to follow-up / 1.1% loss to follow-up; 6% differential attrition when counting those who either died or were lost to follow-up	Yes	Yes	Yes / No	NR/CND	NR/CND	High	Baseline characteristics not similar (more women in the usual care group, more smokers in the intervention group). Inadequate method of handling missing data (completer's analysis). The authors did not describe how mortality and health utilization measures were ascertained.
Aldamiz-Echevarria Iraúrgui et al., 2007[2]	Yes	Yes	Yes	NR/CND	0% / 0%	No	NR/CND	Yes / NA	Yes	Yes	Medium	

Table D1. Risk of bias evaluations and rationale (continued)

Author, Year Trial Name[a]	Randomization Method Adequate?	Allocation Concealment Adequate?	Are Groups Similar at Baseline?	Outcome Assessors Blinded?	Overall Attrition	Differential Attrition	Does High Attrition Rate Raise Concern for Bias?	Intervention Fidelity Adequate?	ITT Analysis?	Appropriate Method for Handling Missing Data?	Utilization Outcomes: Valid, Reliable, Consistent?	Health and Social Outcomes: Valid, Reliable, Consistent?	Risk of Bias	Rationale for Any High or Unclear Risk of Bias Ratings
Angermann et al., 2012[3]	Yes	NR/CND	Yes	Yes	0% for mortality and utilization outcomes; no QoL available for those who died or did not complete a follow-up phone call (58%)	NA for mortality/ utilization; unclear for QoL	No	NR/CND	Yes	Yes	Yes	Yes	Medium	
Barth et al., 2001[4]	NR/CND	NR/CND	Yes	NR/CND	0%	NA	No	NR/CND	Unclear or NR	NA	Unclear	Yes	High	High risk of selection bias; unclear how the 34 participants were recruited from the overall population. Methods used to measure utilization outcomes were not described.

D-2

Table D1. Risk of bias evaluations and rationale (continued)

Author, Year Trial Name[a]	Randomization Method Adequate?	Allocation Concealment Adequate?	Are Groups Similar at Baseline?	Outcome Assessors Blinded?	Overall Attrition	Differential Attrition	Does High Attrition Rate Raise Concern for Bias?	Intervention Fidelity Adequate?	ITT Analysis? Appropriate Method for Handling Missing Data?	Utilization Outcomes: Valid, Reliable, Consistent?	Health and Social Outcomes: Valid, Reliable, Consistent?	Risk of Bias Rationale for Any High or Unclear Risk of Bias Ratings
Benatar et al, 2003[5]	NR/CND	NR/CND	Yes, for age, sex, race, NYHA, EF; higher proportions with DM, ACEI use, BB use in NTM group	NR/CND	0% (3 ms)	0% (3 ms)	No	NR/CND	Unclear or NR; NA for 3 ms; NR beyond that	NR/CND	Yes	Unclear (utilization outcomes); Medium (QoL); Rated unclear for utilization outcomes; ascertainment NR. Measures for QoL, psychological distress, and self-efficacy more clearly described and used validated measures. Masking of outcome assessors NR. Methods or randomization and allocation concealment NR. Although study reports that all randomized patients completed at least 3 months, no flow chart or data included to report attrition over the course of the study. Whether ITT analysis used NR. Unclear how missing data handled (and how much there was) beyond 3 months. Potential COI with senior author as developer of the hardware and software.

Table D1. Risk of bias evaluations and rationale (continued)

Author, Year Trial Name[a]	Randomization Method Adequate?	Allocation Concealment Adequate?	Are Groups Similar at Baseline?	Outcome Assessors Blinded?	Overall Attrition	Differential Attrition	Does High Attrition Rate Raise Concern for Bias?	Intervention Fidelity Adequate?	ITT Analysis?	Appropriate Method for Handling Missing Data?	Utilization Outcomes: Valid, Reliable, Consistent?	Health and Social Outcomes: Valid, Reliable, Consistent?	Risk of Bias	Rationale for Any High or Unclear Risk of Bias Ratings
Cabezas et al., 2006[6]	NR/CND	NR/CND	Yes	NR/CND	0%; no QoL outcomes for 13% who died at 6 months / 0%; 10% when including deaths at 6 months		No	NR/CND	Unclear or NR	NA	Yes	Yes	Medium	
Dar et al., 2009[7]	Yes	Yes	Yes	NR/CND	0% / 0%		No	Yes	Yes	Yes	Yes	Yes	Medium	
Davis et al., 2012[8]	NR/CND	NR/CND	Yes	Yes	13% / 0%		No	NR/CND	Yes	Yes	Yes	Yes	Medium	
Dendale et al., 2012[9]	NR/CND	Yes	Yes	Yes	0% / 0%		No	NR/CND	Yes	NA	NR	Yes	Unclear	Unclear fidelity- study reports that 76% of the GPs logged into the website at least once during the study. Unclear if the GPs could receive patient alerts outside of the website. It is unclear how utilization outcomes were measured; no specific information is given.
Domingues et al., 2011[10]	NR/CND	NR/CND	Yes	NR/CND	4% / 3%		No	Yes	Yes	No	Yes	NA	Medium	

D-4

Table D1. Risk of bias evaluations and rationale (continued)

Author, Year Trial Name[a]	Randomi-zation Method Adequate?	Allo-cation Conceal-ment Ad-equate?	Are Groups Similar at Base-line?	Outcome Asse-ssors Blinded?	Overall Attrition / Differential Attrition	Does High Attrition Rate Raise Concern for Bias?	Inter-vention Fidelity Ad-equate?	ITT Ana-lysis? Appro-priate Method for Handling Missing Data?	Utiliz-ation Out-comes: Valid, Reliable, Con-sistent?	Health and Social Out-comes: Valid, Reliable, Cons-istent?	Risk of Bias	Rationale for Any High or Unclear Risk of Bias Ratings
Ducharme et al., 2005[11]	Yes	Yes	Yes	Yes for QoL, No for utilization outcomes.	0% / 0%	NA	Yes	Yes / NA	Yes	Yes	Low	
Duffy et al., 2010[12]	No	No	NR/CND	NR/CND	NR/CND / NR/CND	Unclear or NR / NR	Yes	Unclear or NR / NA	unclear	Yes	High	Sample characteristics not given for separate arms; in the text, noted that there were no differences. Unclear if the database used to capture healthcare utilization is comprehensive or based on only nurse input of known utilization. Control arm poorly described and received nearly as many home visits as the intervention group.

Table D1. Risk of bias evaluations and rationale (continued)

Author, Year Trial Name[a]	Randomization Method Adequate?	Allocation Concealment Adequate?	Are Groups Similar at Baseline?	Outcome Assessors Blinded?	Overall Attrition / Differential Attrition	Does High Attrition Rate Raise Concern for Bias?	Intervention Fidelity Adequate?	ITT Analysis? / Appropriate Method for Handling Missing Data?	Utilization Outcomes: Valid, Reliable, Consistent?	Health and Social Outcomes: Valid, Reliable, Consistent?	Risk of Bias / Rationale for Any High or Unclear Risk of Bias Ratings
Dunagan et al., 2005[13]	Yes	NR/CND	Yes	Yes	0% for utilization outcomes; see Risk of bias/Rationale for rating column for QoL 0% for utilization outcomes; see Risk of bias/Rationale for rating column for QoL	No	NR/CND	Yes NA for utilization outcomes; no for QoL outcomes	Yes	Yes	Medium
Ekman et al., 1998[14]	Yes	Yes	For most characteristics, however more patients in usual care group had AF	NR/CND	0% NA	No	NR/CND	Yes NA	Yes	Yes	Medium

D-6

Table D1. Risk of bias evaluations and rationale (continued)

Author, Year Trial Name[a]	Randomization Method Adequate?	Allocation Concealment Adequate?	Are Groups Similar at Baseline?	Outcome Assessors Blinded?	Overall Attrition	Differential Attrition	Does High Attrition Rate Raise Concern for Bias?	Intervention Fidelity Adequate?	ITT Analysis?	Appropriate Method for Handling Missing Data?	Utilization Outcomes: Valid, Reliable, Consistent?	Health and Social Outcomes: Valid, Reliable, Consistent?	Risk of Bias	Rationale for Any High or Unclear Risk of Bias Ratings
Goldberg et al., 2003[15]	NR/CND	NR/CND	Yes	Yes	11.4%	CND, but article reports that there was no difference between groups in % of patients who failed to complete 6 months	No	Yes	Yes	NR/CND for utilization (likely censored); completers analysis for health and social outcomes	Yes	Yes	Medium	
Holland et al., 2007[16]	Yes	NR/CND	No	NR/CND	1%	0%	No	Yes	Yes	NA	Yes	Yes	Medium	
Jaarsma et al., 1999[17]	NR/CND	NR/CND	Yes	No	5% "non-response" rate; 17% of sample died	0% for loss to follow-up	No	NR/CND	Unclear		Yes	Yes	Medium	
Jerant et al., 2001[18]	Yes	Yes	Yes	No	0%	0%	No	No	Yes		Yes	Yes	High	
Jerant et al., 2003[19]						0%			NA					Small study (37 participants) that suffers from concerns regarding intervention fidelity. Authors note that at least one technical problem affected 76% of all telemonitoring encounters.

Table D1. Risk of bias evaluations and rationale (continued)

Author, Year Trial Name[a]	Randomization Method Adequate?	Allocation Concealment Adequate?	Are Groups Similar at Baseline?	Outcome Assessors Blinded?	Overall Attrition	Differential Attrition	Does High Attrition Rate Raise Concern for Bias?	Intervention Fidelity Adequate?	ITT Analysis?	Appropriate Method for Handling Missing Data?	Utilization Outcomes: Valid, Reliable, Consistent?	Health and Social Outcomes: Valid, Reliable, Consistent?	Risk of Bias / Rationale for Any High or Unclear Risk of Bias Ratings
Kasper et al., 2002[20]	Yes	NR/CND	Yes	Yes	0%	0%	No	Yes	Yes	NA	Yes	Yes	Low
Kimmelstiel et al., 2004[21]	NR/CND	NR/CND	Yes	Yes	4.5% due to death at 12 weeks	NR	No	Yes	Yes	NA	Yes	Yes	Medium
Koelling et al., 2005[22]	Yes	Yes	Yes	Yes	0.0%	0.0%	No	Yes	Yes	NA	Yes	Yes	Low
Kwok et al., 2007[23]	Yes	NR/CND	No	Yes for functional status; unclear for utilization rates	2.8%	1.5%	No	NR/CND	Yes	NR/CND	Yes	Yes	Medium
Laramee et al., 2003[24] RCT	Yes	NR/CND	Yes, for most, but some differences for PVD, class I and II NYHA, prior CHF admissions, and readmission risk factors	No	8.7%	8.8%	No	NR/CND	No		Yes	Yes	Medium

Table D1. Risk of bias evaluations and rationale (continued)

Author, Year Trial Name[a]	Randomization Method Adequate?	Allocation Concealment Adequate?	Are Groups Similar at Baseline?	Outcome Assessors Blinded?	Overall Attrition	Differential Attrition	Does High Attrition Rate Raise Concern for Bias?	Intervention Fidelity Adequate?	ITT Analysis? / Appropriate Method for Handling Missing Data?	Utilization Outcomes: Valid, Reliable, Consistent?	Health and Social Outcomes: Valid, Reliable, Consistent?	Risk of Bias / Rationale for Any High or Unclear Risk of Bias Ratings
Linne et al., 2006[25]	Yes	Yes	Yes, for most characteristics	Yes	2.6%	1.4%	No	NR/CND	Yes / NR/CND	NR/CND	NR/CND	Unclear Unclear risk of bias, mainly due to inadequate reporting of information to allow complete assessment of risk of measurement bias. Groups similar at baseline Unclear how missing data handled, but very few subjects had missing outcome data (2/108 and 4/122 refused to participate further in the control and intervention groups, respectively), so likely minimal potential impact. They were likely censored in the survival analysis. Unclear risk of measurement bias: authors only report that they used "an administrative system, PAS, ... to verify all-cause readmissions and deaths within 6 months from discharge." Study conducted in Sweden, and no additional information about validity and reliability of that system's readmission and death information.

D-9

Table D1. Risk of bias evaluations and rationale (continued)

Author, Year Trial Name[a]	Randomization Method Adequate?	Allocation Concealment Adequate?	Are Groups Similar at Baseline?	Outcome Assessors Blinded?	Overall Attrition / Differential Attrition	Does High Attrition Rate Raise Concern for Bias?	Intervention Fidelity Adequate?	ITT Analysis? / Appropriate Method for Handling Missing Data?	Utilization Outcomes: Valid, Reliable, Consistent?	Health and Social Outcomes: Valid, Reliable, Consistent?	Risk of Bias / Rationale for Any High or Unclear Risk of Bias Ratings
Liu et al., 2012[26]	Yes	NR/CND	Yes	Yes	0.00% / 0%	No	NR/CND	Yes / NA	Yes	Yes	Low
McDonald et al., 2001[27] McDonald et al., 2002[28] Ledwidge et al., 2003[29]	NR/CND	NR/CND	Yes	NR/CND	0% / 0%	No	NR/CND	Yes / NA	Unclear	Unclear for mortality; Yes for social outcomes	Unclear — Unclear measurement bias. Method of outcome assessment (measurement of mortality and utilization) not described and unclear.
Naylor et al., 2004[30]	Yes	Yes	Yes	Yes	20.5% / 1.4%	No	NR/CND	Yes / Yes	Yes	Yes	Low
Nucifora et al., 2006[31]	NR/CND	NR/CND	No	NR/CND	0% lost to follow-up; 11% died / 0% NA for missing data; 6% for deaths	No	NR/CND	Yes / Yes	Yes	Yes	Medium
Oddone et al., 1999[32]	NR/CND	NR/CND	Yes	Yes	NR/CND / NR	Unclear or NR	Unclear or Yes	Unclear or NR / Unclear or NR	Yes	Yes	Medium
Pekmezaris et al., 2012[33]	Yes	NR/CND	Yes	NR/CND	0% / 0%	No	Yes	Yes / Yes	Yes	NA	Medium

Table D1. Risk of bias evaluations and rationale (continued)

Author, Year Trial Name[a]	Randomization Method Adequate?	Allocation Concealment Adequate?	Are Groups Similar at Baseline?	Outcome Assessors Blinded?	Overall Attrition / Differential Attrition	Does High Attrition Rate Raise Concern for Bias?	Intervention Fidelity Adequate?	ITT Analysis? / Appropriate Method for Handling Missing Data?	Utilization Outcomes: Valid, Reliable, Consistent?	Health and Social Outcomes: Valid, Reliable, Consistent?	Risk of Bias / Rationale for Any High or Unclear Risk of Bias Ratings
Pugh et al., 2001[34]	NR/CND	NR/CND	Yes	NR/CND	10% due to withdrew; 29% died or withdrew; 1%	No	NR/CND	Unclear or NR; No	Unclear	Yes	High. Patients who withdrew or who died appear to be excluded from the readmission/ utilization analysis. Unclear if 11 patients who died had also experienced a readmission or ER visit during study. NR whether those who withdrew were contacted and asked about health care utilization. Randomization and allocation concealment not described.
Rainville et al., 1999[35]	Yes	NR/CND	No	NR/CND	14% died; no loss to follow-up reported after randomization; 0% for loss to follow-up; 17% for death	Yes	NR/CND	Unclear or NR; No	Yes	Yes	Medium
Rich et al., 1993[36]	NR/CND	NR/CND	Yes	NR/CND	0%; 0%	No	NR/CND	Unclear or NR; NA	Yes	NA	Medium

Table D1. Risk of bias evaluations and rationale (continued)

Author, Year Trial Name[a]	Randomization Method Adequate?	Allocation Concealment Adequate?	Are Groups Similar at Baseline?	Outcome Assessors Blinded?	Overall Attrition / Differential Attrition	Does High Attrition Rate Raise Concern for Bias?	Intervention Fidelity Adequate?	ITT Analysis? / Appropriate Method for Handling Missing Data?	Utilization Outcomes: Valid, Reliable, Consistent?	Health and Social Outcomes: Valid, Reliable, Consistent?	Risk of Bias / Rationale for Any High or Unclear Risk of Bias Ratings
Rich et al., 1995[37]	Yes	Yes	No	NR/CND	0% / 0%	No	NR/CND	Yes / NA	Unclear	Yes	Medium
Riegel et al., 2002[38]	No	NR/CND	No	NR/CND	0% for outcomes of interest (acute care resources) / NA	No	Yes	Unclear or NR / NA	Yes	NA	Medium

Table D1. Risk of bias evaluations and rationale (continued)

Author, Year Trial Name[a]	Randomization Method Adequate?	Allocation Concealment Adequate?	Are Groups Similar at Baseline?	Outcome Assessors Blinded?	Overall Attrition	Differential Attrition	Does High Attrition Rate Raise Concern for Bias?	Intervention Fidelity Adequate?	ITT Analysis?	Appropriate Method for Handling Missing Data?	Utilization Outcomes: Valid, Reliable, Consistent?	Health and Social Outcomes: Valid, Reliable, Consistent?	Risk of Bias	Rationale for Any High or Unclear Risk of Bias Ratings
Riegel et al., 2004[39]	Yes	NR/CND	No	NR/CND	31.8%	1.5%	Yes	Yes	Yes for utilization outcome; no for self-care/social outcomes (those were completer's analysis)	No	NR/CND	NR/CND for mortality; Yes for self-care measures	High	High risk of selection bias, measurement bias, and confounding. Over 30% of sample dropped out, high attrition; methods of handling missing data NR for utilization outcomes. Unclear how utilization outcomes were ascertained, and unclear how complete data was for utilization outcomes (focus of study on self-care and social support outcomes). Masking of outcome assessors NR. Several baseline differences between groups: fewer married in intervention group, fewer retired, fewer with stage 3/4 NYHA when collapsing those groups (57% vs. 69%), fewer with COPD and history of MI.
Riegel et al., 2006[40]	NR/CND	Yes	Yes	Yes	0.0%	0.0%	No	Yes	Yes	NA	Yes	Yes	Medium	

D-13

Table D1. Risk of bias evaluations and rationale (continued)

Author, Year Trial Name[a]	Randomization Method Adequate?	Allocation Concealment Adequate?	Are Groups Similar at Baseline?	Outcome Assessors Blinded?	Overall Attrition Differential Attrition	Does High Attrition Rate Raise Concern for Bias?	Intervention Fidelity Adequate?	ITT Analysis? Appropriate Method for Handling Missing Data?	Utilization Outcomes: Valid, Reliable, Consistent?	Health and Social Outcomes: Valid, Reliable, Consistent?	Risk of Bias Rationale for Any High or Unclear Risk of Bias Ratings
Schwarz et al., 2008[41]	NR/CND	NR/CND	No	NR/CND	21% including death, nursing home and withdrawal from study; appears that mortality and utilization outcomes were available for full sample. 8%	No	Yes	Yes Yes	Yes	Yes	Medium

Table D1. Risk of bias evaluations and rationale (continued)

Author, Year Trial Name[a]	Randomization Method Adequate?	Allocation Concealment Adequate?	Are Groups Similar at Baseline?	Outcome Assessors Blinded?	Overall Attrition	Differential Attrition	Does High Attrition Rate Raise Concern for Bias?	Intervention Fidelity Adequate?	ITT Analysis? Appropriate Method for Handling Missing Data?	Utilization Outcomes: Valid, Reliable, Consistent?	Health and Social Outcomes: Valid, Reliable, Consistent?	Risk of Bias	Rationale for Any High or Unclear Risk of Bias Ratings
Sethares et al., 2004[42]	NR/CND	NR/CND	Yes	Mixed (yes for readmission, no for QoL for the intervention group)	20.5%	CND	Yes	NR/CND	No / No	Yes	Yes	High	High risk of selection bias and confounding. Completers analysis, 18/88 post-randomization exclusions due to death (10) or missing data (8); analysis only included 70 subjects who did not die and not lost to follow-up. Unclear why more detailed assessments of the 10 deaths not included in analysis. No reporting of which groups the 18 post-randomization exclusions were in to allow determination of differential attrition. The

Table D1. Risk of bias evaluations and rationale (continued)

Author, Year Trial Name[a]	Randomization Method Adequate?	Allocation Concealment Adequate?	Are Groups Similar at Baseline?	Outcome Assessors Blinded?	Overall Attrition / Differential Attrition	Does High Attrition Rate Raise Concern for Bias?	Intervention Fidelity Adequate?	ITT Analysis? / Appropriate Method for Handling Missing Data?	Utilization Outcomes: Valid, Reliable, Consistent?	Health and Social Outcomes: Valid, Reliable, Consistent?	Risk of Bias / Rationale for Any High or Unclear Risk of Bias Ratings
Sethares et al., 2004[42] (continued)											10 deaths, if adequately assessed for readmission and attributed to appropriate study groups, could significantly change results, since only 6 people readmitted in intervention group and 12 in control group. Inadequate handling of missing data; methods of randomization and allocation concealment NR
Stewart et al., 1998[43]	No	NR/CND	Yes	NR/CND	NR/CND; appears to be mortality and utilization outcomes on all participants / NA	Unclear or Yes / NR		Yes / NA	Yes	Yes	Medium

Table D1. Risk of bias evaluations and rationale (continued)

Author, Year Trial Name[a]	Randomization Method Adequate?	Allocation Concealment Adequate?	Are Groups Similar at Baseline?	Outcome Assessors Blinded?	Overall Attrition / Differential Attrition	Does High Attrition Rate Raise Concern for Bias?	Intervention Fidelity Adequate?	ITT Analysis? / Appropriate Method for Handling Missing Data?	Utilization Outcomes: Valid, Reliable, Consistent?	Health and Social Outcomes: Valid, Reliable, Consistent?	Risk of Bias / Rationale for Any High or Unclear Risk of Bias Ratings
Stewart et al., 1999[44]	Yes	Yes	Yes	Yes	NR/CND; 10% of the intervention group withdrew and unclear how missing data handled / 10% of intervention group withdrew; attrition NR for usual care group	No	NR/CND	Yes / Unclear	Yes	Yes	Medium
Stromberg et al., 2003[45]	Yes	Yes	Yes, for most (but more with HTN in intervention group and fewer with DM)	Yes	0% lost to follow-up; 15% died before 3 months / 0% lost to follow-up; 18% for deaths by 3 months	No	Yes	Yes / Yes	Yes	Yes	Low / Patients who died were censored in analysis.

Table D1. Risk of bias evaluations and rationale (continued)

Author, Year Trial Name[a]	Randomization Method Adequate?	Allocation Concealment Adequate?	Are Groups Similar at Baseline?	Outcome Assessors Blinded?	Overall Attrition / Differential Attrition	Does High Attrition Rate Raise Concern for Bias?	Intervention Fidelity Adequate?	ITT Analysis? / Appropriate Method for Handling Missing Data?	Utilization Outcomes: Valid, Reliable, Consistent?	Health and Social Outcomes: Valid, Reliable, Consistent?	Risk of Bias / Rationale for Any High or Unclear Risk of Bias Ratings
Thompson et al., 2005[46]	NR/CND	NR/CND	No	Yes	0% for utilization outcomes; 57% for QoL / 0% for utilization outcomes; NR/CND for QoL	Yes (QoL only)	Yes	Yes / No (no for QoL only)	Yes	Yes	High — Study used cluster randomization according to treating GP, resulting in important baseline differences between groups; analysis done at patient level. Higher proportion of diabetes (27% vs. 14%) and lower proportion of medication use for ACEIs, BBs, Aspirin, and warfarin at time of hospital discharge for control group than intervention group. Thus, control group at higher risk of readmissions and death than intervention group. QoL outcome data have high risk of bias due to very high attrition, with fewer than half of subjects returning questionnaire.

Table D1. Risk of bias evaluations and rationale (continued)

Author, Year Trial Name[a]	Randomization Method Adequate?	Allocation Concealment Adequate?	Are Groups Similar at Baseline?	Outcome Assessors Blinded?	Overall Attrition	Differential Attrition	Does High Attrition Rate Raise Concern for Bias?	Intervention Fidelity Adequate?	ITT Analysis? / Appropriate Method for Handling Missing Data?	Utilization Outcomes: Valid, Reliable, Consistent?	Health and Social Outcomes: Valid, Reliable, Consistent?	Risk of Bias / Rationale for Any High or Unclear Risk of Bias Ratings
Triller et al., 2008[47]	Yes	Yes	Yes	NR/CND	0%	NA	No	No	Yes / NA	Unclear	No	Unclear — No information provided on method used to measure readmission and other utilization outcomes. Neither type of QoL measured nor QoL scale used are described, making validity of those data unclear. Only 53% of sample received full 3 visits from a pharmacist. Unclear fidelity.
Tsuyuki et al., 2004[48]	Yes	NR/CND	Yes	No	2.5% 0.8%		No	NR/CND	Yes / NR/CND	Yes	Yes	Medium
Wakefield et al., 2008[49] Wakefield et al., 2009[50]	NR/CND	NR/CND	Yes	NR/CND	0% for readmission and mortality		No	Unclear	Yes / NA	Yes	Yes	Medium

D-19

Table D1. Risk of bias evaluations and rationale (continued)

Author, Year Trial Name[a]	Randomization Method Adequate?	Allocation Concealment Adequate?	Are Groups Similar at Baseline?	Outcome Assessors Blinded?	Overall Attrition Differential Attrition	Does High Attrition Rate Raise Concern for Bias?	Intervention Fidelity Adequate?	ITT Analysis? Appropriate Method for Handling Missing Data?	Utilization Outcomes: Valid, Reliable, Consistent?	Health and Social Outcomes: Valid, Reliable, Consistent?	Risk of Bias Rationale for Any High or Unclear Risk of Bias Ratings
Woodend et al., 2008[51]	NR/CND	NR/CND	No	NR/CND	NR/CND at eligible time points NR/CND	Unclear or NR/CND NR	NR/CND	Yes NR/CND	No	unclear	High Fewer patients in telemonitoring group had angina compared with usual care. Loss to follow-up and death reported for 12 months, unclear if these were included in data analysis for earlier time points or excluded. At 12 months, 22% of the intervention group also received home visits. Utilization outcomes assessed by self-report only. Not clear if attempt made to account for utilization among those lost to follow-up or who were later found to have died.

[a] Three studies involved crossover designs or contamination: Duffy et al., 2010,[12] Pekmezaris et al., 2012[33] and Woodend et al., 2008.[51]

Abbreviations: ACEI = ACE inhibitor; AF = atrial fibrillation; BB = beta-blocker; CND = cannot determine; COI = conflict of interest; COPD = chronic obstructive pulmonary disease; DM = diabetes mellitus; EF = ejection fraction; ER = emergency room; GP = general practitioner; CHF = congestive heart failure; HTN = hypertension; ITT = intent-to-treat; MI = myocardial infarction; Ms = months; NA = not applicable; NR = not reported; NTM = no telemonitoring; NYHA = New York Heart Association functional classification; PVD = peripheral vascular disease; QoL = quality of life; RoB = risk of bias; vs. = versus

Appendix D References

1. Albert NM, Buchsbaum R, Li J. Randomized study of the effect of video education on heart failure healthcare utilization, symptoms, and self-care behaviors. Patient Educ Couns. 2007 Dec;69(1-3):129-39. PMID: 17913440.

2. Aldamiz-Echevarría Iraúrgui B, Muñiz J, Rodríguez-Fernández JA, et al. [Randomized controlled clinical trial of a home care unit intervention to reduce readmission and death rates in patients discharged from hospital following admission for heart failure]. Rev Esp Cardiol. 2007(9):914-22. PMID: CN-00612373.

3. Angermann CE, Stork S, Gelbrich G, et al. Mode of action and effects of standardized collaborative disease management on mortality and morbidity in patients with systolic heart failure: the Interdisciplinary Network for Heart Failure (INH) study. Circ Heart Fail. 2012 Jan;5(1):25-35. PMID: 21956192.

4. Barth V. A nurse-managed discharge program for congestive heart failure patients: outcomes and costs. Home Health Care Manag Pract. 2001(6):436-43. PMID: CN-00773514.

5. Benatar D, Bondmass M, Ghitelman J, et al. Outcomes of chronic heart failure. Arch Intern Med. 2003 Feb 10;163(3):347-52. PMID: 12578516.

6. Lopez Cabezas C, Falces Salvador C, Cubi Quadrada D, et al. Randomized clinical trial of a postdischarge pharmaceutical care program vs regular follow-up in patients with heart failure. Farm Hosp. 2006 Nov-Dec;30(6):328-42. PMID: 17298190.

7. Dar O, Riley J, Chapman C, et al. A randomized trial of home telemonitoring in a typical elderly heart failure population in North West London: results of the Home-HF study. Eur J Heart Fail. 2009(3):319-25. PMID: CN-00681894.

8. Davis KK, Mintzer M, Dennison Himmelfarb CR, et al. Targeted intervention improves knowledge but not self-care or readmissions in heart failure patients with mild cognitive impairment. Eur J Heart Fail. 2012 Sep;14(9):1041-9. PMID: 22736737.

9. Dendale P, De Keulenaer G, Troisfontaines P, et al. Effect of a telemonitoring-facilitated collaboration between general practitioner and heart failure clinic on mortality and rehospitalization rates in severe heart failure: the TEMA-HF 1 (TElemonitoring in the MAnagement of Heart Failure) study. Eur J Heart Fail. 2012 Mar;14(3):333-40. PMID: 22045925.

10. Domingues FB, Clausell N, Aliti GB, et al. Education and telephone monitoring by nurses of patients with heart failure: randomized clinical trial. Arq Bras Cardiol. 2011 Mar;96(3):233-9. PMID: 21308343.

11. Ducharme A, Doyon O, White M, et al. Impact of care at a multidisciplinary congestive heart failure clinic: a randomized trial. CMAJ. 2005 Jul 5;173(1):40-5. PMID: 15997043.

12. Duffy JR, Hoskins LM, Dudley-Brown S. Improving outcomes for older adults with heart failure: a randomized trial using a theory-guided nursing intervention. J Nurs Care Qual. 2010 Jan-Mar;25(1):56-64. PMID: 19512945.

13. Dunagan WC, Littenberg B, Ewald GA, et al. Randomized trial of a nurse-administered, telephone-based disease management program for patients with heart failure. J Card Fail. 2005 Jun;11(5):358-65. PMID: 15948086.

14. Ekman I, Andersson B, Ehnfors M, et al. Feasibility of a nurse-monitored, outpatient-care programme for elderly patients with moderate-to-severe, chronic heart failure. Eur Heart J. 1998 Aug;19(8):1254-60. PMID: 9740348.

15. Goldberg LR, Piette JD, Walsh MN, et al. Randomized trial of a daily electronic home monitoring system in patients with advanced heart failure: the Weight Monitoring in Heart Failure (WHARF) trial. Am Heart J. 2003 Oct;146(4):705-12. PMID: 14564327.

16. Holland R, Brooksby I, Lenaghan E, et al. Effectiveness of visits from community pharmacists for patients with heart failure: HeartMed randomised controlled trial. BMJ. 2007 May 26;334(7603):1098. PMID: 17452390.

17. Jaarsma T, Halfens R, Huijer Abu-Saad H, et al. Effects of education and support on self-care and resource utilization in patients with heart failure. Eur Heart J. 1999 May;20(9):673-82. PMID: 10208788.

18. Jerant AF, Azari R, Nesbitt TS. Reducing the cost of frequent hospital admissions for congestive heart failure: a randomized trial of a home telecare intervention. Med Care. 2001 Nov;39(11):1234-45. PMID: 11606877.

19. Jerant AF, Azari R, Martinez C, et al. A randomized trial of telenursing to reduce hospitalization for heart failure: patient-centered outcomes and nursing indicators. Home Health Care Serv Q. 2003;22(1):1-20. PMID: 12749524.

20. Kasper EK, Gerstenblith G, Hefter G, et al. A randomized trial of the efficacy of multidisciplinary care in heart failure outpatients at high risk of hospital readmission. J Am Coll Cardiol. 2002 Feb 6;39(3):471-80. PMID: 11823086.

21. Kimmelstiel C, Levine D, Perry K, et al. Randomized, controlled evaluation of short- and long-term benefits of heart failure disease management within a diverse provider network: the SPAN-CHF trial. Circulation. 2004 Sep 14;110(11):1450-5. PMID: 15313938.

22. Koelling TM, Johnson ML, Cody RJ, et al. Discharge education improves clinical outcomes in patients with chronic heart failure. Circulation. 2005 Jan 18;111(2):179-85. PMID: 15642765.

23. Kwok T, Lee J, Woo J, et al. A randomized controlled trial of a community nurse-supported hospital discharge programme in older patients with chronic heart failure. J Clin Nurs. 2008 Jan;17(1):109-17. PMID: 18088263.

24. Laramee AS, Levinsky SK, Sargent J, et al. Case management in a heterogeneous congestive heart failure population: a randomized controlled trial. Arch Intern Med. 2003 Apr 14;163(7):809-17. PMID: 12695272.

25. Linne AB, Liedholm H. Effects of an interactive CD-program on 6 months readmission rate in patients with heart failure - a randomised, controlled trial [NCT00311194]. BMC Cardiovasc Disord. 2006;6:30. PMID: 16796760.

26. Liu MH, Wang CH, Huang YY, et al. Edema index-guided disease management improves 6-month outcomes of patients with acute heart failure. Int Heart J. 2012;53(1):11-7. PMID: 22398670.

27. McDonald K, Ledwidge M, Cahill J, et al. Elimination of early rehospitalization in a randomized, controlled trial of multidisciplinary care in a high-risk, elderly heart failure population: the potential contributions of specialist care, clinical stability and optimal angiotensin-converting enzyme inhibitor dose at discharge. Eur J Heart Fail. 2001 Mar;3(2):209-15. PMID: 11246059.

28. McDonald K, Ledwidge M, Cahill J, et al. Heart failure management: multidisciplinary care has intrinsic benefit above the optimization of medical care. J Card Fail. 2002 Jun;8(3):142-8. PMID: 12140806.

29. Ledwidge M, Barry M, Cahill J, et al. Is multidisciplinary care of heart failure cost-beneficial when combined with optimal medical care? Eur J Heart Fail. 2003(3):381-9. PMID: CN-00456908.

30. Naylor MD, Brooten DA, Campbell RL, et al. Transitional care of older adults hospitalized with heart failure: a randomized, controlled trial. J Am Geriatr Soc. 2004 May;52(5):675-84. PMID: 15086645.

31. Nucifora G, Albanese MC, De Biaggio P, et al. Lack of improvement of clinical outcomes by a low-cost, hospital-based heart failure management programme. J Cardiovasc Med (Hagerstown). 2006 Aug;7(8):614-22. PMID: 16858241.

32. Oddone EZ, Weinberger M, Giobbie-Hurder A, et al. Enhanced access to primary care for patients with congestive heart failure. Veterans Affairs Cooperative Study Group on Primary Care and Hospital Readmission. Eff Clin Pract. 1999 Sep-Oct;2(5):201-9. PMID: 10623052.

33. Pekmezaris R, Mitzner I, Pecinka KR, et al. The impact of remote patient monitoring (telehealth) upon Medicare beneficiaries with heart failure. Telemed J E Health. 2012 Mar;18(2):101-8. PMID: 22283360.

34. Pugh LC, Havens DS, Xie S, et al. Case management for elderly persons with heart failure: the quality of life and cost outcomes. Medsurg Nurs. 2001;10(2):71-8.

35. Rainville EC. Impact of pharmacist interventions on hospital readmissions for heart failure. Am J Health Syst Pharm. 1999 Jul 1;56(13):1339-42. PMID: 10683133.

36. Rich MW, Vinson JM, Sperry JC, et al. Prevention of readmission in elderly patients with congestive heart failure: results of a prospective, randomized pilot study. J Gen Intern Med. 1993 Nov;8(11):585-90. PMID: 8289096.

37. Rich MW, Beckham V, Wittenberg C, et al. A multidisciplinary intervention to prevent the readmission of elderly patients with congestive heart failure. N Engl J Med. 1995 Nov 2;333(18):1190-5. PMID: 7565975.

38. Riegel B, Carlson B, Kopp Z, et al. Effect of a standardized nurse case-management telephone intervention on resource use in patients with chronic heart failure. Arch Intern Med. 2002 Mar 25;162(6):705-12. PMID: 11911726.

39. Riegel B, Carlson B. Is individual peer support a promising intervention for persons with heart failure? J Cardiovasc Nurs. 2004 May-Jun;19(3):174-83. PMID: 15191260.

40. Riegel B, Carlson B, Glaser D, et al. Randomized controlled trial of telephone case management in Hispanics of Mexican origin with heart failure. J Card Fail. 2006 Apr;12(3):211-9. PMID: 16624687.

41. Schwarz KA, Mion LC, Hudock D, et al. Telemonitoring of heart failure patients and their caregivers: a pilot randomized controlled trial. Prog Cardiovasc Nurs. 2008 Winter;23(1):18-26. PMID: 18326990.

42. Sethares KA, Elliott K. The effect of a tailored message intervention on heart failure readmission rates, quality of life, and benefit and barrier beliefs in persons with heart failure. Heart Lung. 2004 Jul-Aug;33(4):249-60. PMID: 15252415.

43. Stewart S, Pearson S, Horowitz JD. Effects of a home-based intervention among patients with congestive heart failure discharged from acute hospital care. Arch Intern Med. 1998 May 25;158(10):1067-72. PMID: 9605777.

44. Stewart S, Marley JE, Horowitz JD. Effects of a multidisciplinary, home-based intervention on unplanned readmissions and survival among patients with chronic congestive heart failure: a randomised controlled study. Lancet. 1999 Sep 25;354(9184):1077-83. PMID: 10509499.

45. Stromberg A, Martensson J, Fridlund B, et al. Nurse-led heart failure clinics improve survival and self-care behaviour in patients with heart failure: results from a prospective, randomised trial. Eur Heart J. 2003 Jun;24(11):1014-23. PMID: 12788301.

46. Thompson DR, Roebuck A, Stewart S. Effects of a nurse-led, clinic and home-based intervention on recurrent hospital use in chronic heart failure. Eur J Heart Fail. 2005 Mar 16;7(3):377-84. PMID: 15718178.

47. Triller DM, Hamilton RA. Effect of pharmaceutical care services on outcomes for home care patients with heart failure. Am J Health Syst Pharm. 2007 Nov 1;64(21):2244-9. PMID: 17959576.

48. Tsuyuki RT, Fradette M, Johnson JA, et al. A multicenter disease management program for hospitalized patients with heart failure. J Card Fail. 2004 Dec;10(6):473-80. PMID: 15599837.

49. Wakefield BJ, Ward MM, Holman JE, et al. Evaluation of home telehealth following hospitalization for heart failure: a randomized trial. Telemed J E Health. 2008 Oct;14(8):753-61. PMID: 18954244.

50. Wakefield BJ, Holman JE, Ray A, et al. Outcomes of a home telehealth intervention for patients with heart failure. J Telemed Telecare. 2009;15(1):46-50. PMID: 19139220.

51. Woodend AK, Sherrard H, Fraser M, et al. Telehome monitoring in patients with cardiac disease who are at high risk of readmission. Heart Lung. 2008 Jan-Feb;37(1):36-45. PMID: 18206525.

Appendix E. Meta-Analysis and Forest Plots of Individual Trials

Figure E1. All-cause readmission for transitional care interventions compared with usual care, by intervention category and outcome timing: Meta-analysis and forest plot of individual trials

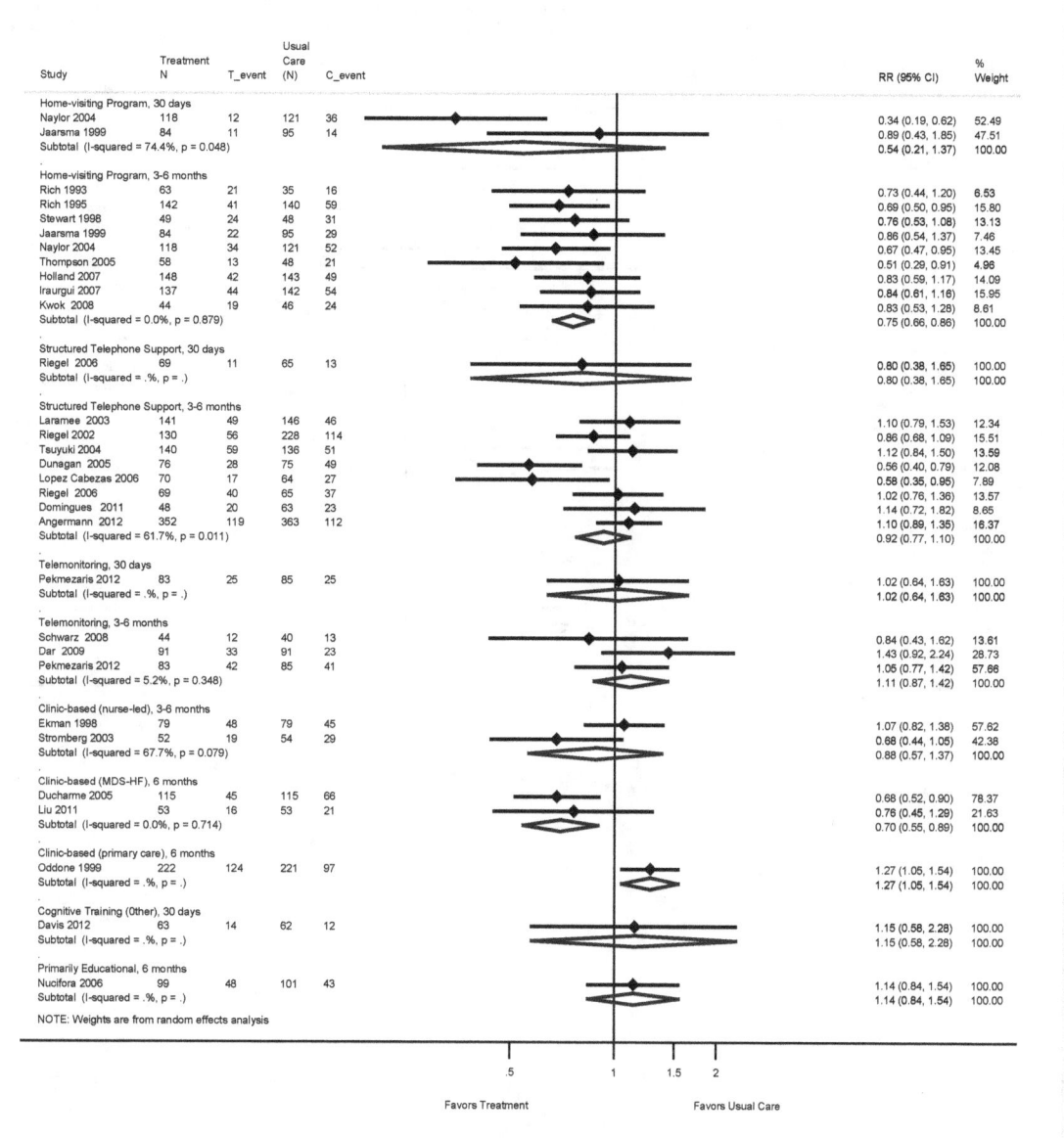

NOTE: Weights are from random effects analysis

Figure E2. HF-specific readmission for transitional care interventions compared with usual care, by intervention category and outcome timing: Meta-analysis and forest plot of individual trials

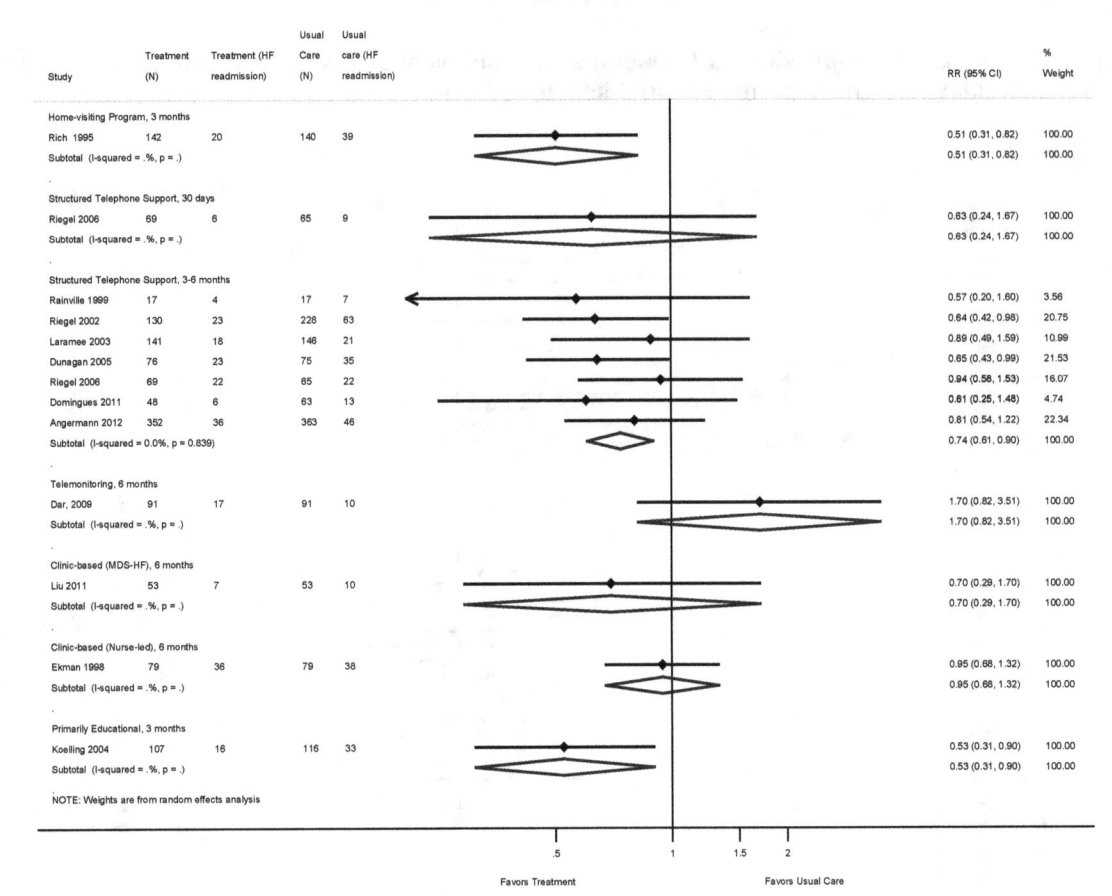

Study	Treatment (N)	Treatment (HF readmission)	Usual Care (N)	Usual care (HF readmission)		RR (95% CI)	% Weight
Home-visiting Program, 3 months							
Rich 1995	142	20	140	39		0.51 (0.31, 0.82)	100.00
Subtotal (I-squared = .%, p = .)						0.51 (0.31, 0.82)	100.00
Structured Telephone Support, 30 days							
Riegel 2006	69	6	65	9		0.63 (0.24, 1.67)	100.00
Subtotal (I-squared = .%, p = .)						0.63 (0.24, 1.67)	100.00
Structured Telephone Support, 3-6 months							
Rainville 1999	17	4	17	7		0.57 (0.20, 1.60)	3.56
Riegel 2002	130	23	228	63		0.64 (0.42, 0.98)	20.75
Laramee 2003	141	18	146	21		0.89 (0.49, 1.59)	10.99
Dunagan 2005	76	23	75	35		0.65 (0.43, 0.99)	21.53
Riegel 2006	69	22	65	22		0.94 (0.58, 1.53)	16.07
Domingues 2011	48	6	63	13		0.61 (0.25, 1.48)	4.74
Angermann 2012	352	36	363	46		0.81 (0.54, 1.22)	22.34
Subtotal (I-squared = 0.0%, p = 0.839)						0.74 (0.61, 0.90)	100.00
Telemonitoring, 6 months							
Dar, 2009	91	17	91	10		1.70 (0.82, 3.51)	100.00
Subtotal (I-squared = .%, p = .)						1.70 (0.82, 3.51)	100.00
Clinic-based (MDS-HF), 6 months							
Liu 2011	53	7	53	10		0.70 (0.29, 1.70)	100.00
Subtotal (I-squared = .%, p = .)						0.70 (0.29, 1.70)	100.00
Clinic-based (Nurse-led), 6 months							
Ekman 1998	79	36	79	38		0.95 (0.68, 1.32)	100.00
Subtotal (I-squared = .%, p = .)						0.95 (0.68, 1.32)	100.00
Primarily Educational, 3 months							
Koelling 2004	107	16	116	33		0.53 (0.31, 0.90)	100.00
Subtotal (I-squared = .%, p = .)						0.53 (0.31, 0.90)	100.00

NOTE: Weights are from random effects analysis

.5   1   1.5   2

Favors Treatment   Favors Usual Care

Figure E3. Composite all-cause readmission or death for transitional care interventions compared with usual care, by intervention category and outcome timing: Meta-analysis and forest plot of individual trials

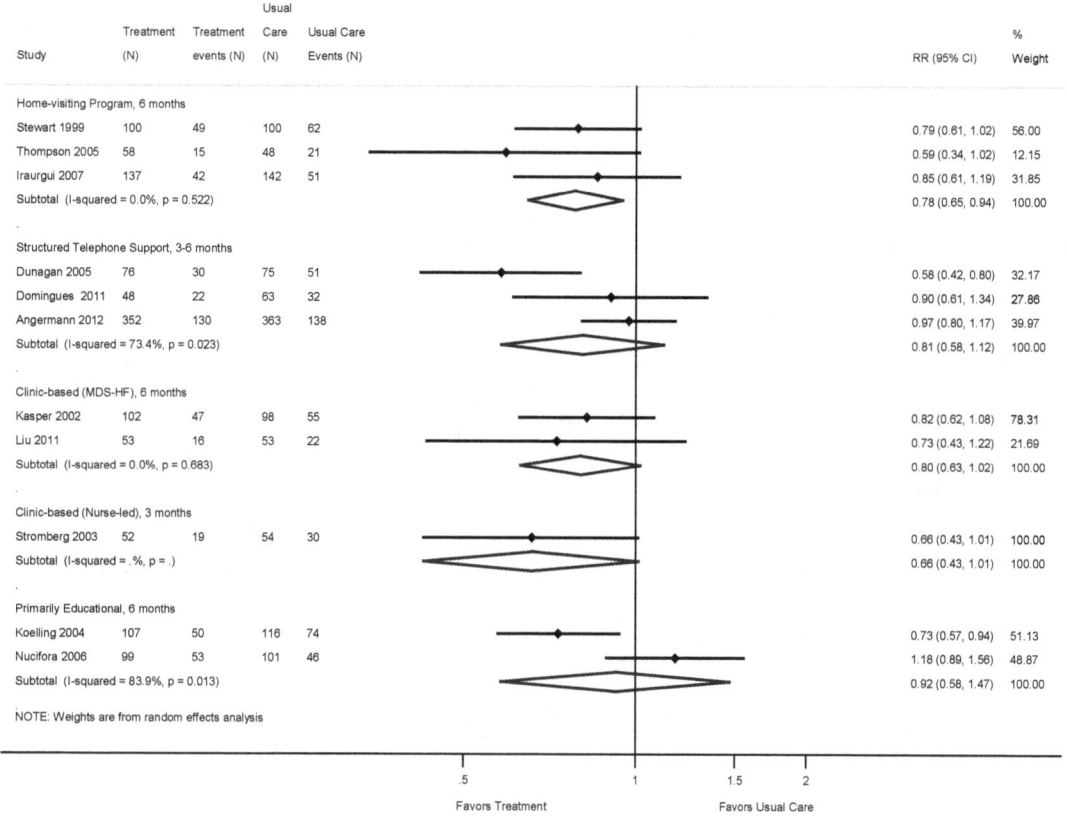

Study	Treatment (N)	Treatment events (N)	Usual Care (N)	Usual Care Events (N)	RR (95% CI)	% Weight
Home-visiting Program, 6 months						
Stewart 1999	100	49	100	62	0.79 (0.61, 1.02)	56.00
Thompson 2005	58	15	48	21	0.59 (0.34, 1.02)	12.15
Iraurgui 2007	137	42	142	51	0.85 (0.61, 1.19)	31.85
Subtotal (I-squared = 0.0%, p = 0.522)					0.78 (0.65, 0.94)	100.00
Structured Telephone Support, 3-6 months						
Dunagan 2005	76	30	75	51	0.58 (0.42, 0.80)	32.17
Domingues 2011	48	22	63	32	0.90 (0.61, 1.34)	27.86
Angermann 2012	352	130	363	138	0.97 (0.80, 1.17)	39.97
Subtotal (I-squared = 73.4%, p = 0.023)					0.81 (0.58, 1.12)	100.00
Clinic-based (MDS-HF), 6 months						
Kasper 2002	102	47	98	55	0.82 (0.62, 1.08)	78.31
Liu 2011	53	16	53	22	0.73 (0.43, 1.22)	21.69
Subtotal (I-squared = 0.0%, p = 0.683)					0.80 (0.63, 1.02)	100.00
Clinic-based (Nurse-led), 3 months						
Stromberg 2003	52	19	54	30	0.66 (0.43, 1.01)	100.00
Subtotal (I-squared = .%, p = .)					0.66 (0.43, 1.01)	100.00
Primarily Educational, 6 months						
Koelling 2004	107	50	116	74	0.73 (0.57, 0.94)	51.13
Nucifora 2006	99	53	101	46	1.18 (0.89, 1.56)	48.87
Subtotal (I-squared = 83.9%, p = 0.013)					0.92 (0.58, 1.47)	100.00

NOTE: Weights are from random effects analysis

.5   1   1.5   2

Favors Treatment   Favors Usual Care

Figure E4. Mean hospital days per person (of subsequent readmissions) for home-visiting programs compared with usual care over 3 months

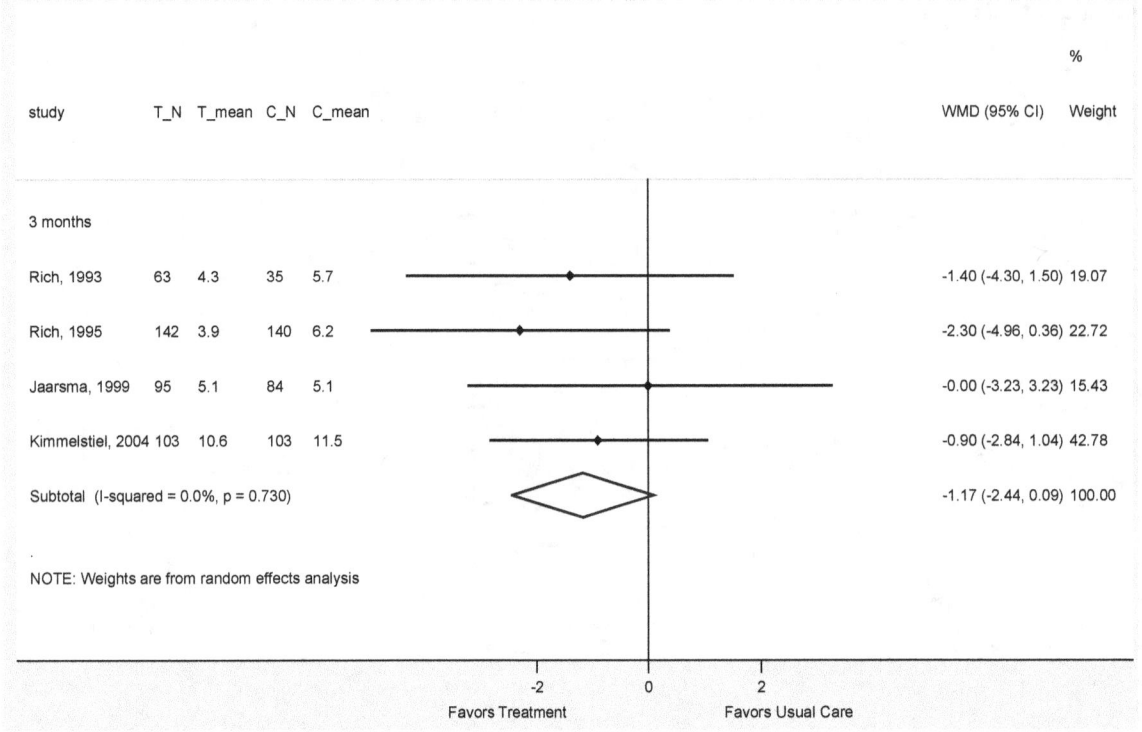

Figure E5. Total hospital days per group (of subsequent readmissions) for structured telephone support interventions compared with usual care, by outcome timing: Meta-analysis and forest plot of individual trials

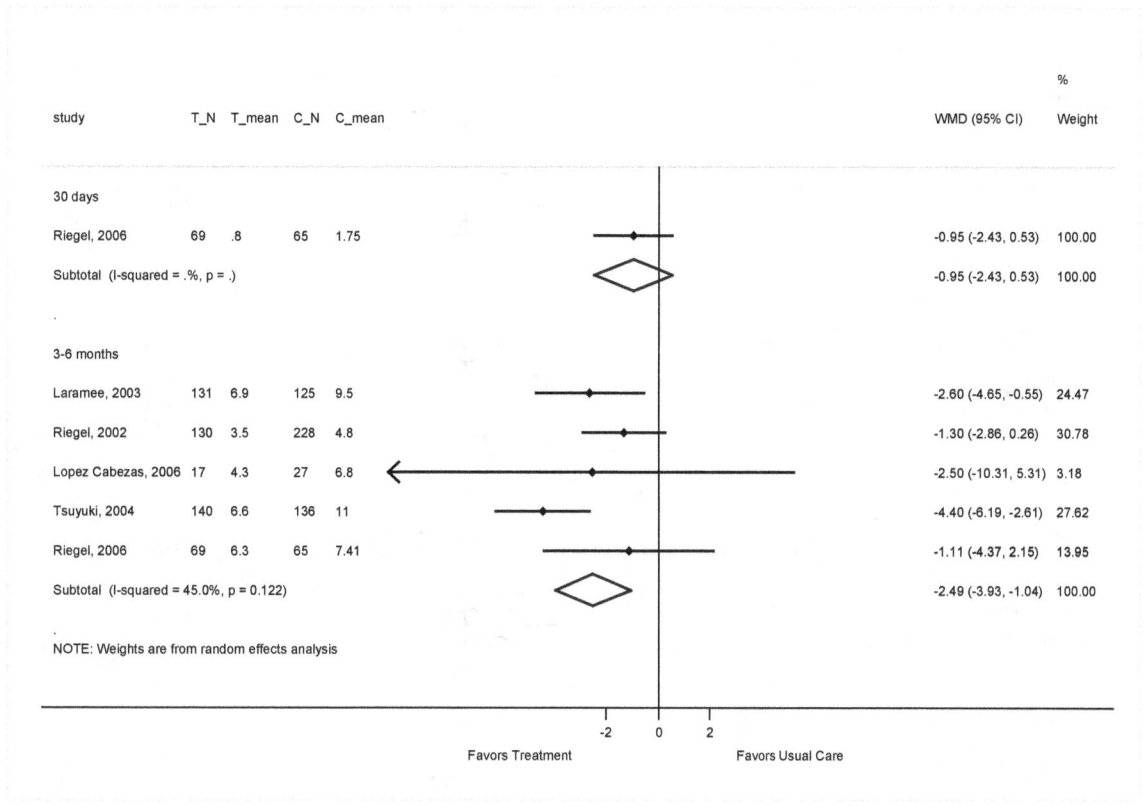

Figure E6. Mortality among patients receiving transitional care interventions compared with usual care, by intervention category and outcome timing: Meta-analysis and forest plot of individual trials

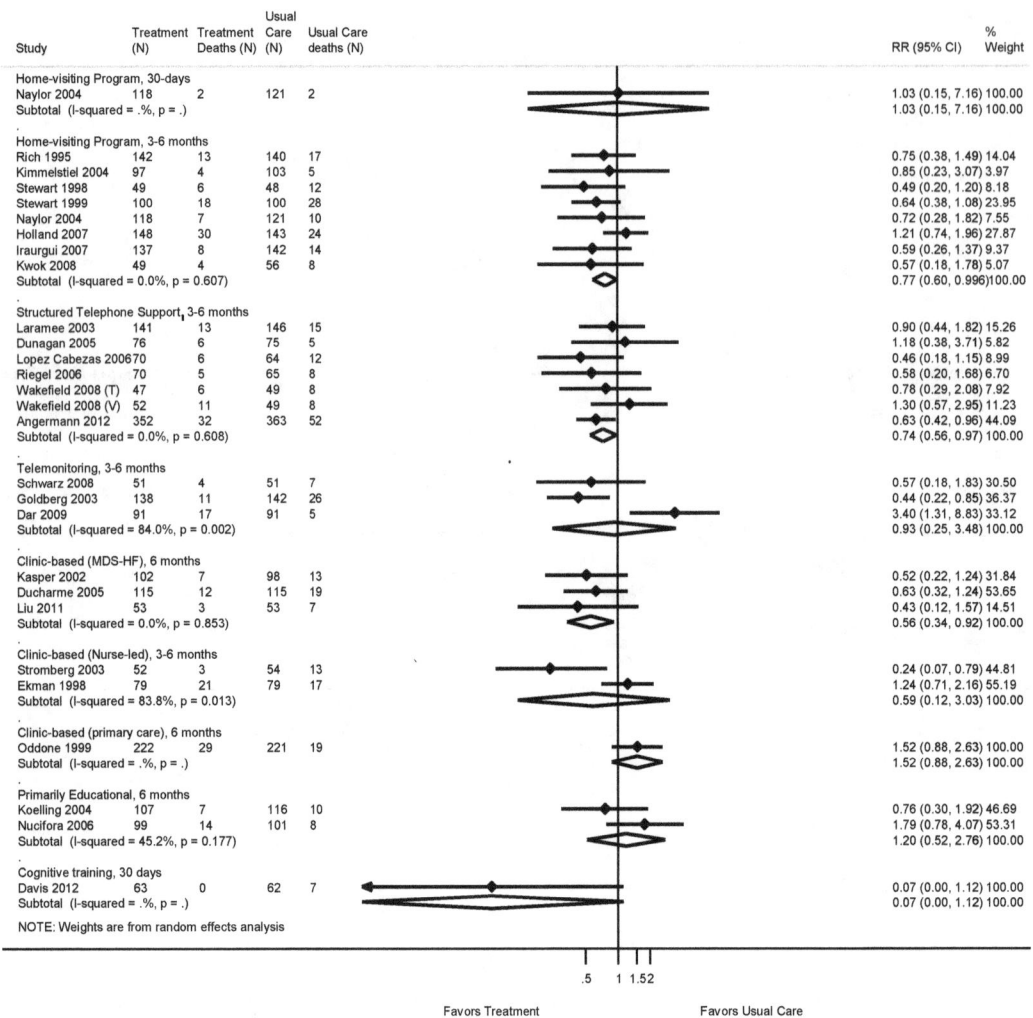

Note: For the trial by Wakefield et al., we include the telephone care arm here (not the videophone arm).[1]

Figure E7. Difference in mean MLWHFQ scores for home-visiting programs compared with usual care, by outcome timing

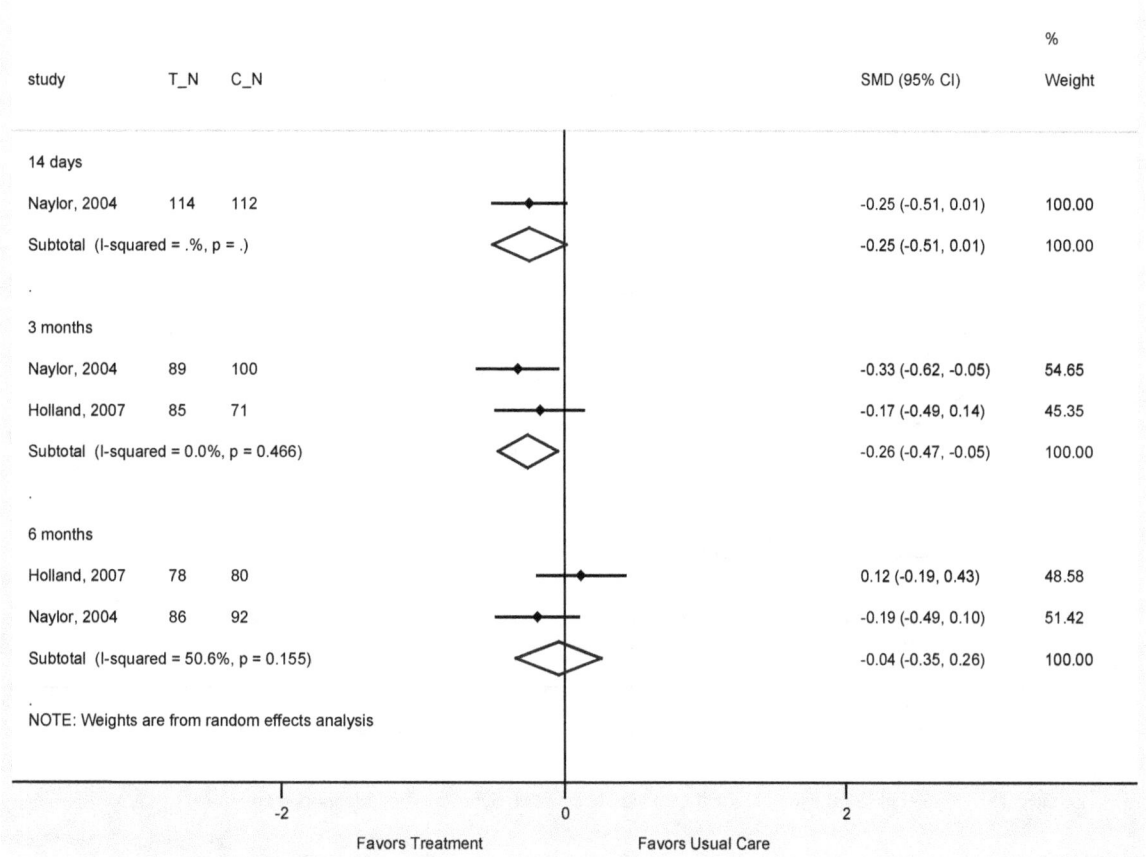

study	T_N	C_N	SMD (95% CI)	% Weight
14 days				
Naylor, 2004	114	112	-0.25 (-0.51, 0.01)	100.00
Subtotal (I-squared = .%, p = .)			-0.25 (-0.51, 0.01)	100.00
3 months				
Naylor, 2004	89	100	-0.33 (-0.62, -0.05)	54.65
Holland, 2007	85	71	-0.17 (-0.49, 0.14)	45.35
Subtotal (I-squared = 0.0%, p = 0.466)			-0.26 (-0.47, -0.05)	100.00
6 months				
Holland, 2007	78	80	0.12 (-0.19, 0.43)	48.58
Naylor, 2004	86	92	-0.19 (-0.49, 0.10)	51.42
Subtotal (I-squared = 50.6%, p = 0.155)			-0.04 (-0.35, 0.26)	100.00

NOTE: Weights are from random effects analysis

Favors Treatment   Favors Usual Care

Note: Naylor and colleagues transformed MLWHFQ scores to ordinal scales (assigning a score of 0 to patients who died to account for missing data and grouping other scores into quartiles ranging from 1 to 5); thus, although they measured quality of life with the same instrument, the scale differed from that used in other trials.[2]

Figure E8. Difference in mean MLWHFQ scores for structured telephone support interventions compared with usual care, by outcome timing

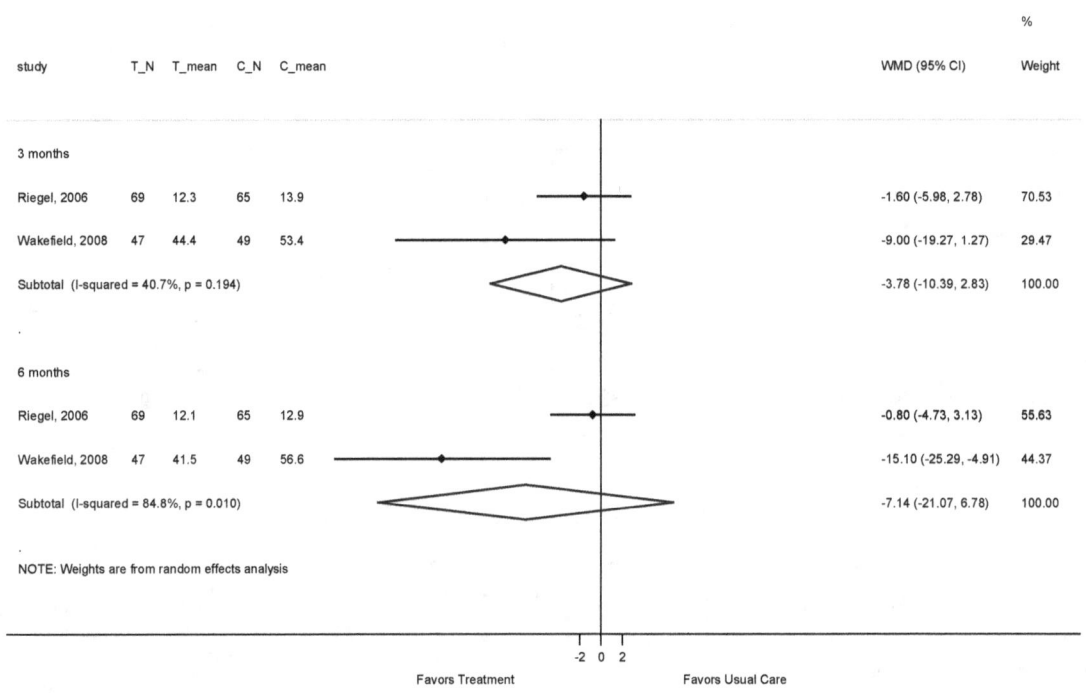

Note: For the trial by Wakefield et al., we include the telephone care arm here (not the videophone arm).[1]

Figure E9. All-cause readmissions for home-visiting programs compared with usual care, by intensity and outcome timing: Meta-analysis and forest plot of individual trials

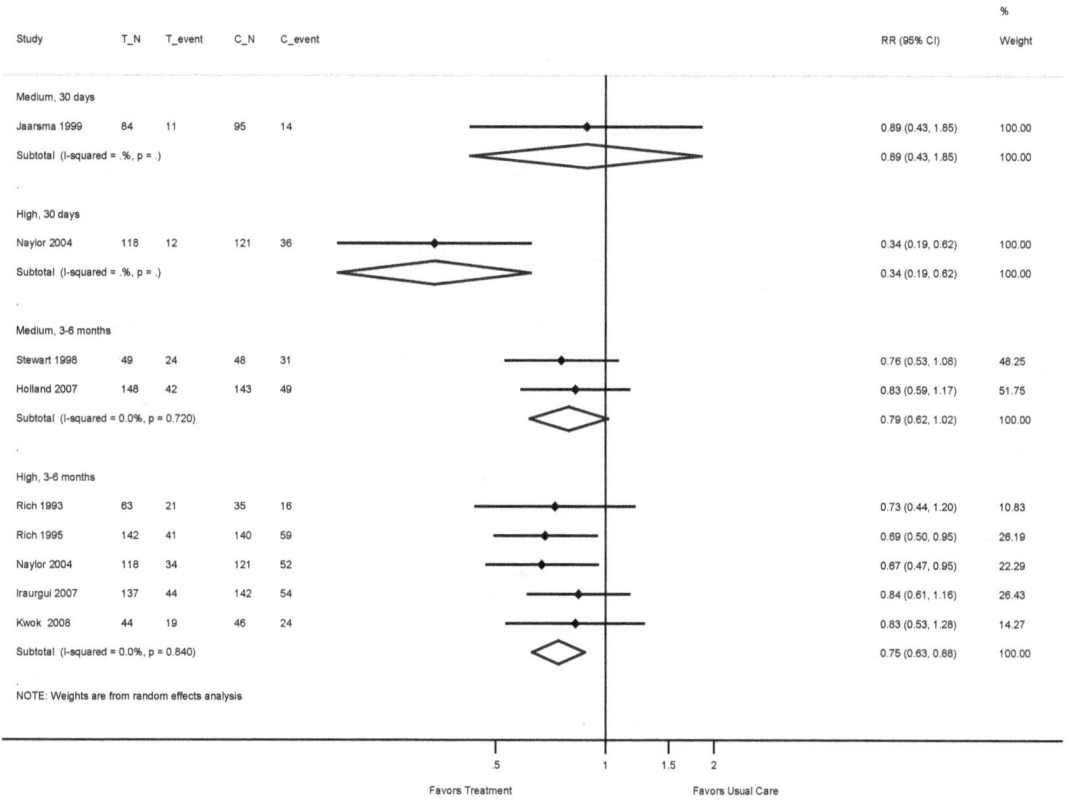

Study	T_N	T_event	C_N	C_event	RR (95% CI)	% Weight
Medium, 30 days						
Jaarsma 1999	84	11	95	14	0.89 (0.43, 1.85)	100.00
Subtotal (I-squared = .%, p = .)					0.89 (0.43, 1.85)	100.00
High, 30 days						
Naylor 2004	118	12	121	36	0.34 (0.19, 0.62)	100.00
Subtotal (I-squared = .%, p = .)					0.34 (0.19, 0.62)	100.00
Medium, 3-6 months						
Stewart 1998	49	24	48	31	0.76 (0.53, 1.08)	48.25
Holland 2007	148	42	143	49	0.83 (0.59, 1.17)	51.75
Subtotal (I-squared = 0.0%, p = 0.720)					0.79 (0.62, 1.02)	100.00
High, 3-6 months						
Rich 1993	63	21	35	16	0.73 (0.44, 1.20)	10.83
Rich 1995	142	41	140	59	0.69 (0.50, 0.95)	26.19
Naylor 2004	118	34	121	52	0.67 (0.47, 0.95)	22.29
Iraurgui 2007	137	44	142	54	0.84 (0.61, 1.16)	26.43
Kwok 2008	44	19	46	24	0.83 (0.53, 1.28)	14.27
Subtotal (I-squared = 0.0%, p = 0.840)					0.75 (0.63, 0.88)	100.00

NOTE: Weights are from random effects analysis

Favors Treatment   Favors Usual Care

Figure E10. Mortality for home-visiting programs compared with usual care, by intensity and outcome timing: Meta-analysis and forest plot of individual trials

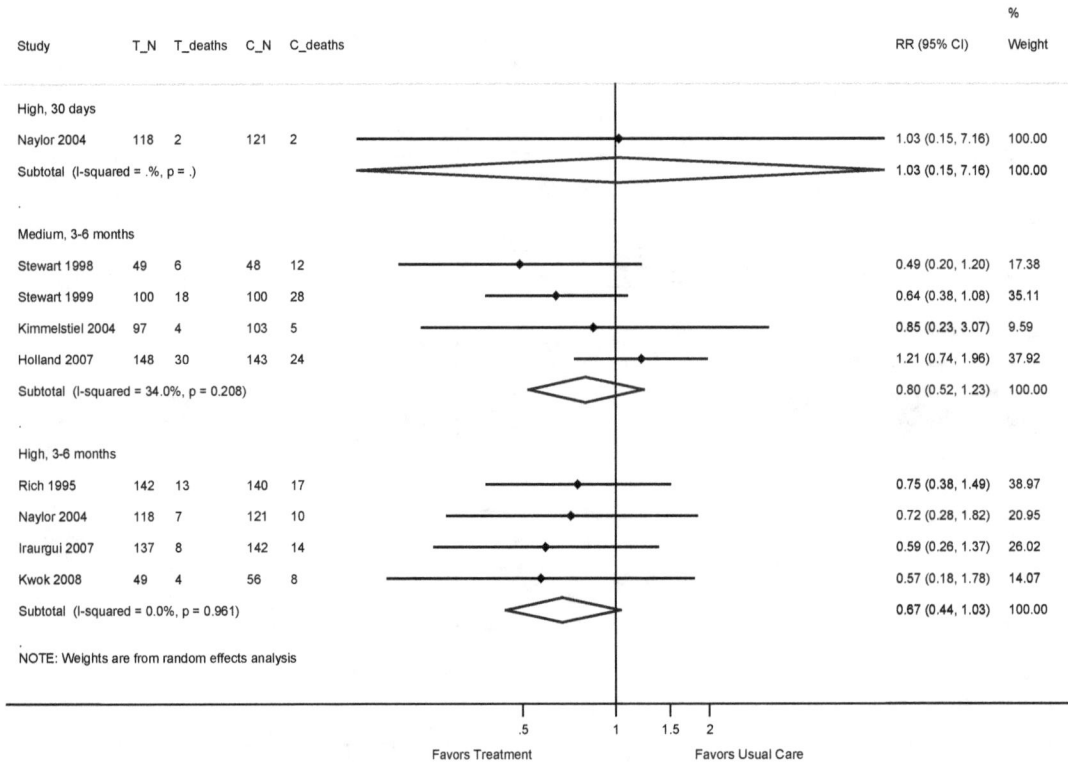

Study	T_N	T_deaths	C_N	C_deaths	RR (95% CI)	% Weight
High, 30 days						
Naylor 2004	118	2	121	2	1.03 (0.15, 7.16)	100.00
Subtotal (I-squared = .%, p = .)					1.03 (0.15, 7.16)	100.00
Medium, 3-6 months						
Stewart 1998	49	6	48	12	0.49 (0.20, 1.20)	17.38
Stewart 1999	100	18	100	28	0.64 (0.38, 1.08)	35.11
Kimmelstiel 2004	97	4	103	5	0.85 (0.23, 3.07)	9.59
Holland 2007	148	30	143	24	1.21 (0.74, 1.96)	37.92
Subtotal (I-squared = 34.0%, p = 0.208)					0.80 (0.52, 1.23)	100.00
High, 3-6 months						
Rich 1995	142	13	140	17	0.75 (0.38, 1.49)	38.97
Naylor 2004	118	7	121	10	0.72 (0.28, 1.82)	20.95
Iraurgui 2007	137	8	142	14	0.59 (0.26, 1.37)	26.02
Kwok 2008	49	4	56	8	0.57 (0.18, 1.78)	14.07
Subtotal (I-squared = 0.0%, p = 0.961)					0.67 (0.44, 1.03)	100.00

NOTE: Weights are from random effects analysis

.5   1   1.5   2

Favors Treatment   Favors Usual Care

Figure E11. All-cause readmissions for structured telephone support interventions compared with usual care, by intensity and outcome timing: Meta-analysis and forest plot of individual trials

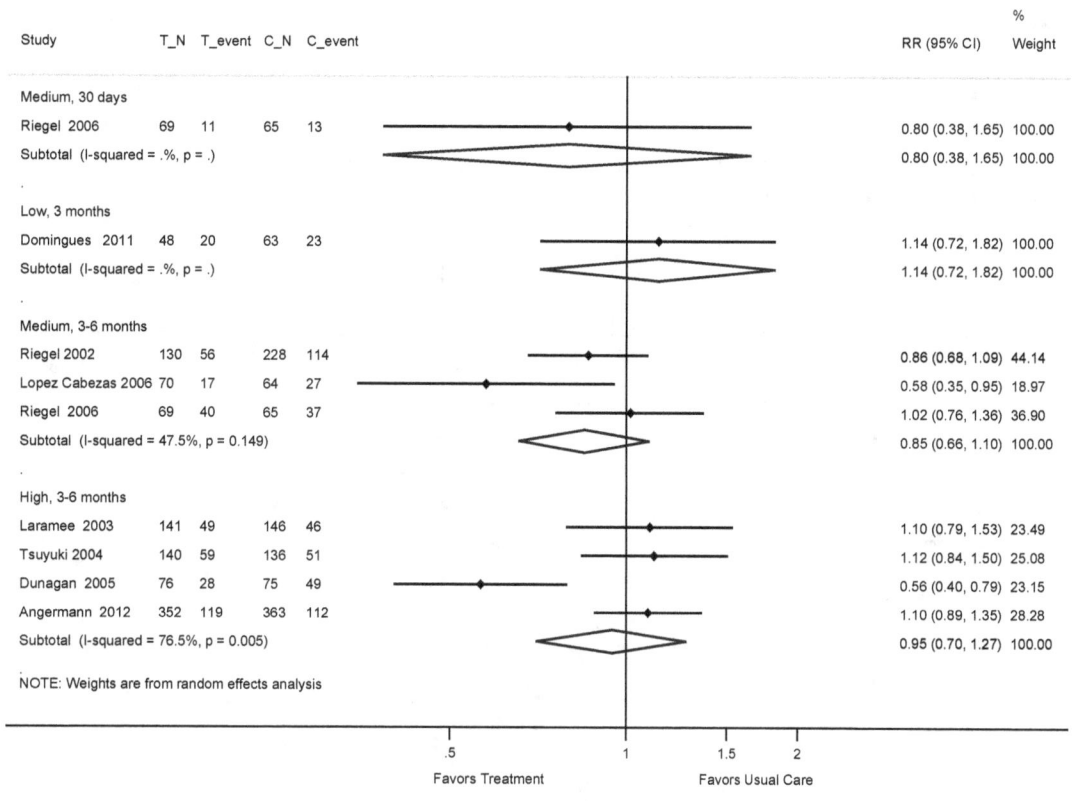

Study	T_N	T_event	C_N	C_event	RR (95% CI)	% Weight
Medium, 30 days						
Riegel 2006	69	11	65	13	0.80 (0.38, 1.65)	100.00
Subtotal (I-squared = .%, p = .)					0.80 (0.38, 1.65)	100.00
Low, 3 months						
Domingues 2011	48	20	63	23	1.14 (0.72, 1.82)	100.00
Subtotal (I-squared = .%, p = .)					1.14 (0.72, 1.82)	100.00
Medium, 3-6 months						
Riegel 2002	130	56	228	114	0.86 (0.68, 1.09)	44.14
Lopez Cabezas 2006	70	17	64	27	0.58 (0.35, 0.95)	18.97
Riegel 2006	69	40	65	37	1.02 (0.76, 1.36)	36.90
Subtotal (I-squared = 47.5%, p = 0.149)					0.85 (0.66, 1.10)	100.00
High, 3-6 months						
Laramee 2003	141	49	146	46	1.10 (0.79, 1.53)	23.49
Tsuyuki 2004	140	59	136	51	1.12 (0.84, 1.50)	25.08
Dunagan 2005	76	28	75	49	0.56 (0.40, 0.79)	23.15
Angermann 2012	352	119	363	112	1.10 (0.89, 1.35)	28.28
Subtotal (I-squared = 76.5%, p = 0.005)					0.95 (0.70, 1.27)	100.00

NOTE: Weights are from random effects analysis

.5   1   1.5   2

Favors Treatment   Favors Usual Care

Figure E12. Mortality for structured telephone support interventions compared with usual care, by intensity and outcome timing: Meta-analysis and forest plot of individual trials

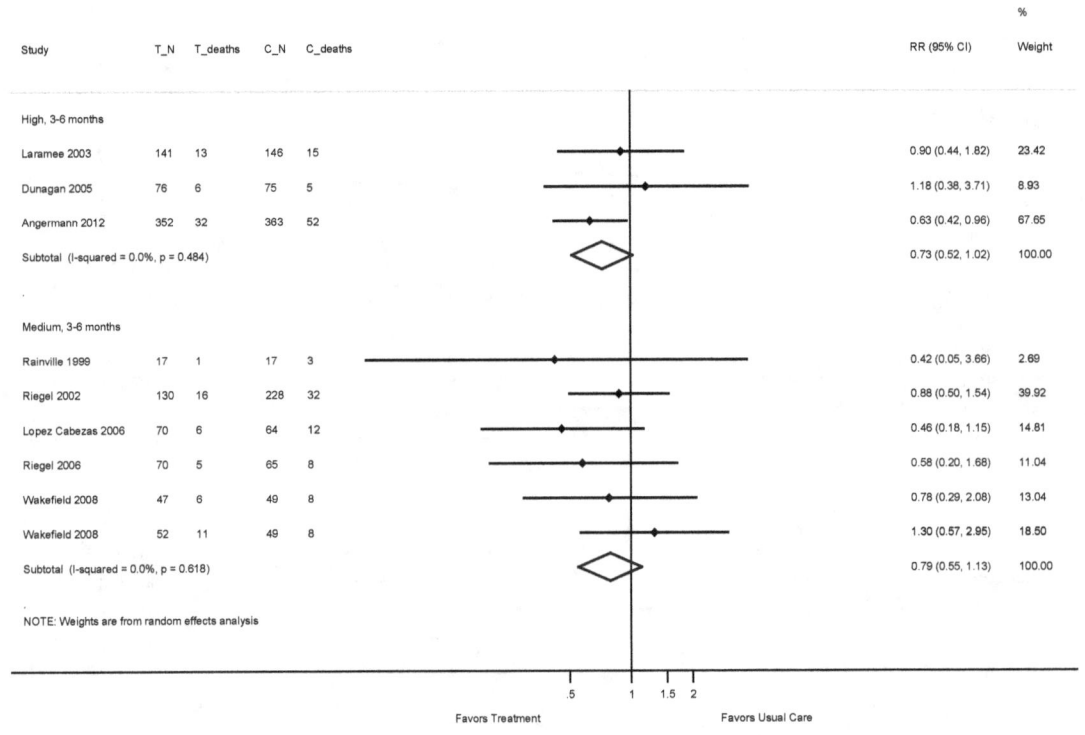

Study	T_N	T_deaths	C_N	C_deaths	RR (95% CI)	% Weight
High, 3-6 months						
Laramee 2003	141	13	146	15	0.90 (0.44, 1.82)	23.42
Dunagan 2005	76	6	75	5	1.18 (0.38, 3.71)	8.93
Angermann 2012	352	32	363	52	0.63 (0.42, 0.96)	67.65
Subtotal (I-squared = 0.0%, p = 0.484)					0.73 (0.52, 1.02)	100.00
Medium, 3-6 months						
Rainville 1999	17	1	17	3	0.42 (0.05, 3.66)	2.69
Riegel 2002	130	16	228	32	0.88 (0.50, 1.54)	39.92
Lopez Cabezas 2006	70	6	64	12	0.46 (0.18, 1.15)	14.81
Riegel 2006	70	5	65	8	0.58 (0.20, 1.68)	11.04
Wakefield 2008	47	6	49	8	0.78 (0.29, 2.08)	13.04
Wakefield 2008	52	11	49	8	1.30 (0.57, 2.95)	18.50
Subtotal (I-squared = 0.0%, p = 0.618)					0.79 (0.55, 1.13)	100.00

NOTE: Weights are from random effects analysis

.5   1   1.5   2

Favors Treatment   Favors Usual Care

Figure E13. All-cause readmissions for home-visiting programs compared with usual care, by delivery personnel and outcome timing: Meta-analysis and forest plot of individual trials

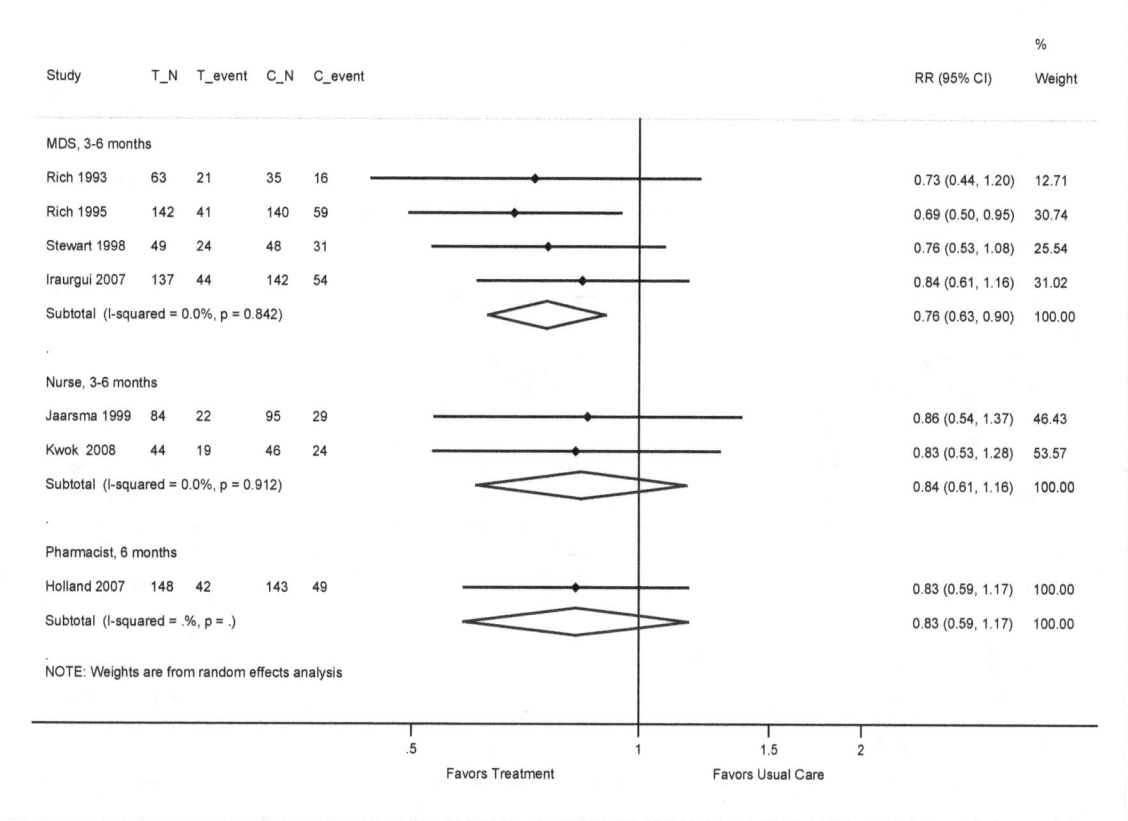

Figure E14. Mortality for home-visiting programs compared with usual care, by delivery personnel and outcome timing: Meta-analysis and forest plot of individual trials

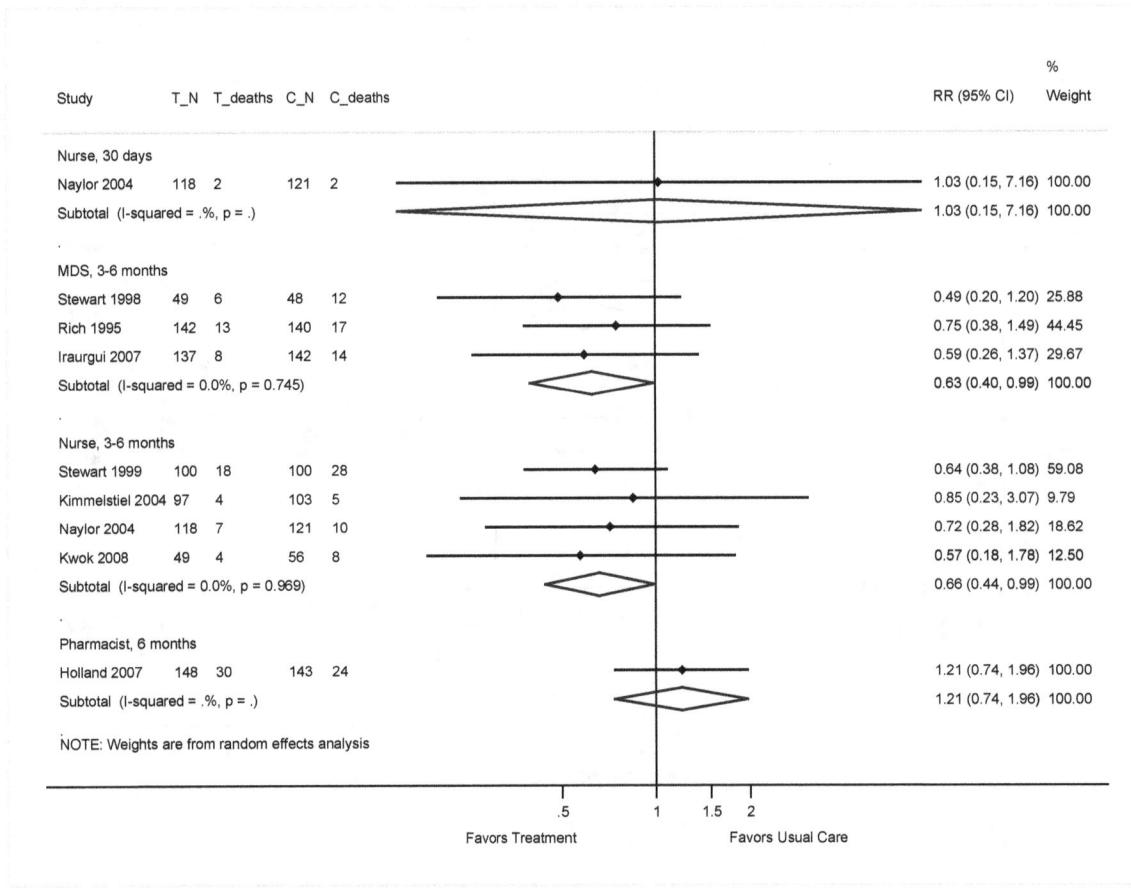

Study	T_N	T_deaths	C_N	C_deaths	RR (95% CI)	% Weight
Nurse, 30 days						
Naylor 2004	118	2	121	2	1.03 (0.15, 7.16)	100.00
Subtotal (I-squared = .%, p = .)					1.03 (0.15, 7.16)	100.00
MDS, 3-6 months						
Stewart 1998	49	6	48	12	0.49 (0.20, 1.20)	25.88
Rich 1995	142	13	140	17	0.75 (0.38, 1.49)	44.45
Iraurgui 2007	137	8	142	14	0.59 (0.26, 1.37)	29.67
Subtotal (I-squared = 0.0%, p = 0.745)					0.63 (0.40, 0.99)	100.00
Nurse, 3-6 months						
Stewart 1999	100	18	100	28	0.64 (0.38, 1.08)	59.08
Kimmelstiel 2004	97	4	103	5	0.85 (0.23, 3.07)	9.79
Naylor 2004	118	7	121	10	0.72 (0.28, 1.82)	18.62
Kwok 2008	49	4	56	8	0.57 (0.18, 1.78)	12.50
Subtotal (I-squared = 0.0%, p = 0.969)					0.66 (0.44, 0.99)	100.00
Pharmacist, 6 months						
Holland 2007	148	30	143	24	1.21 (0.74, 1.96)	100.00
Subtotal (I-squared = .%, p = .)					1.21 (0.74, 1.96)	100.00

NOTE: Weights are from random effects analysis

.5   1   1.5   2

Favors Treatment   Favors Usual Care

Figure E15. All-cause readmission for structured telephone support interventions compared with usual care, by delivery personnel and outcome timing: Meta-analysis and forest plot of individual trials

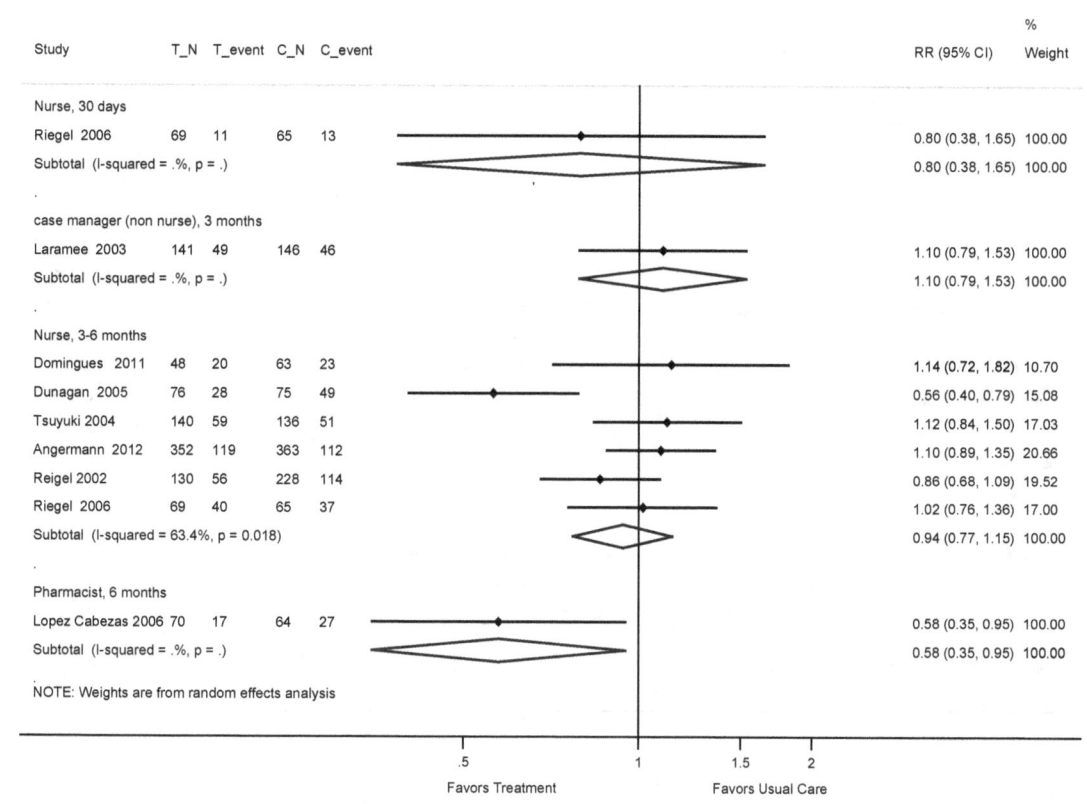

Figure E16. Mortality for structured telephone support interventions compared with usual care, by delivery personnel and outcome timing: Meta-analysis and forest plot of individual trials

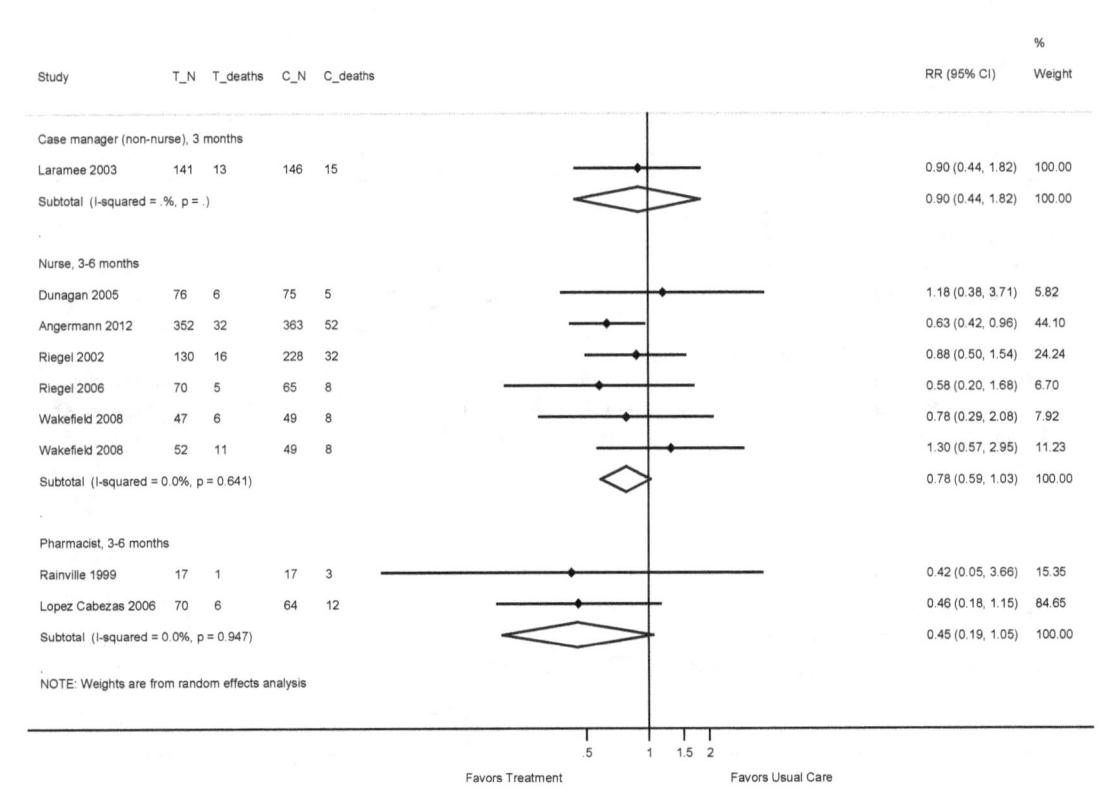

Study	T_N	T_deaths	C_N	C_deaths	RR (95% CI)	% Weight
Case manager (non-nurse), 3 months						
Laramee 2003	141	13	146	15	0.90 (0.44, 1.82)	100.00
Subtotal (I-squared = .%, p = .)					0.90 (0.44, 1.82)	100.00
Nurse, 3-6 months						
Dunagan 2005	76	6	75	5	1.18 (0.38, 3.71)	5.82
Angermann 2012	352	32	363	52	0.63 (0.42, 0.96)	44.10
Riegel 2002	130	16	228	32	0.88 (0.50, 1.54)	24.24
Riegel 2006	70	5	65	8	0.58 (0.20, 1.68)	6.70
Wakefield 2008	47	6	49	8	0.78 (0.29, 2.08)	7.92
Wakefield 2008	52	11	49	8	1.30 (0.57, 2.95)	11.23
Subtotal (I-squared = 0.0%, p = 0.641)					0.78 (0.59, 1.03)	100.00
Pharmacist, 3-6 months						
Rainville 1999	17	1	17	3	0.42 (0.05, 3.66)	15.35
Lopez Cabezas 2006	70	6	64	12	0.46 (0.18, 1.15)	84.65
Subtotal (I-squared = 0.0%, p = 0.947)					0.45 (0.19, 1.05)	100.00

NOTE: Weights are from random effects analysis

.5　1　1.5　2

Favors Treatment　　　Favors Usual Care

Figure E17. All-cause readmission for structured telephone support interventions compared with usual care, by method of communication and outcome timing: Meta-analysis and forest plot of individual trials

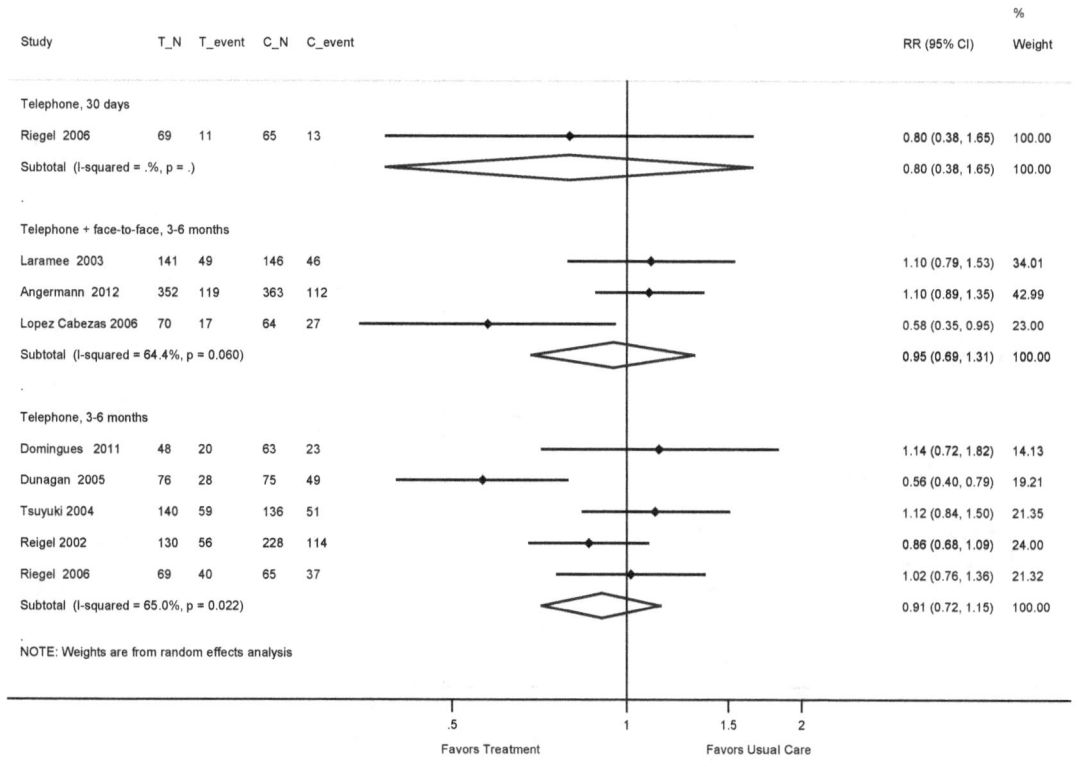

Figure E18. Mortality for structured telephone support interventions, by method of communication and outcome timing: Meta-analysis and forest plot of individual trials

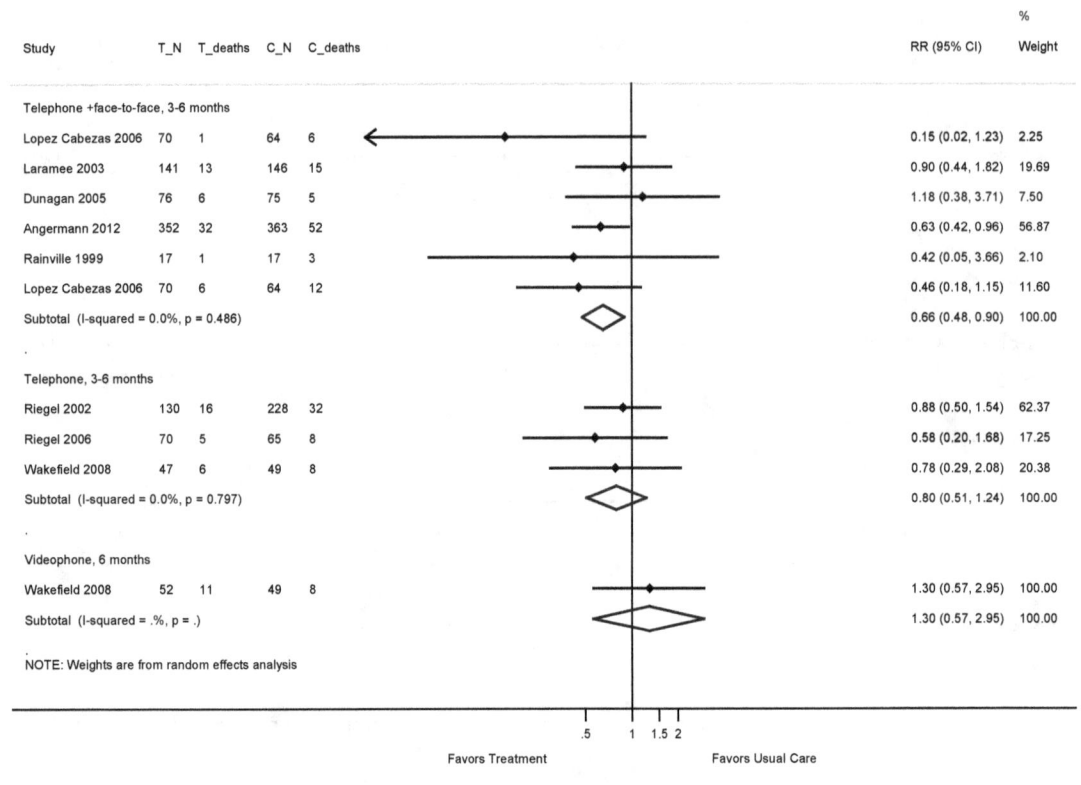

Study	T_N	T_deaths	C_N	C_deaths	RR (95% CI)	% Weight
Telephone +face-to-face, 3-6 months						
Lopez Cabezas 2006	70	1	64	6	0.15 (0.02, 1.23)	2.25
Laramee 2003	141	13	146	15	0.90 (0.44, 1.82)	19.69
Dunagan 2005	76	6	75	5	1.18 (0.38, 3.71)	7.50
Angermann 2012	352	32	363	52	0.63 (0.42, 0.96)	56.87
Rainville 1999	17	1	17	3	0.42 (0.05, 3.66)	2.10
Lopez Cabezas 2006	70	6	64	12	0.46 (0.18, 1.15)	11.60
Subtotal (I-squared = 0.0%, p = 0.486)					0.66 (0.48, 0.90)	100.00
Telephone, 3-6 months						
Riegel 2002	130	16	228	32	0.88 (0.50, 1.54)	62.37
Riegel 2006	70	5	65	8	0.58 (0.20, 1.68)	17.25
Wakefield 2008	47	6	49	8	0.78 (0.29, 2.08)	20.38
Subtotal (I-squared = 0.0%, p = 0.797)					0.80 (0.51, 1.24)	100.00
Videophone, 6 months						
Wakefield 2008	52	11	49	8	1.30 (0.57, 2.95)	100.00
Subtotal (I-squared = .%, p = .)					1.30 (0.57, 2.95)	100.00

NOTE: Weights are from random effects analysis

Favors Treatment   Favors Usual Care

Appendix E References

1. Wakefield BJ, Holman JE, Ray A, et al. Outcomes of a home telehealth intervention for patients with heart failure. J Telemed Telecare. 2009;15(1):46-50. PMID: 19139220.

2. Naylor MD, Brooten DA, Campbell RL, et al. Transitional care of older adults hospitalized with heart failure: a randomized, controlled trial. J Am Geriatr Soc. 2004 May;52(5):675-84. PMID: 15086645.

Appendix F. Meta-Analysis and Forest Plots of Individual Trials: Sensitivity Analyses

Figure F1. All-cause readmission for transitional care interventions compared with usual care, by intervention category and outcome timing: Sensitivity analysis of including trials rated as having high or unclear ROB

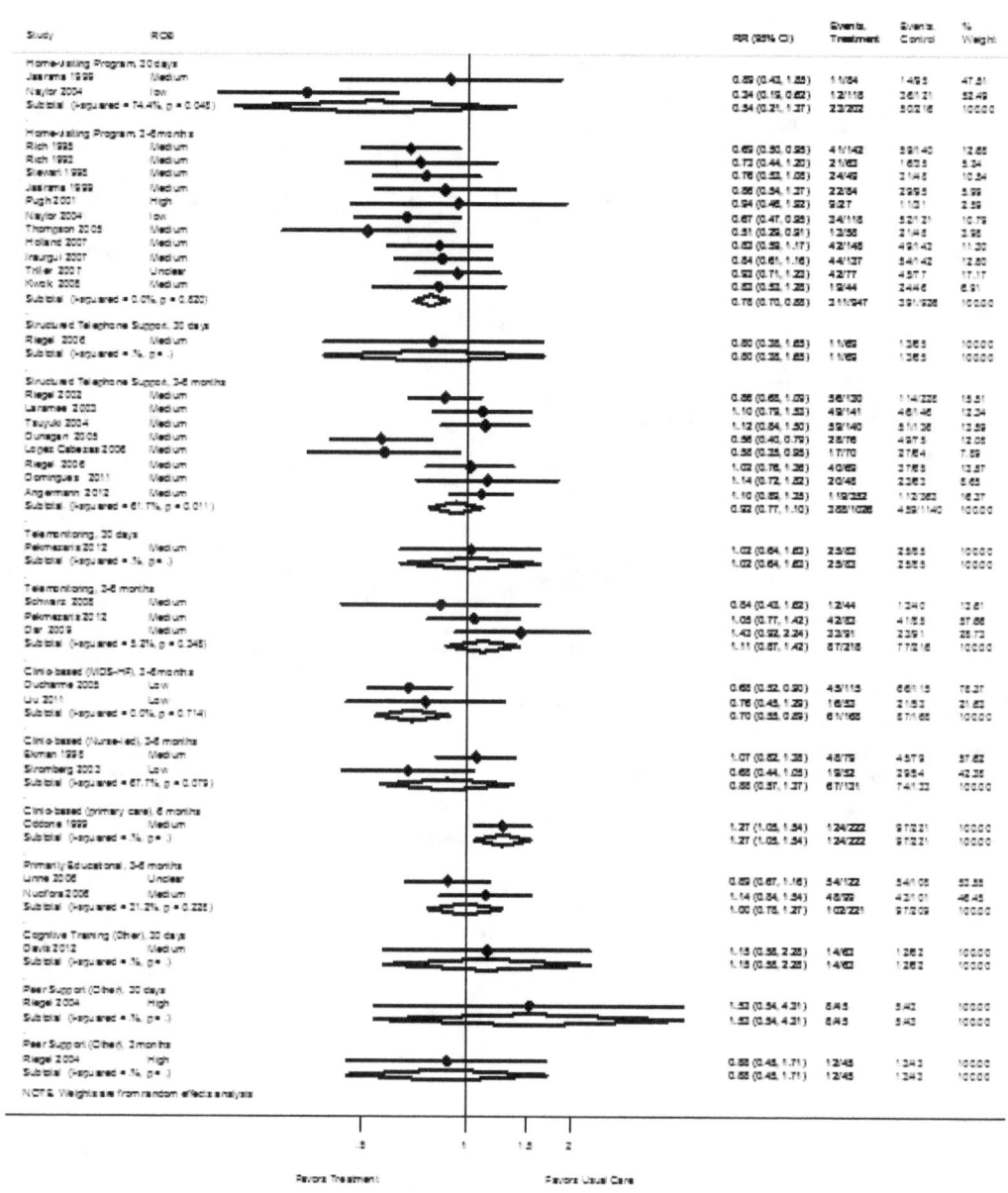

Figure F2. HF readmissions for transitional care interventions compared with usual care, by intervention category and outcome timing: Sensitivity analysis including trials rated as having high or unclear ROB

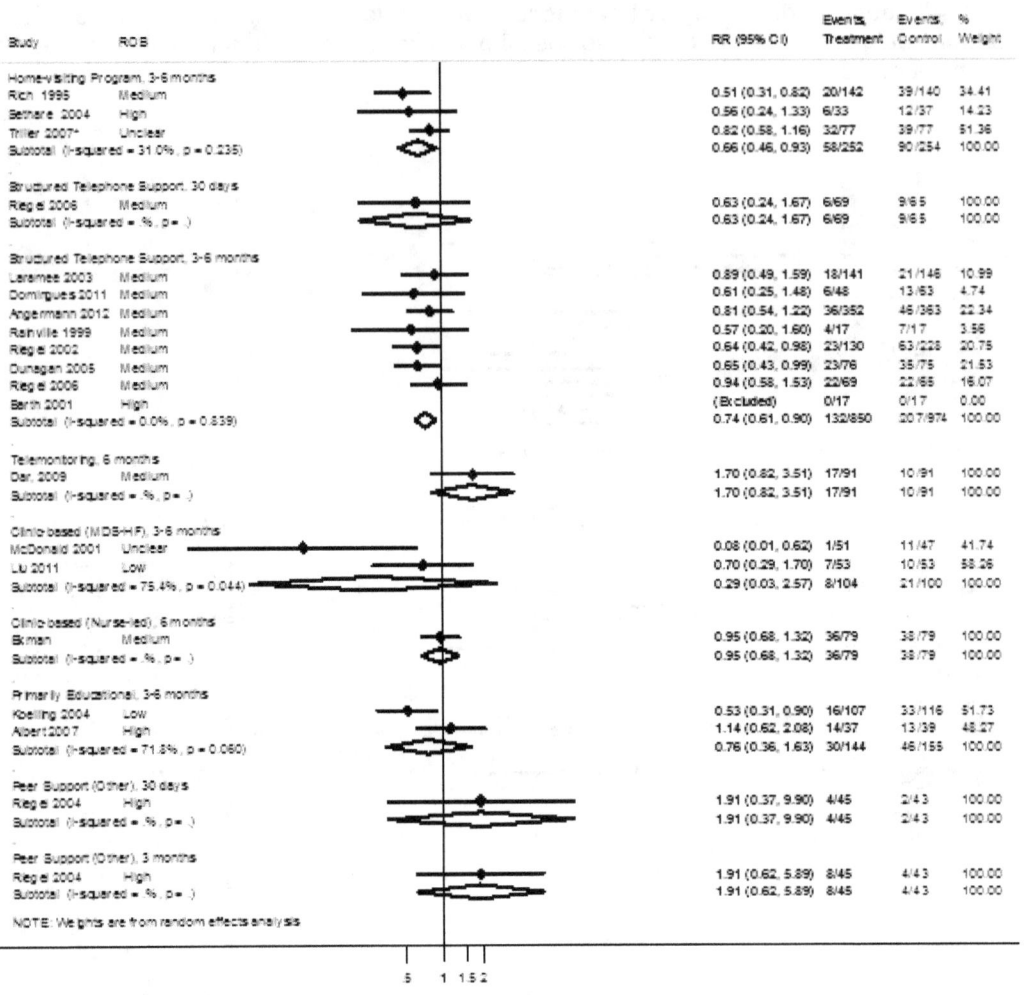

Study	ROB	RR (95% CI)	Events Treatment	Events Control	% Weight
Home-visiting Program, 3-6 months					
Rich 1995	Medium	0.51 (0.31, 0.82)	20/142	39/140	34.41
Bethare 2004	High	0.56 (0.24, 1.33)	6/33	12/37	14.23
Triller 2007*	Unclear	0.82 (0.58, 1.16)	32/77	39/77	51.36
Subtotal (I-squared = 31.0%, p = 0.235)		0.66 (0.46, 0.93)	58/252	90/254	100.00
Structured Telephone Support, 30 days					
Riegel 2006	Medium	0.63 (0.24, 1.67)	6/69	9/65	100.00
Subtotal (I-squared = .%, p = .)		0.63 (0.24, 1.67)	6/69	9/65	100.00
Structured Telephone Support, 3-6 months					
Laramee 2003	Medium	0.89 (0.49, 1.59)	18/141	21/146	10.99
Domingues 2011	Medium	0.61 (0.25, 1.48)	6/48	13/53	4.74
Angermann 2012	Medium	0.81 (0.54, 1.22)	36/352	46/363	22.34
Rainville 1999	Medium	0.57 (0.20, 1.60)	4/17	7/17	3.56
Riegel 2002	Medium	0.64 (0.42, 0.98)	23/130	63/228	20.75
Dunagan 2005	Medium	0.65 (0.43, 0.99)	23/76	35/75	21.53
Riegel 2006	Medium	0.94 (0.58, 1.53)	22/69	22/65	16.07
Barth 2001	High	(Excluded)	0/17	0/17	0.00
Subtotal (I-squared = 0.0%, p = 0.839)		0.74 (0.61, 0.90)	132/850	207/974	100.00
Telemonitoring, 6 months					
Dar, 2009	Medium	1.70 (0.82, 3.51)	17/91	10/91	100.00
Subtotal (I-squared = .%, p = .)		1.70 (0.82, 3.51)	17/91	10/91	100.00
Clinic-based (MDS-HF), 3-6 months					
McDonald 2001	Unclear	0.08 (0.01, 0.62)	1/51	11/47	41.74
Liu 2011	Low	0.70 (0.29, 1.70)	7/53	10/53	58.26
Subtotal (I-squared = 75.4%, p = 0.044)		0.29 (0.03, 2.57)	8/104	21/100	100.00
Clinic-based (Nurse-led), 6 months					
Ekman	Medium	0.95 (0.68, 1.32)	36/79	38/79	100.00
Subtotal (I-squared = .%, p = .)		0.95 (0.68, 1.32)	36/79	38/79	100.00
Primarily Educational, 3-6 months					
Koelling 2004	Low	0.53 (0.31, 0.90)	16/107	33/116	51.73
Albert 2007	High	1.14 (0.62, 2.08)	14/37	13/39	48.27
Subtotal (I-squared = 71.8%, p = 0.060)		0.76 (0.36, 1.63)	30/144	46/155	100.00
Peer Support (Other), 30 days					
Riegel 2004	High	1.91 (0.37, 9.90)	4/45	2/43	100.00
Subtotal (I-squared = .%, p = .)		1.91 (0.37, 9.90)	4/45	2/43	100.00
Peer Support (Other), 3 months					
Riegel 2004	High	1.91 (0.62, 5.89)	8/45	4/43	100.00
Subtotal (I-squared = .%, p = .)		1.91 (0.62, 5.89)	8/45	4/43	100.00

NOTE: Weights are from random effects analysis

.5   1   1.5 2

Favors Treatment   Favors Usual Care

Figure F3. Composite all-cause readmission or death for transitional care interventions compared with usual care, by intervention category and outcome timing: Sensitivity analysis including trials rated as having high or unclear ROB

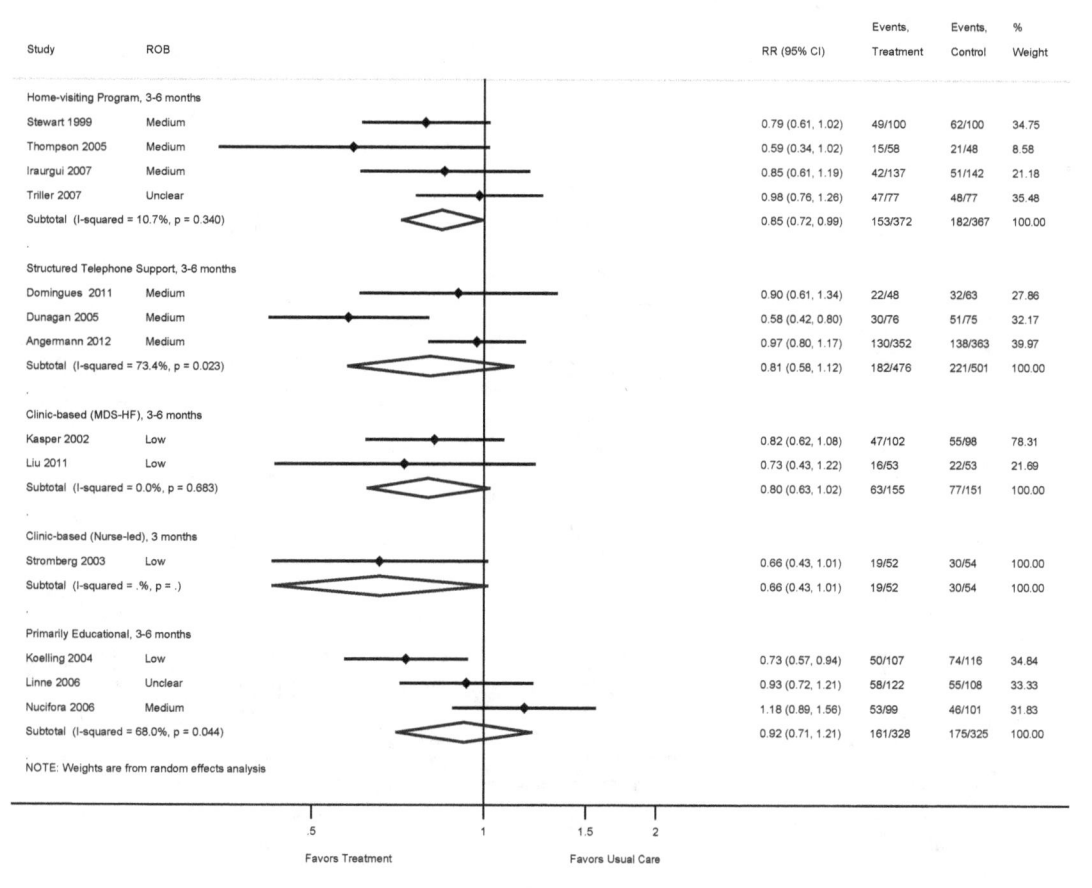

Study	ROB	RR (95% CI)	Events, Treatment	Events, Control	% Weight
Home-visiting Program, 3-6 months					
Stewart 1999	Medium	0.79 (0.61, 1.02)	49/100	62/100	34.75
Thompson 2005	Medium	0.59 (0.34, 1.02)	15/58	21/48	8.58
Iraurgui 2007	Medium	0.85 (0.61, 1.19)	42/137	51/142	21.18
Triller 2007	Unclear	0.98 (0.76, 1.26)	47/77	48/77	35.48
Subtotal (I-squared = 10.7%, p = 0.340)		0.85 (0.72, 0.99)	153/372	182/367	100.00
Structured Telephone Support, 3-6 months					
Domingues 2011	Medium	0.90 (0.61, 1.34)	22/48	32/63	27.86
Dunagan 2005	Medium	0.58 (0.42, 0.80)	30/76	51/75	32.17
Angermann 2012	Medium	0.97 (0.80, 1.17)	130/352	138/363	39.97
Subtotal (I-squared = 73.4%, p = 0.023)		0.81 (0.58, 1.12)	182/476	221/501	100.00
Clinic-based (MDS-HF), 3-6 months					
Kasper 2002	Low	0.82 (0.62, 1.08)	47/102	55/98	78.31
Liu 2011	Low	0.73 (0.43, 1.22)	16/53	22/53	21.69
Subtotal (I-squared = 0.0%, p = 0.683)		0.80 (0.63, 1.02)	63/155	77/151	100.00
Clinic-based (Nurse-led), 3 months					
Stromberg 2003	Low	0.66 (0.43, 1.01)	19/52	30/54	100.00
Subtotal (I-squared = .%, p = .)		0.66 (0.43, 1.01)	19/52	30/54	100.00
Primarily Educational, 3-6 months					
Koelling 2004	Low	0.73 (0.57, 0.94)	50/107	74/116	34.84
Linne 2006	Unclear	0.93 (0.72, 1.21)	58/122	55/108	33.33
Nucifora 2006	Medium	1.18 (0.89, 1.56)	53/99	46/101	31.83
Subtotal (I-squared = 68.0%, p = 0.044)		0.92 (0.71, 1.21)	161/328	175/325	100.00

NOTE: Weights are from random effects analysis

.5   1   1.5   2

Favors Treatment   Favors Usual Care

Figure F4. Mortality for transitional care interventions compared with usual care, by intervention category and outcome timing: Sensitivity analysis including trials rated as having high or unclear ROB

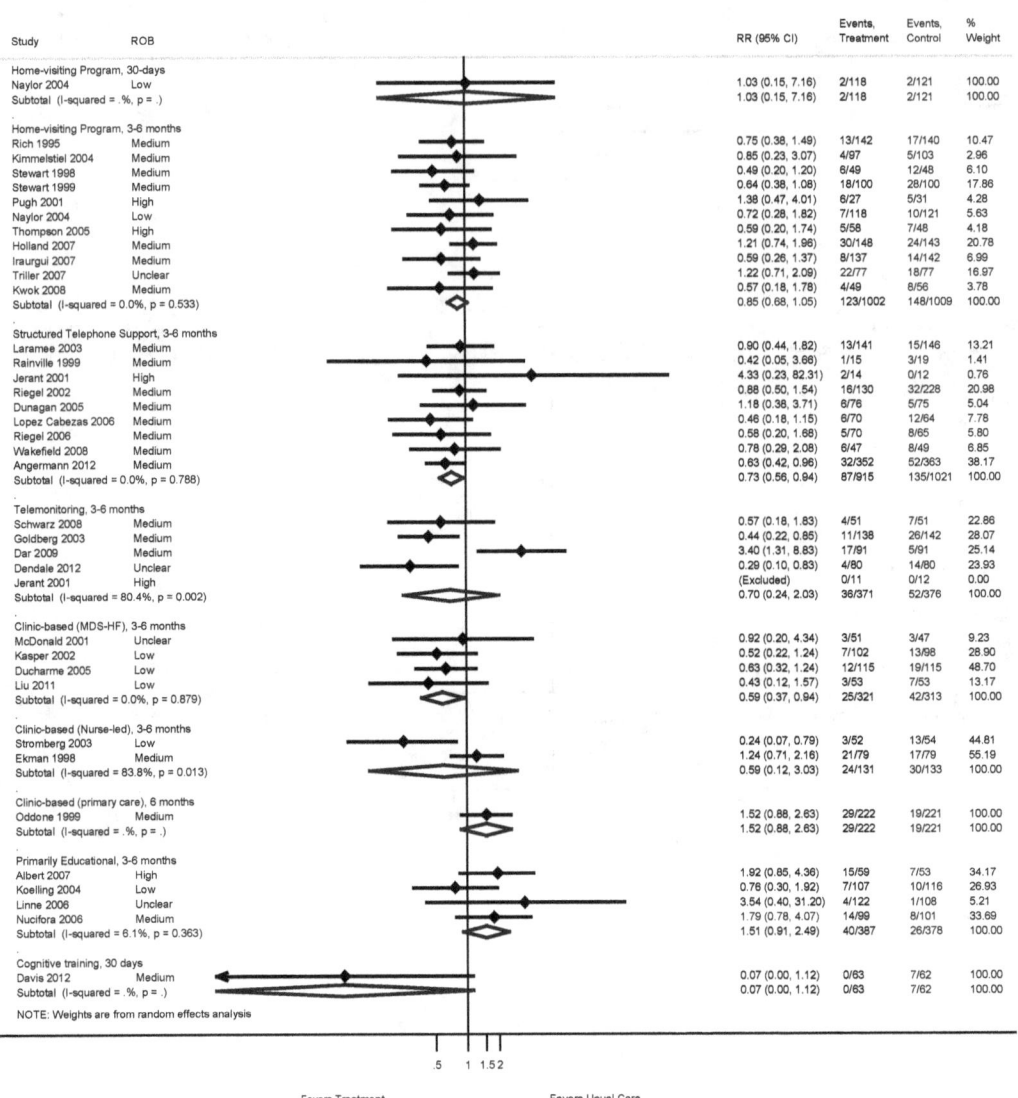

Note: For the trial by Wakefield et al., we include the telephone care arm here (not the videophone arm).[1]

Appendix F Reference

1.   Wakefield BJ, Holman JE, Ray A, et al. Outcomes of a home telehealth intervention for patients with heart failure. J Telemed Telecare. 2009;15(1):46-50. PMID: 19139220.

Appendix G. Strength of Evidence Tables

Table G1. All-cause readmission (number of people readmitted): Strength of evidence

Intervention Category; Time-point	Number of Studies; Subjects	Study Limitations	Consistency	Directness	Precision	Findings and Direction[a] [Magnitude] of Effect RR (95% CI)	Strength of Evidence
Home-visiting; 30 days	2; 418	Low	Consistent[b]	Direct	Imprecise	High intensity (1 trial): 0.34 (0.19 to 0.62) Lower intensity (1 trial): 0.89 (0.43 to 1.85)	Low[b]
Home-visiting; 3 to 6 months	9; 1,563	Low	Consistent	Direct	Precise	0.75 (0.68 to 0.86)	High[c]
Structured telephone support; 30 days	1; 134	Low	Unknown	Direct	Imprecise	0.80 (0.38 to 1.65)	Insufficient
Structured telephone support; 3 to 6 months	8; 2,166	Low	Consistent	Direct	Imprecise	0.92 (0.77 to 1.10)	Moderate
Tele-monitoring; 30 days	1; 168	Low	Unknown	Direct	Imprecise	1.02 (0.64 to 1.63)	Insufficient
Tele-monitoring; 3 to 6 months	3; 434	Low	Consistent[d]	Direct	Imprecise	1.11 (0.87 to 1.42)	Moderate
Clinic-based (nurse-led); 3 to 6 months	2; 264	Low	Inconsistent	Direct	Imprecise	0.88 (0.57 to 1.37)	Low
Clinic-based (MDS-HF); 3 to 6 months	2; 336	Low	Consistent	Direct	Precise	0.70 (0.55 to 0.89)	High
Clinic-based (Primary Care); 3 to 6 months	1; 443	Low	Unknown	Direct	Precise	1.27 (1.05 to 1.54)	Insufficient
Primarily Educational; 3 to 6 months	1; 200	Low	Unknown	Direct	Imprecise	1.14 (0.84 to 1.54)	Insufficient
Cognitive Training; 30 days	1; 125	Low	Unknown	Direct	Imprecise	1.15 (0.71 to 2.28)	Insufficient

[a] For RR, values less than one favor the intervention group.

[b] For home-visiting programs, reduction in 30-day all-cause readmission differed by intervention intensity. The one trial assessing a higher intensity intervention showed efficacy[1] while the one trial assessing a lower intensity intervention did not show efficacy.[2] In grading the SOE, we considered results of similar interventions at other time-points. The low SOE refers to the overall assessment that the higher intensity home-visiting program reduced all-cause readmission while the lower intensity intervention did not.

[c] Two additional trials reported on the total number of readmissions per group (rather than people readmitted): In one trial (N=200), patients receiving home visits had fewer unplanned readmissions (68) than those receiving usual care (118) (p = 0.031).[3] In another trial (N=200), all-cause readmission did not differ between patients receiving home visits and those receiving usual care (measured as mean readmissions per patient-year alive: RR, 0.89; p=0.61).[4]

[d] Four telemonitoring studies reported the total number of readmissions per group (rather than the number of people readmitted); all-cause readmission did not differ between patients receiving telemonitoring and those receiving usual care at 30 days,[5] 3 months,[6] or 6 months.[5,7,8]

Abbreviations: CI = confidence interval; MDS-HF = multidisciplinary heart failure; N = trial sample size; RCT = randomized controlled trial; RR = relative risk

Table G2. HF-specific readmission (number of people readmitted): Strength of evidence

Intervention Category; Time-point	Number of Studies; Subjects	Study Limitations	Consistency	Directness	Precision	Findings and Direction [Magnitude] of Effect[a] RR (95% CI)	Strength of Evidence
Home-visiting; 3 to 6 months	1; 282	Low	Consistent[b]	Direct	Imprecise	0.51 (0.31 to 0.82)	Moderate[b]
Structured telephone support; 30 days	1; 134	Low	Unknown	Direct	Imprecise	0.63 (0.24 to 1.87)	Insufficient
Structured telephone support; 3 to 6 months	7; 1790	Low	Consistent	Direct	Precise	0.74 (0.61 to 0.90)	High
Tele-monitoring; 3 to 6 months	1; 182	Low	Consistent[c]	Direct	Imprecise	1.70 (0.82 to 3.51)	Moderate[c]
Clinic-based (Nurse-led); 3 to 6 months	1; 158	Low	Unknown	Direct	Imprecise	0.95 (0.68 to 1.32)	Insufficient
Clinic-based (MDS-HF); 3 to 6 months	1; 106	Low	Unknown	Direct	Imprecise	0.70 (0.29 to 1.70)	Insufficient
Primarily Educational; 3 months	1; 223	Low	Unknown	Direct	Precise	0.53 (0.31 to 0.90)	Insufficient

[a] For RR, values less than one favor the intervention group

[b] Although one trial reported total number of people readmitted per group, we considered the findings consistent due to the fact that one other trial reported on the number of readmissions per group and found a similar effect: patients receiving home visits had fewer total HF readmissions than did patients receiving usual care (measured as readmissions per patient year alive, RR, 0.54; p<0.001; N=200).[4]

[c] Although one trial reported total number of people readmitted per group, we considered the findings consistent due to the fact that two other trial reported on the number of readmissions per group neither study found a difference between the intervention and control group two groups.[7,8]

Abbreviations: CI = confidence interval; HF = heart failure; MDS-HF = multidisciplinary heart failure; N = trial sample size; RR = relative risk.

Table G3. Composite all-cause readmission or death: Strength of evidence

Intervention Category; Time-point	Number of Studies; Subjects	Study Limitations	Consistency	Directness	Precision	Findings and Direction [Magnitude] of Effect[a]	Strength of Evidence
Home-visiting; 30 days	1; 239	Low	Unknown	Direct	Imprecise	HR (SE): 0.869 (0.033) vs. 0.737 (0.041)	Low[b]
Home-visiting; 3 to 6 months	4; 824	Low	Consistent	Direct	Imprecise	3 trials (N=585): RR (95% CI): - 0.78 (0.65 to 0.94) 1 trial (N=239): HR (SE): 0.600 (0.047) vs. 0.444 (0.047)	Moderate
Structured telephone support; 3 to 6 months	3; 977	Low	Inconsistent	Direct	Imprecise	RR (95% CI): 0.81 (0.58 to 1.12)	Low
Clinic-based (Nurse-led); 3 to 6 months	1; 106	Low	Unknown	Direct	Imprecise	RR (95% CI): 0.66 (0.43 to 1.01)	Insufficient
Clinic-based (MDS-HF); 3 to 6 months	2; 306	Low	Consistent	Direct	Imprecise	RR (95% CI): 0.80 (0.43 to 1.01)	Moderate
Primarily Educational; 3 to 6 months	2; 423	Low	Inconsistent	Direct	Imprecise	RR (95% CI): 0.92 (0.58 to 1.47)	Low

[a] For RRs, values less than one favor the intervention group.

[b] Although evidence was limited to 1 trial, consistency for the 30-day outcome was unknown, and evidence was imprecise, we upgraded the SOE because this intervention category has demonstrated efficacy for this outcome at different time points—thus, increasing our confidence in the results of this single trial.

Abbreviations: CI = confidence interval; HR = hazard ratio; MDS-HF = multidisciplinary heart failure; N = trial sample size; SE = standard error; SOE = strength of evidence.

Table G4. Emergency room or acute care visits

Intervention Category; Time-point	Number of Studies; Subjects	Study Limitations	Consistency	Directness	Precision	Findings and Direction [Magnitude] of Effect[a]	Strength of Evidence
Home-visiting; 30 days	1; 179	Medium	Unknown	Direct	Imprecise	% of subjects with ER visits, (intervention vs. control): 5% vs. 4%, p-value NR	Insufficient
Home-visiting; 3 to 6 months	1; 179	Medium	Unknown	Direct	Imprecise	% of subjects with ER visits (intervention vs. control): 17% vs. 22%, p-value NR	Insufficient
Home-visiting; 3 to 6 months	1; 97	Medium	Unknown	Direct	Imprecise	Total ER visits per group (intervention vs. control): 48 vs. 87 visits, p=0.05	Insufficient
Structured telephone support; 3 to 6 months	1; 111	Medium	Unknown	Direct	Imprecise	Total ER visits per group: RR (95% CI): 0.66 (0.21 to 2.05)	Insufficient
Structured telephone support; 3 to 6 months	2; 634	Medium	Consistent	Direct	Imprecise	% of patients with at least one ER visit (intervention vs. control): 22.1 vs. 27.9, p=0.266 Mean ER visits per person (intervention vs. control): 0.14 vs. 0.11, p=0.58	Low
Telemonitoring 3 to 6 months	2; 284	Medium	Unknown	Direct	Imprecise	Average ER visits per patient (intervention vs. control): 0.34 vs. 0.38, p=0.73 Total ER visits per group (intervention vs. control): 20 vs. 32, p-value NR	Insufficient
Clinic-based (MDS-HF); 3 to 6 months	1; 230	Medium	Unknown	Direct	Imprecise	Number of patients per group with ER visits: HR (95% CI): 0.97 (0.70 to 1.36)	Insufficient
Primarily Educational; 3 to 6 months	1; 76	Medium	Unknown	Direct	Imprecise	% of patients per group seen in ER (intervention vs. control): 38 vs. 33, p=0.68	Insufficient

[a] For RRs and HRs, values less than 1.0 favor the intervention group.

Abbreviations: CI = confidence interval; ER = emergency room; HR = hazard ratio; MDS-HF = multidisciplinary heart failure; NR = not reported; RR = relative risk.

Table G5. Hospital days (of subsequent readmissions)

Intervention Category; Time-point	Number of Studies; Subjects	Study Limitations	Consistency	Directness	Precision	Findings and Direction [Magnitude] of Effect[a]	Strength of Evidence
Home-visiting; 30 days	1; 179	Medium	Unknown	Direct	Imprecise	Mean number of readmission days per person readmitted (SD) (intervention vs. control): 2.2 (7) vs. 2.3 (7)	Insufficient
Home-visiting; 3 months	4; 765	Medium	Consistent	Direct	Imprecise	Difference in total hospital days per group: WMD (95% CI): -1.17 (-2.44 to 0.09)	Low
Home-visiting; 6 months	3; 403	Medium	Consistent	Direct	Imprecise	Total hospital days (intervention vs. control, p=value): 261 vs. 452, p=0.05; 875 vs. 1476, p=0.04; 108 vs. 459, p≤0.01	Low
Structured telephone support; 30 days	1; 134	Medium	Unknown	Direct	Imprecise	WMD (95% CI): -0.95 (-2.43 to 0.53)	Insufficient
Structured telephone support; 3 to 6 months	5; 1,068	Medium	Consistent	Direct	Precise	WMD (95% CI): -2.49 (-3.93 to -1.04)	Moderate
Telemonitoring 30 days	1; 168	Medium	Unknown	Direct	Imprecise	Mean length of hospital stay per patient readmitted (SD) (intervention vs. control): 1.9 (4.4) vs. 1.8 (12.2)	Insufficient
Telemonitoring 3 to 6 months	2; 350	Medium	Unknown	Direct	Imprecise	Mean length of hospital stay per patient readmitted (SD) (intervention vs. control): 4.9 (8.2) vs. 4.8 (10.2); Median duration of readmission hospital stay (intervention vs. control): 17 vs. 13 days, p=0.99	Insufficient

Table G5. Hospital days (of subsequent readmissions) (continued)

Intervention Category; Time-point	Number of Studies; Subjects	Study Limitations	Consistency	Directness	Precision	Findings and Direction [Magnitude] of Effect[a]	Strength of Evidence
Clinic-based (Nurse-led); 3 to 6 months	2; 260	Medium	Inconsistent	Direct	Imprecise	Total hospital days per group (intervention vs. control): 350 vs. 592, p=0.045 Mean hospital days per patient readmitted (SD) (intervention vs. control): 26 (19) vs. 18 (19); p-value NS per investigators	Insufficient
Clinic-based (MDS-HF); 3 to 6 months	1; 230	Medium	Unknown	Direct	Imprecise	Total hospital days per patient (intervention vs. control): Hazard ratio (95% CI): 0.61 (0.39 to 0.95)	Insufficient
Clinic-based (primary-care); 3 to 6 months	1; 443	Medium	Unknown	Direct	Precise	Mean hospital days per patient readmitted (intervention vs. control): 9.1 vs. 7.3, p=0.04	Insufficient
Primarily Educational; 3 to 3 months	1; 200	Medium	Unknown	Direct	Imprecise	Mean length of hospital stay per person readmitted: 20 vs. 15 days, p-value NS per authors	Insufficient

[a] Negative values favor the intervention group (for WMD).

Abbreviations: CI = confidence interval; HR = hazard ratio; MDS-HF = multidisciplinary heart failure; NS = not significant; SD = standard deviation; WMD = weighted mean difference.

Table G6. Quality of life (MLWHFQ) by outcome timing – home-visiting programs versus usual care: Strength of evidence

Intervention Category; Time-point	Number of Studies; Subjects Analyzed	Study Limitations	Consistency	Directness	Precision	Findings and Direction [Magnitude] of Effect[a]	Strength of Evidence
Home-visiting; 14 days	1; 226	Medium	Unknown	Direct	Imprecise	No difference in mean MLWHFQ score at 14 days	Insufficient
Home-visiting; 3 months	3; 345	Medium	Consistent	Direct	Imprecise	2 trials: SMD (95% CI): -0.26 (-0.47 to -0.05).[1,9] One trial (N=200): mean MLWHFQ (change from baseline, intervention vs. control): -19 vs. -1, p=0.04.[3]	Low
Home-visiting; 6 months	2; 384	Medium	Inconsistent	Direct	Imprecise	Difference in mean score at 6 months: SMD (95% CI): -0.04 (-0.35 to 0.26)	Insufficient
Structured telephone support; 3 months	3; 331	Medium	Consistent	Direct	Imprecise	Difference in mean scores at 3 months: WMD (95% CI): -0.26 (-0.47 to -0.05)	Low
Structured telephone support; 6 months	3; 331	Medium	Consistent	Direct	Imprecise	Difference in mean scores at 6 months: WMD (95% CI): -0.19 (-0.49 to 0.10)	Low
Telemonitoring 3 months	1; 102	Medium	Unknown	Direct	Imprecise	Difference in mean scores at 3 months: 27.4 vs. 27.3, p=0.99	Insufficient
Clinic-based Interventions 6 months	1; 200	Medium	Unknown	Direct	Imprecise	MLWHFQ change from baseline: -28.3 vs. -15.7, p=0.01	Insufficient
Primarily Educational 6 months	2; 372	Medium	Inconsistent	Direct	Imprecise	One trial (N=223): mean MLWHFQ (SD) (intervention vs. control): 14 (20) vs. 10 (16), p<0.0001]. Another trial (N=149): mean MLWHFQ (SD) (intervention vs. control): 41 (22) vs. 42 (25), p-value NR.	Insufficient

[a] For SMDs and WMDs, negative values favor the intervention group.

G-7

Abbreviations: CI = confidence interval; MLWHFQ = Minnesota Living With Heart Failure Questionnaire; N = trial sample size; NR = not reported; SD = standard deviation; SMD = standardized mean difference; vs. = versus; WMD = weighted mean difference.

Table G7. Mortality: Strength of evidence

Intervention Category; Time-point	Number of Studies; Subjects	Study Limitations	Consistency	Directness	Precision	Findings and Direction [Magnitude] of Effect RR (95% CI)[a]	Strength of Evidence
Home-visiting; 30 days	1; 239	Low	Unknown	Direct	Imprecise	1.03 (0.15 to 7.16)	Insufficient
Home-visiting; 3 to 6 months	8; 1693	Low	Consistent	Direct	Imprecise[b]	0.77 (0.60 to 0.996)	Moderate
Structured telephone support; 3 to 6 months	7; 2011	Low	Consistent	Direct	Imprecise	0.74 (0.56 to 0.97)	Moderate
Telemonitoring 3 to 6 months	3; 564	Low	Inconsistent	Direct	Imprecise	0.93 (0.25 to 3.48)	Low
Clinic-based (Nurse-led); 3 to 6 months	2; 264	Low	Unknown	Direct	Imprecise	0.59 (0.12 to 3.03)	Low
Clinic-based (MDS-HF); 6 months	3; 536	Low	Consistent	Direct	Imprecise[b]	0.56 (0.34 to 0.92)	Moderate
Clinic-based (primary care); 6 months	1; 443	Low	Unknown	Direct	Imprecise	1.52 (0.88 to 2.63)	Insufficient
Primarily Educational; 3 to 6 months	2; 423	Low	Inconsistent	Direct	Imprecise	1.20 (0.52 to 2.76)	Low
Cognitive Training 30 days	1; 125	Low	Unknown	Direct	Imprecise	0.07 (0.00 to 1.12)	Insufficient

[a] RR less than one favor the intervention.

[b] Although the findings are statistically significant, the confidence intervals around these estimates are wide, making it difficult to determine the true magnitude of effect for these mortality outcomes (compared to usual care). For this reason, we have called these estimates "imprecise."

Abbreviations: CI = confidence interval; MDS-HF = multidisciplinary heart failure; RR = relative risk

G-8

Appendix G References

1. Naylor MD, Brooten DA, Campbell RL, et al. Transitional care of older adults hospitalized with heart failure: a randomized, controlled trial. J Am Geriatr Soc. 2004 May;52(5):675-84. PMID: 15086645.

2. Jaarsma T, Halfens R, Huijer Abu-Saad H, et al. Effects of education and support on self-care and resource utilization in patients with heart failure. Eur Heart J. 1999 May;20(9):673-82. PMID: 10208788.

3. Stewart S, Marley JE, Horowitz JD. Effects of a multidisciplinary, home-based intervention on unplanned readmissions and survival among patients with chronic congestive heart failure: a randomised controlled study. Lancet. 1999 Sep 25;354(9184):1077-83. PMID: 10509499.

4. Kimmelstiel C, Levine D, Perry K, et al. Randomized, controlled evaluation of short- and long-term benefits of heart failure disease management within a diverse provider network: the SPAN-CHF trial. Circulation. 2004 Sep 14;110(11):1450-5. PMID: 15313938.

5. Jerant AF, Azari R, Martinez C, et al. A randomized trial of telenursing to reduce hospitalization for heart failure: patient-centered outcomes and nursing indicators. Home Health Care Serv Q. 2003;22(1):1-20. PMID: 12749524.

6. Woodend AK, Sherrard H, Fraser M, et al. Telehome monitoring in patients with cardiac disease who are at high risk of readmission. Heart Lung. 2008 Jan-Feb;37(1):36-45. PMID: 18206525.

7. Goldberg LR, Piette JD, Walsh MN, et al. Randomized trial of a daily electronic home monitoring system in patients with advanced heart failure: the Weight Monitoring in Heart Failure (WHARF) trial. Am Heart J. 2003 Oct;146(4):705-12. PMID: 14564327.

8. Dendale P, De Keulenaer G, Troisfontaines P, et al. Effect of a telemonitoring-facilitated collaboration between general practitioner and heart failure clinic on mortality and rehospitalization rates in severe heart failure: the TEMA-HF 1 (TElemonitoring in the MAnagement of Heart Failure) study. Eur J Heart Fail. 2012 Mar;14(3):333-40. PMID: 22045925.

9. Holland R, Brooksby I, Lenaghan E, et al. Effectiveness of visits from community pharmacists for patients with heart failure: HeartMed randomised controlled trial. BMJ. 2007 May 26;334(7603):1098. PMID: 17452390.

www.ingramcontent.com/pod-product-compliance
Lightning Source LLC
Chambersburg PA
CBHW081722170526
45167CB00009B/3666